Basic Current Procedural Terminology and HCPCS Coding

Gail I. Smith, MA, RHIA, CCS-P

2012 Edition

AHIMA PRESS

ISBN 978-1-58426-342-5

AHIMA Product Number AC200612

Claire Blondeau, MBA, Senior Editor
Adrienne Cook, JD, Developmental Editor
Katie Greenock, MS, Editorial and Production Coordinator
Ashley Sullivan, Assistant Editor
Ken Zielske, Director of Publications
Karen Kostick, RHIT, CCS, CCS-P, Reviewer

American Health Information Management Association
233 North Michigan Avenue, 21st Floor
Chicago, Illinois 60601-5809
ahima.org

Contents

About the Author

Gail I. Smith, MA, RHIA, CCS-P, is President of Gail I. Smith Consulting in Cincinnati, Ohio. Prior to launching an independent consulting business in 2011, Gail was an Associate Professor and Director of the Health Information Management (HIM) program at the University of Cincinnati. Before joining the University of Cincinnati, she served as the Director of the HIM program at Cincinnati State Technical and Community College for eighteen years. Before a career in education, Smith held management positions in two Cincinnati hospitals. On a part-time basis, Gail has served as a coding consultant for over 20 years. Her projects include developing content for courses/workshops, delivering presentations, performing coding reviews, and mapping ICD-10-CM/PCS for database conversions.

Gail has served as president of the Ohio Health Information Management Association and received the Professional Achievement Award in 1996 and Distinguished Member Award in 2005. Gail also served on the Board of Directors of the American Health Information Management Association from 2003–2006.

Ms. Smith received her bachelor's degree in HIM from The Ohio State University and her master's degree in education from The College of Mt. St. Joseph in Cincinnati, Ohio.

Preface

This workbook provides basic training and practice in the application of procedural codes from the *Current Procedural Terminology* (CPT) and the *Healthcare Procedure Coding System* (HCPCS). CPT is published by the American Medical Association (AMA). Updated annually on January 1, CPT is a proprietary terminology created and maintained by the AMA. Its purpose is to provide a uniform language for describing and reporting the professional services performed by physicians. HCPCS is maintained by the Centers for Medicare and Medicaid Services (CMS). Its purpose is to provide a system for reporting the medical services received by Medicare beneficiaries. HCPCS is made up of two parts: Level I is composed entirely of the current version of CPT; HCPCS Level II provides codes to represent medical services that are not covered by the CPT system, for example, medical supplies and services performed by healthcare professionals who are not physicians.

Like previous editions, the 2011 edition of *Basic Current Procedural Terminology and HCPCS Coding* is intended for students who have limited knowledge of, or experience in, CPT/HCPCS coding, and also as a resource and review guide for professionals. The instructional materials in this workbook are not specific to any particular practice setting, and they apply to both hospital-based and office-based coding. The exercises provide hands-on experience in coding some of the more common procedures and services performed by physicians and other healthcare professionals.

Many healthcare facilities and providers develop their own systematic methods for assigning CPT codes to frequently performed diagnostic procedures. For this reason, this workbook provides only minimal practice in assigning CPT/HCPCS codes for diagnostic procedures.

The CPT/HCPCS coding process requires coders to apply analytic skills in combination with a practical knowledge of medical science. To become effective coding professionals, students must be able to apply their knowledge of medical terminology, anatomy and physiology, pathophysiology, pharmacology, and medical-surgical techniques. This workbook assumes that students will already have a basic understanding of these subject areas.

The primary objectives of this workbook include the following:

- To provide a basic introduction to the format of CPT codes as well as CPT coding conventions
- To demonstrate different ways to locate CPT codes through the use of the codebook's index

- To identify ways to ensure accurate code assignment through the application of coding guidelines from the AMA and CMS
- To delineate the documentation necessary for code assignment

Specifically, Chapter 1, Introduction to Clinical Coding, discusses the purpose of CPT/HCPCS codes. It also addresses diagnostic coding and the Medicare requirements for claims submission.

Chapter 2, Application of the CPT System, introduces the CPT coding conventions and explains the application of CPT codes for healthcare reimbursement.

Chapter 3, Modifiers, provides an overview of the purpose and use of CPT and HCPCS Level II modifiers.

Chapter 4, Surgery, reviews the coding guidelines associated with the surgical procedures performed to treat illnesses and injuries of the various anatomical systems. It emphasizes the surgical procedures that are performed most commonly in the ambulatory setting (hospital and physician's office).

Chapter 5, Radiology, discusses the claims process for radiology services performed by physicians and hospital-based outpatient providers. The chapter also discusses the principles of radiology code reporting.

Chapter 6, Pathology and Laboratory Services, addresses the code assignment process for common laboratory tests and procedures performed, supervised, or interpreted by pathologists and other physicians.

Chapter 7, Evaluation and Management Services, provides a concise explanation of the evaluation and management section of CPT. The chapter also provides practice exercises designed to address the complexities of assigning evaluation and management codes.

Chapter 8, Medicine, provides a general overview of the procedures and services described in the medicine chapter of the CPT codebook.

Chapter 9, Anesthesia, introduces the codes used by the physicians who provide or supervise anesthesia services.

Chapter 10, HCPCS Level II, reviews the format and usage of HCPCS National Codes and modifiers.

Chapter 11, Reimbursement in the Ambulatory Setting, explains the claims process for ambulatory services, which is based on correct CPT code assignment. This publication introduces CMS's efforts to tie reimbursement to quality measurers. A skills practice at the end of this chapter asks students to review sections of a CMS-1500 form to determine the accuracy of code assignment. This practice reinforces the students' understanding of the CPT/HCPCS coding principles and guidelines discussed in the preceding chapters.

The 2011 edition of *Basic Current Procedural Terminology and HCPCS Coding* has been expanded and updated in several ways. As in previous editions, review exercises are interspersed in each chapter. Appendix C of *Basic Current Procedural Terminology and HCPCS Coding* includes exercises and operative reports. Appendix D includes keys to the chapter review exercises for student reference. Keys to appendix C exercises and operative reports are available in the supplementary materials for instructors.

This book must be used with the 2011 edition of *Current Procedural Terminology* (CPT 2011) (code changes effective January 1, 2011), published by the AMA. The HCPCS Level II codes included in this publication were current as of October 1, 2010. The most current version of the HCPCS Level II codes can be found on the CMS Web site: www.cms.hhs.gov.

Students beginning a CPT course of study should have several additional references to help them assign codes. Suggested references and recommended readings that may be helpful to students are listed in appendix A of this workbook.

Chapter 7 of this publication is based on the evaluation and management documentation guidelines developed jointly by the AMA and CMS in 1997. For additional information on these guidelines or to check for additional revisions, students and educators should visit the CMS Web page at www.cms.hhs.gov.

AHIMA provides supplementary materials for educators who use this workbook in their classes. Materials include lesson plans, keys to practice exercises in Appendix C, PowerPoint slides, and other educational resources. All answer keys are available to instructors in online format from the individual book page in the AHIMA Bookstore (www.ahima.org/orders), and also are posted on the AHIMA Assembly on Education Community of Practice (AOE CoP) Web site. Instructors who are AHIMA members can sign up for this private community by clicking on the help icon within the CoP home page and requesting additional information on becoming an AOE CoP member. An instructor who is not an AHIMA member or a member who is not an instructor may contact the publisher at publications@ahima.org.

Acknowledgments

AHIMA wishes to acknowledge

Rita A. Scichilone, MHSA, RHIA, CCS, CCS-P, CHC;
the late Rita Finnegan, RHIA, CCS; and
Toula Nicholas, RHIT, CCS, CCS-P,

who served as authors of previous editions of *Basic CPT®/HCPCS Coding,* as well as the many internal and external reviewers who have contributed throughout the years to this publication.

Chapter 1
Introduction to Clinical Coding

Several medical terminologies and classification systems are used to document and report information related to healthcare services in the United States. *The International Classification of Diseases, Clinical Modification,* currently in its ninth revision (ICD-9-CM), is used to describe and report the illnesses, conditions, and injuries of patients who require medical services. ICD-9-CM is made up of a series of numerical and alphanumerical codes and code descriptions that represent very specific illnesses and injuries.

Similarly, the services provided by physicians and other healthcare professionals are described and reported by using terminologies and classification systems. The *International Classification of Diseases, Clinical Modification,* provides a system for coding medical procedures performed in the inpatient departments of hospitals, but two other systems, the *Current Procedural Terminology (CPT)* and the *Healthcare Common Procedure Coding System (HCPCS),* apply to the services provided by physicians and other medical providers in hospital-based outpatient departments, physicians' offices, and other ambulatory settings.

Current Procedural Terminology

CPT, published by the American Medical Association (AMA), provides a system for describing and reporting the professional services furnished to patients by physicians and hospital outpatient services.

CPT was initially developed in 1966 and was designed to meet the reporting and communication needs of physicians. The system was adopted for application to the Medicare reimbursement system in 1983. Since that time, CPT has been widely used as the standard for outpatient and ambulatory care procedural coding and reimbursement.

The information represented by CPT codes is also used for several purposes other than reimbursement, including:

- Trending and planning outpatient and ambulatory services
- Benchmarking activities that compare and contrast the services provided by similar nonacute care programs
- Assessing and improving the quality of patient services

The CPT codebook includes several additional appendices and an index of procedures. CPT codebooks and codes are updated annually, with additions, revisions, and deletions becoming effective on January 1 of each year. A new edition of the CPT codebook is published annually, and the new edition should be purchased every year to ensure accurate coding. Healthcare providers are expected to begin using the newest edition for encounters on January 1. There is no longer a grace period during which claims based on out-of-date codes will be accepted.

CPT Category I

The CPT codebook includes a general introduction followed by six main sections that together make up the list of Category I CPT codes:

Evaluation and Management
Anesthesia
Surgery
Radiology
Pathology and Laboratory
Medicine

Specific coding guidelines are provided for each of the main sections.

The Category I codes in each of the main sections are further broken down into subsections and subcategories according to the type of service provided and the body system or disorder involved. For example, code 76645—Ultrasound, breast(s) (unilateral or bilateral) real time with image documentation—appears in the radiology section under the subsection entitled Diagnostic Ultrasound and the subcategory Chest.

Subcategory → Chest

76645 Ultrasound breast(s) (unilateral or bilateral), real time with image documentation

Similar procedures are grouped to form ranges of codes. For example, the range of codes from 19300 through 19307 represents the various types of mastectomy procedures in the subsection covering the integumentary system in the surgery section. The codes in each of the six main sections (or Category I) of the CPT codebook are composed of five digits and are primarily arranged in numerical order within each section. Several coding sections are not in numerical order (for example, 23071). This type of formatting is explained in chapter 2.

CPT Supplementary Codes

CPT also provides three types of supplementary codes: Category II codes, Category III codes, and modifiers. Each of these code sets is listed and explained in a separate section. The Category II and III sections are located after the medicine codes in the codebook. The list of modifiers and the coding guidelines for modifiers are included in appendix A of CPT 2012.

CPT Category II Codes

Category II provides supplementary tracking codes that are designed for use in performance assessment and quality improvement activities. CPT Category II codes are composed of five characters: four numbers and an alphabetic fifth character, capital letter F. Code 1000F, for example, describes a specific aspect of patient history: assessments of patient tobacco use. The following is an example of a Category II code under the Physical Examination subsection:

> Physical Examination
>
> Physical examination codes describe aspects of physical examination or clinical assessment.
>
> 2000F Blood pressure, measured

The assignment of Category II CPT codes is optional. Category II supplementary codes are implemented and released as needed throughout the year. These updates can be obtained by accessing the AMA Web site (http://www.ama-assn.org) and entering the term "category II codes" into the site's search engine.

CPT Category III Codes

CPT Category III includes temporary codes that represent emerging medical technologies, services, and procedures that have not yet been approved for general use by the FDA and so are not otherwise covered by CPT codes. Category III codes give physicians and other healthcare providers and researchers a system for documenting the use of unconventional methods so that their efficacy and outcomes can be tracked. Like CPT Category II codes, Category III codes are composed of five characters: four numbers and an alphabetic fifth character, capital letter T.

Example: Code 0058T, Cryopreservation; reproductive tissue, ovarian

This procedure describes a process where cells or whole tissues are preserved by cooling to low sub-zero temperatures.

Updated Category III codes are released semiannually on January 1 and July 1 via the AMA's CPT Web site. The complete list of temporary codes is published annually in the CPT codebooks.

CPT Modifiers

A third set of supplementary codes known as *modifiers* can be reported along with many of the Category I CPT codes. The two-character modifier codes are appended to Category I five-digit CPT codes to report additional information about any unusual circumstances under which a procedure was performed. The reporting of modifiers is meant to support the medical necessity of procedures that might not otherwise qualify for reimbursement.

Example: Suppose that a surgeon successfully performed a percutaneous transluminal balloon angioplasty to remove a blockage from a patient's renal artery, but later that day it became evident that the artery had become occluded again. If the surgeon who performed the original procedure is not available, another surgeon on call would repeat the procedure to remove the blockage. Code 35471 would be reported by the first surgeon to identify the original angioplasty, and the second surgeon would report 35471–77 to identify the repeat angioplasty.

Most of the two-character modifiers for Category I codes are numerical. (Chapter 3 of this workbook includes a list of the CPT modifiers in CPT 2012.) However, there also are some alphanumeric modifiers to indicate the physical status of patients undergoing anesthesia. These modifiers begin with a capital letter P, as follows:

Anesthesia Modifiers:

P1 A normal healthy patient

P2 A patient with mild systemic disease

P3 A patient with severe systemic disease

P4 A patient with severe systemic disease that is a constant threat to life

P5 A moribund patient who is not expected to survive without the operation

P6 A declared brain-dead patient whose organs are being removed for donor purposes

(Chapter 2 of this workbook provides additional guidelines for applying CPT codes, and chapter 3 discusses modifiers in more detail.)

Healthcare Common Procedure Coding System

The Health Care Financing Administration (HCFA) developed the original version of the *HCFA Common Procedure Coding System* (HCPCS) in 1983. HCPCS was designed to represent the physician and nonphysician services provided to Social Security beneficiaries under the federal Medicare program. HCFA's name was changed to the Centers for Medicare and Medicaid Services (CMS) in 2001. The official name of the coding system was also changed, and the system is now called the Healthcare Common Procedure Coding System. CMS is the division of the U.S. Department of Health and Human Services that administers the Medicare program and the federal portion of the Medicaid program.

The purpose of HCPCS as implemented in 1985 was to fulfill the operational needs of the Medicare reimbursement system. Originally, HCPCS codes applied only to the services provided by physicians to Medicare patients. Since 1986, however, the federal government has required that physicians use HCPCS codes to report services provided to Medicaid patients as well. Moreover, with the passage of the Omnibus Reconciliation Act of 1986, hospitals are also required to report HCPCS codes on reimbursement claims for ambulatory surgery services, as well as radiology and other diagnostic services provided to Medicare and Medicaid patients.

HCPCS codes enable providers and suppliers to accurately communicate information about the services they provide. Analysis of HCPCS data also helps Medicare carriers to establish financial controls that prevent expense escalation. Finally, the information from coded claims facilitates uniform application of Medicare and Medicaid coverage and reimbursement policies.

HCPCS includes two separate levels of codes. Level I is based on the current edition of CPT. Level II is made up of the National Codes that represent the medical supplies and services not included in CPT.

HCPCS Level I (CPT)

Copyrighted and published by the AMA, Level I of HCPCS consists of five-digit Category I CPT codes. Level I HCPCS codes are used by physicians to report services such as hospital visits, surgical procedures, radiological procedures, supervisory services, and other medical services. Hospitals also use Level I codes to report hospital-based outpatient services, such as laboratory and radiological procedures and ambulatory services, to Medicare and other third-party payers. Level I codes represent approximately 80 percent of the HCPCS codes submitted for reimbursement each year.

HCPCS Level II

Known as the National Codes, HCPCS Level II codes were developed by CMS for use in reporting medical services not covered in CPT. Level II codes are provided for injectable drugs, ambulance services, prosthetic devices, and selected provider services.

Level II codes are made up of five characters: The first character is a capital Arabic letter, and the following four characters are numbers. Examples of HCPCS Level II codes include the following:

A4550	Surgical trays
E1625	Water softening system, for hemodialysis
J0475	Injection, Baclofen, 10 mg

Like Level I (CPT) codes, HCPCS Level II codes are updated annually. A list of current Level II codes can be requested from the U.S. Government Printing Office or any local Medicare carrier. Several commercial publishing companies distribute the National Codes in book form, adding enhancements such as indexes and cross-references to make them more user-friendly than the government-issued lists. In addition, an electronic file containing the most current version of the HCPCS Level II codes can be downloaded from the CMS Web site at http://www.cms.gov/HCPCSReleaseCodeSets. (HCPCS Level II codes are discussed in more detail in chapter 10 of this workbook.)

International Classification of Diseases, Ninth Revision, Clinical Modification (ICD-9-CM)

The *International Classification of Diseases, Ninth Revision, Clinical Modification* (ICD-9-CM), is based on an international classification system originally developed and maintained by the World Health Organization (WHO). The purpose of the international version of the ICD is the classification and reporting of morbidity data (illnesses and injuries) and mortality data (fatalities) from around the world. ICD-9 was modified for use in the United States and was first released as ICD-9-CM in 1979.

Currently, ICD-9-CM diagnosis codes are required for Medicare and private third-party payers to support medical necessity of procedures and services. By definition, medical necessity is the determination that a service or procedure rendered is reasonable and necessary for the diagnosis or treatment of an illness or injury.

The official version of ICD-9-CM is published in three volumes. Volume 1 contains the main list of diagnostic codes in tabular format. The codes are organized into chapters according to body system. For example, chapter 1 covers the codes for Infectious and Parasitic Diseases. Volume 2 provides an alphabetic index of diseases and injuries that help coding professionals locate the appropriate code listings in the tabular list. Volume 3 includes procedural codes in tabular format and an alphabetic index for procedures. Only inpatient acute-care hospitals use ICD-9-CM volume 3 to report procedures for reimbursement.

Like CPT and HCPCS, ICD-9-CM codes are reevaluated and appropriate revisions are implemented on a regular basis. ICD-9-CM code updates are now released by the federal government twice each year, on April 1 and October 1. October 1, 2011 was the last major update of ICD-9-CM because of the transition to ICD-10-CM. Any further revisions to ICD-9-CM will only be for a new disease and/or procedure representing new technology. Updated ICD-9-CM codes are also available electronically from the National Center for Health Statistics Web site. Several commercial publishers, however, offer enhanced print versions of the classification. The yearly editions of these codebooks are usually released during the summer and incorporate the official ICD-9-CM changes that will become effective on October 1 of the same year.

To ensure complete and accurate coding, healthcare providers must update or replace their ICD-9-CM codebooks as new codes are implemented and existing codes are amended or deleted. In addition, encoders and other coding software must also be updated at least yearly.

ICD-9-CM Diagnostic Codes

ICD-9-CM diagnostic codes represent the reasons why patients require and seek medical care. Each numerical code represents a specific symptom, condition, injury, or disease. ICD-9-CM diagnostic codes in the main classification (codes 001 through 999) consist of three, four, or five digits. The first three numbers represent a specific diagnosis, and one or two additional numbers may follow a decimal point after the three-number code to provide information that is more specific.

> **Example:** Code 562.13 represents a diagnosis of diverticulitis of the colon with intestinal hemorrhaging. The first three numbers (562) indicate a diagnosis of diverticula of the intestine; the number 1 after the decimal point represents the location of the diverticula, the colon; and the fifth digit represents the most specific diagnosis: diverticulitis of colon with hemorrhage.

Supplementary ICD-9-CM Codes

ICD-9-CM includes two supplementary classifications consisting of alphanumeric codes that provide additional information about the patient and the circumstances surrounding the patient's illness or injury. V codes represent the various factors that may influence the patient's health status and contact with health services. E codes represent the external factors that cause injuries and poisonings.

Diagnostic Coding

The Central Office on ICD-9-CM maintains the official coding guidelines for diagnostic coding. The guidelines require ICD-9-CM code assignments to be as specific as possible and to be supported by health record documentation. The guidelines also require the reporting of as many codes as necessary to completely describe the patient's condition. Guidelines also establish the order in which multiple codes are to be reported. The ICD-9-CM codebook also provides detailed advice on assigning codes correctly.

Every claim for outpatient services must contain at least one ICD-9-CM code, but care must be taken to report every applicable code in the sequence specified in the official coding guidelines. Medicare and most other third-party payers reject claims that report incomplete ICD-9-CM codes.

Coding professionals must thoroughly understand and carefully follow the *Official ICD-9-CM Coding Guidelines for Outpatient Services* (reference the CDC website) published by the National Center for Health Statistics (NCHS). Official ICD-9-CM coding advice is also published by the American Hospital Association (AHA) in its quarterly publication, *Coding Clinic*. The official coding guidelines for ICD-9-CM are available from the Central Office on ICD-9-CM of the AHA as well as from the CMS Web site.

The following examples illustrate correct and incorrect code assignments for a patient with a diagnosis of Type 2 diabetes.

Example:

250.00	Diabetes mellitus without mention of complication, Type 2 or unspecified type, not stated as uncontrolled	**Correct**
250.0	Diabetes mellitus without mention of complication, Type 2 or unspecified type, not stated as uncontrolled	**Incorrect**
250	Diabetes mellitus without mention of complication, Type 2 or unspecified type, not stated as uncontrolled	**Incorrect**

Basic ICD-10-CM/PCS and ICD-9-CM Coding, 2012 Edition, by Lou Ann Schraffenberger, MBA, RHIA, CCS, CCS-P, provides a more detailed discussion of the basics of ICD-10-CM/PCS and ICD-9-CM coding. A new edition of the workbook with updated codes is released by the American Health Information Management Association every summer.)

International Classification of Diseases, Tenth Revision, Clinical Modification (ICD-10-CM)

On January 16, 2009, the U.S. Department of Health and Human Services (HHS) published a Final Rule for the adoption of ICD-10-CM and ICD-10-PCS code sets to replace the 30-year-old ICD-9-CM code sets. The compliance date for the two classification sets was established as October 1, 2013. The adoption of ICD-10-CM (diagnoses) will affect all components of the healthcare industry. However, the adoption of ICD-10-PCS will affect only those components of the healthcare industry that currently utilize Volume 3 of ICD-9-CM to report inpatient procedures.

The use of ICD-10-CM will offer greater detail and granularity and will greatly enhance HHS's capability to measure quality outcomes, such as the quality performance measures used in the hospital pay-for-reporting programs. The following table provides a brief example of the difference between ICD-9-CM and ICD-10-CM diagnosis codes.

ICD-9-CM Code	ICD-10-CM Code
682.6 Cellulitis, leg	L03.115 Cellulitis, lower limb, right

Documentation for Reimbursement

Health record documentation continues to play a pivotal role in the accurate and complete collection of health services data. The documentation records pertinent facts, findings, and observations about an individual's health history, including past and current illnesses, examinations, tests, treatments, and outcomes. By chronologically documenting the patient's care, the health record becomes an important element in the provision of high-quality healthcare and serves as the source document for code assignment.

The following general principles of health record documentation, developed jointly by the AMA and CMS, apply to the records maintained for all types of medical and surgical services:

- The health record should be complete and legible.
- The documentation of each patient encounter should include:
  - —The reason for the encounter and the patient's relevant history, physical examination findings, and prior diagnostic test results
  - —A patient assessment, clinical impression, or diagnosis
  - —A plan for care
  - —The date of the encounter and the identity of the observer
- The rationale for ordering diagnostic and other ancillary services should be documented or easily inferred.
- Past and present diagnoses should be accessible to the treating and consulting physicians.
- Appropriate health risk factors should be identified.
- The patient's progress and response to treatment and any revision in the treatment plan and diagnoses should be documented.
- The CPT and ICD-9-CM codes reported on health insurance claim forms or billing statements should be supported by documentation in the health record.

Additional documentation guidelines pertinent to evaluation and management (E/M) services are discussed in chapter 7 of this book. (Various links pertinent to the information discussed in this chapter are listed in the Web resources in appendix A of this workbook.)

The Medicare Program

The Social Security Act of 1965 and its subsequent amendments established the federal regulations that govern Medicare. The Medicare program is organized into two separate sections: Part A, which pays for the cost of hospital and facility care, and Part B, which covers the physician services and durable medical equipment that are not paid for under Part A. Medicare regulations require the collection of several types of coded information on reimbursement claims for services provided to Medicare beneficiaries:

- ICD-9-CM diagnostic and ICD-9-CM procedural codes for inpatient hospital services
- ICD-9-CM diagnostic codes and HCPCS procedural codes for hospital outpatient services, including laboratory and radiology procedures
- ICD-9-CM diagnostic codes and HCPCS procedural codes (regardless of the service location) for medical services provided by physicians and allied health professionals (psychologists, nurse practitioners, social workers, licensed therapists, and dietitians)

Health Insurance Portability and Accountability Act (HIPAA) Administrative Simplification

The intent of the federal government's simplification mandate is to streamline and standardize the electronic filing and processing of health insurance claims; to save money; and to provide better service to providers, insurers, and patients.

HIPAA Transaction and Code Set Standards

Before the implementation of HIPAA transaction and code set standards, healthcare providers and health plans used various formats when performing daily electronic transactions, which led to confusion. HIPAA requirements specify that all electronic data interchange formats be standardized. These standards apply to any health plan, clearinghouse, and any healthcare providers that transmit health information in electronic form in connection with defined transactions. HIPAA also requires the standardization of the reporting of medical procedures with industry-established and -maintained codes. These are codes used by healthcare providers to identify what procedures, services, and diagnoses pertain to any specific encounter. The following code sets have been approved for use by HIPAA:

- International Classification of Diseases, Ninth Edition, Clinical Modification (ICD-9-CM)
- Current Procedural Terminology (CPT)
- Healthcare Common Procedure Coding System (HCPCS)
- Current Dental Terminology (CDT)
- National Drug Codes (NDC)

Claims Submission

Reimbursement claims for medical services provided to beneficiaries of commercial and government-sponsored health insurance programs may be submitted in electronic or paper form. Electronic claims, however, must follow the standards developed by the Accredited Standards Committee (ASC) and mandated by HIPAA. ASC Standard X12 applies exclusively to electronic claims. Effective in early 2012, all covered entities must implement the 5010 version of the standard. The 5010 standards pave the way for use of ICD-10-CM and ICD-10-PCS codes for data submission.

CMS-1500 Claim Form

The CMS-1500 form shown in figure 1.1 is the standard billing document used for physician claims submitted on paper for Medicare Part B reimbursement. Providers also use this form for paper claims submitted to many private health insurance companies and Medicaid agencies. Medicare does not distribute blank forms. Forms may be purchased at the U.S. Government Printing Office.

Up to four diagnostic codes may be reported in field location 21 of this form; information on the service or procedure provided is reported in field location 24. Up to six CPT/HCPCS codes may be reported in column D of field location 24; in column E, the diagnostic codes are linked with the related HCPCS codes by placing a number (1, 2, 3, or 4) to show which diagnostic code is related to the procedure. Coding professionals must be sure that any association of ICD-9-CM diagnostic codes with HCPCS procedure codes is logical and appropriate.

Example: Patient's chief complaint is lower leg pain. The physician orders a lower leg x-ray and an EKG. The lower leg pain is linked with the x-ray, but there is no logical symptom or diagnosis to link with the EKG. Review of the health record may reveal an existing condition, such as premature ventricular contractions, or a symptom, such as tachycardia. Documentation must support the procedure or service provided; otherwise, the claim will be denied.

Figure 1.1. Sample CMS-1500 form

1500

HEALTH INSURANCE CLAIM FORM

APPROVED BY NATIONAL UNIFORM CLAIM COMMITTEE 08/05

PICA | PICA

CARRIER

1. MEDICARE (Medicare #) | MEDICAID (Medicaid #) | TRICARE CHAMPUS (Sponsor's SSN) | CHAMPVA (Member ID#) | GROUP HEALTH PLAN (SSN or ID) | FECA BLK LUNG (SSN) | OTHER (ID)

1a. INSURED'S I.D. NUMBER (For Program in Item 1)

2. PATIENT'S NAME (Last Name, First Name, Middle Initial)

3. PATIENT'S BIRTH DATE MM DD YY SEX M F

4. INSURED'S NAME (Last Name, First Name, Middle Initial)

5. PATIENT'S ADDRESS (No., Street)

6. PATIENT RELATIONSHIP TO INSURED Self Spouse Child Other

7. INSURED'S ADDRESS (No., Street)

CITY STATE

8. PATIENT STATUS Single Married Other

CITY STATE

ZIP CODE TELEPHONE (Include Area Code) ( )

Employed Full-Time Student Part-Time Student

ZIP CODE TELEPHONE (Include Area Code) ( )

9. OTHER INSURED'S NAME (Last Name, First Name, Middle Initial)

10. IS PATIENT'S CONDITION RELATED TO:

11. INSURED'S POLICY GROUP OR FECA NUMBER

a. OTHER INSURED'S POLICY OR GROUP NUMBER

a. EMPLOYMENT? (Current or Previous) YES NO

a. INSURED'S DATE OF BIRTH MM DD YY SEX M F

b. OTHER INSURED'S DATE OF BIRTH MM DD YY SEX M F

b. AUTO ACCIDENT? YES NO PLACE (State)

b. EMPLOYER'S NAME OR SCHOOL NAME

c. EMPLOYER'S NAME OR SCHOOL NAME

c. OTHER ACCIDENT? YES NO

c. INSURANCE PLAN NAME OR PROGRAM NAME

d. INSURANCE PLAN NAME OR PROGRAM NAME

10d. RESERVED FOR LOCAL USE

d. IS THERE ANOTHER HEALTH BENEFIT PLAN? YES NO *If yes*, return to and complete item 9 a-d.

READ BACK OF FORM BEFORE COMPLETING & SIGNING THIS FORM.

12. PATIENT'S OR AUTHORIZED PERSON'S SIGNATURE I authorize the release of any medical or other information necessary to process this claim. I also request payment of government benefits either to myself or to the party who accepts assignment below.

SIGNED ______ DATE ______

13. INSURED'S OR AUTHORIZED PERSON'S SIGNATURE I authorize payment of medical benefits to the undersigned physician or supplier for services described below.

SIGNED ______

PATIENT AND INSURED INFORMATION

14. DATE OF CURRENT: MM DD YY ILLNESS (First symptom) OR INJURY (Accident) OR PREGNANCY(LMP)

15. IF PATIENT HAS HAD SAME OR SIMILAR ILLNESS. GIVE FIRST DATE MM DD YY

16. DATES PATIENT UNABLE TO WORK IN CURRENT OCCUPATION FROM MM DD YY TO MM DD YY

17. NAME OF REFERRING PROVIDER OR OTHER SOURCE

17a.

17b. NPI

18. HOSPITALIZATION DATES RELATED TO CURRENT SERVICES FROM MM DD YY TO MM DD YY

19. RESERVED FOR LOCAL USE

20. OUTSIDE LAB? YES NO $ CHARGES

21. DIAGNOSIS OR NATURE OF ILLNESS OR INJURY (Relate Items 1, 2, 3 or 4 to Item 24E by Line)

1. ___ . ___

2. ___ . ___

3. ___ . ___

4. ___ . ___

22. MEDICAID RESUBMISSION CODE ORIGINAL REF. NO.

23. PRIOR AUTHORIZATION NUMBER

24. A. DATE(S) OF SERVICE From MM DD YY To MM DD YY	B. PLACE OF SERVICE	C. EMG	D. PROCEDURES, SERVICES, OR SUPPLIES (Explain Unusual Circumstances) CPT/HCPCS MODIFIER	E. DIAGNOSIS POINTER	F. $ CHARGES	G. DAYS OR UNITS	H. EPSDT Family Plan	I. ID. QUAL.	J. RENDERING PROVIDER ID. #
1								NPI	
2								NPI	
3								NPI	
4								NPI	
5								NPI	
6								NPI	

25. FEDERAL TAX I.D. NUMBER SSN EIN

26. PATIENT'S ACCOUNT NO.

27. ACCEPT ASSIGNMENT? (For govt. claims, see back) YES NO

28. TOTAL CHARGE $

29. AMOUNT PAID $

30. BALANCE DUE $

31. SIGNATURE OF PHYSICIAN OR SUPPLIER INCLUDING DEGREES OR CREDENTIALS (I certify that the statements on the reverse apply to this bill and are made a part thereof.)

SIGNED DATE

32. SERVICE FACILITY LOCATION INFORMATION

a. NPI b.

33. BILLING PROVIDER INFO & PH # ( )

a. NPI b.

PHYSICIAN OR SUPPLIER INFORMATION

NUCC Instruction Manual available at: www.nucc.org

APPROVED OMB-0938-0999 FORM CMS-1500 (08/05)

Medicare and many commercial third-party payers establish coverage limits for certain services. Reimbursement claims for services with coverage limits (for example, inpatient psychiatric care) must include sufficient diagnostic information to support the medical necessity of the services provided. This diagnostic information is communicated in the form of ICD-9-CM codes.

Medicare policies include two types of coverage limits: national coverage decisions (NCDs) and local coverage determinations (LCDs). These policies include decisions on items and services that are reasonable and necessary for the diagnosis or treatment of an illness or injury. For example, a Medicare policy may deny coverage for cosmetic surgical procedures. CMS establishes contractual arrangements with the private insurance companies (referred to as carriers), intermediaries, and Program Safeguard Contractors who process Medicare claims in local geographic regions. These contractors are responsible for making coverage decisions for Medicare beneficiaries, and the contractors base their decisions on established national coverage requirements for specific medical supplies and services. For cases that are not covered by existing national policies, contractors may make LCDs at their own discretion. A list of the Medicare coverage policies can be found on the CMS Web site. The following policy is an example of a LCD.

Example: CPT code 43235—Upper gastrointestinal endoscopy including esophagus, stomach, and either the duodenum and/or jejunum (commonly referred to as an esophagogastroduodenoscopy [EGD]) is covered by Medicare only with an appropriate ICD-9-CM diagnosis code submitted on the claim, such as:

211.0 Benign neoplasm of esophagus
230.2 Carcinoma in situ of stomach

CMS-1450 Claim Form (UB-04)

The CMS-1450 form (UB-04) (figure 1.2), is used primarily by hospitals for both outpatient and inpatient services. This form is used to submit claims for Medicare Part A services. It is also used by other third-party payers to report claims for outpatient and inpatient services provided by hospitals and ambulatory surgery centers (ASCs). Further information on UB-04 can be found at the Web site of the National Uniform Billing Committee: http://www.nubc.org.

Completion and coding instructions can be found in the Medicare Claims Processing Manual.

Figure 1.2. Sample UB-04 (CMS-1450) form

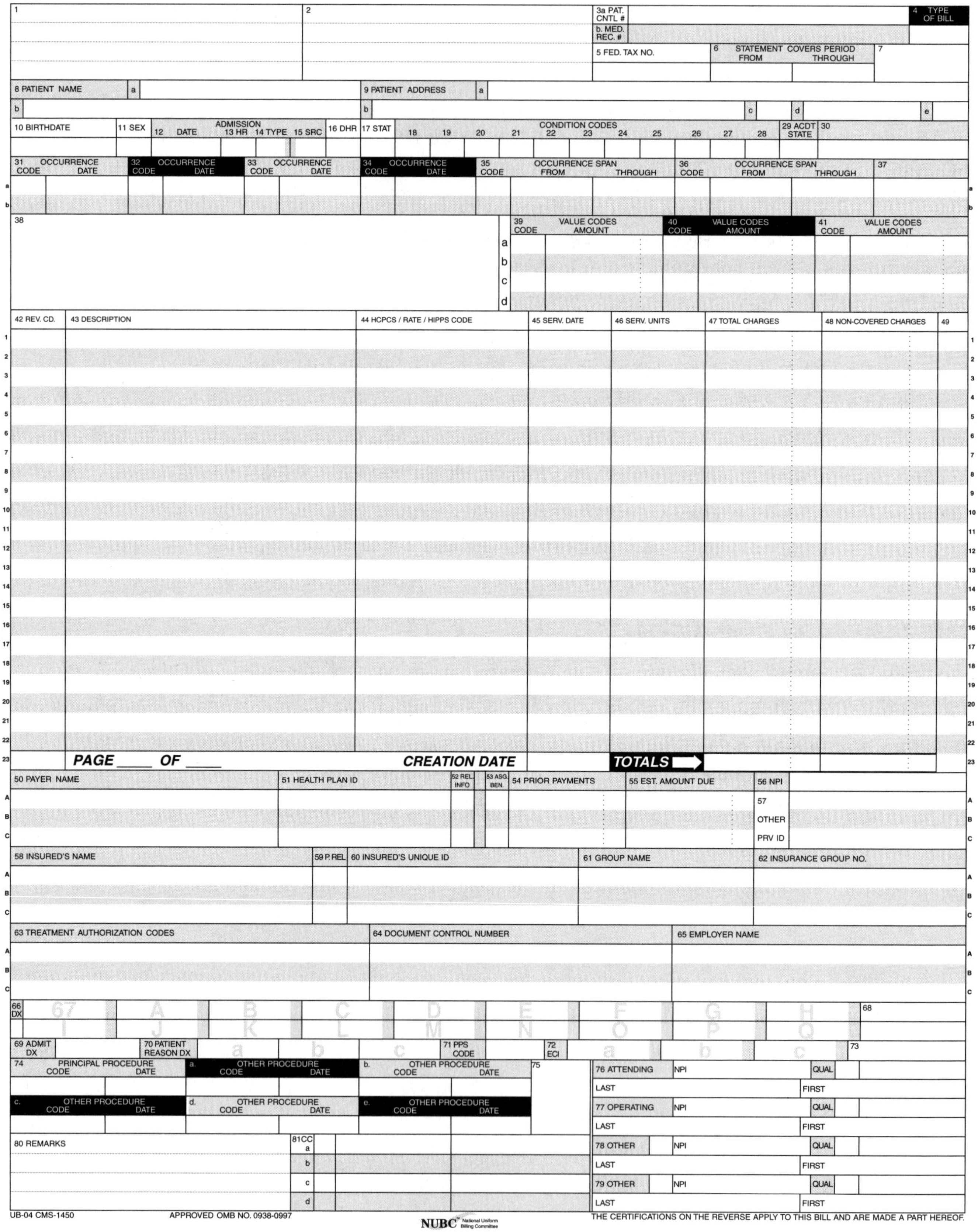

1 | 2 | 3a PAT. CNTL # | b. MED. REC. # | 4 TYPE OF BILL

5 FED. TAX NO. | 6 STATEMENT COVERS PERIOD FROM THROUGH | 7

8 PATIENT NAME a b | 9 PATIENT ADDRESS a b c d e

10 BIRTHDATE | 11 SEX | ADMISSION 12 DATE 13 HR 14 TYPE 15 SRC | 16 DHR | 17 STAT | CONDITION CODES 18 19 20 21 22 23 24 25 26 27 28 | 29 ACDT STATE | 30

31 OCCURRENCE CODE DATE | 32 OCCURRENCE CODE DATE | 33 OCCURRENCE CODE DATE | 34 OCCURRENCE CODE DATE | 35 OCCURRENCE SPAN CODE FROM THROUGH | 36 OCCURRENCE SPAN CODE FROM THROUGH | 37

38 | 39 VALUE CODES CODE AMOUNT | 40 VALUE CODES CODE AMOUNT | 41 VALUE CODES CODE AMOUNT

42 REV. CD. | 43 DESCRIPTION | 44 HCPCS / RATE / HIPPS CODE | 45 SERV. DATE | 46 SERV. UNITS | 47 TOTAL CHARGES | 48 NON-COVERED CHARGES | 49

PAGE ____ OF ____ | CREATION DATE | TOTALS

50 PAYER NAME | 51 HEALTH PLAN ID | 52 REL. INFO | 53 ASG. BEN. | 54 PRIOR PAYMENTS | 55 EST. AMOUNT DUE | 56 NPI | 57 OTHER PRV ID

58 INSURED'S NAME | 59 P. REL | 60 INSURED'S UNIQUE ID | 61 GROUP NAME | 62 INSURANCE GROUP NO.

63 TREATMENT AUTHORIZATION CODES | 64 DOCUMENT CONTROL NUMBER | 65 EMPLOYER NAME

66 DX | 67 A B C D E F G H I J K L M N O P Q | 68

69 ADMIT DX | 70 PATIENT REASON DX a b c | 71 PPS CODE | 72 ECI a b c | 73

74 PRINCIPAL PROCEDURE CODE DATE | a. OTHER PROCEDURE CODE DATE | b. OTHER PROCEDURE CODE DATE | 75

c. OTHER PROCEDURE CODE DATE | d. OTHER PROCEDURE CODE DATE | e. OTHER PROCEDURE CODE DATE

76 ATTENDING NPI QUAL LAST FIRST

77 OPERATING NPI QUAL LAST FIRST

78 OTHER NPI QUAL LAST FIRST

79 OTHER NPI QUAL LAST FIRST

80 REMARKS | 81CC a b c d

UB-04 CMS-1450 APPROVED OMB NO. 0938-0997 NUBC National Uniform Billing Committee THE CERTIFICATIONS ON THE REVERSE APPLY TO THIS BILL AND ARE MADE A PART HEREOF.

Exercise 1.1 Introduction

Unless otherwise noted, all answers can be found in appendix D of this book. Answers to selected exercises are located in the Instructor's Guide and available only to faculty of educational programs.

Review each of the following questions, and write the appropriate answers in the spaces provided.

1. What organizations are responsible for updating CPT codes and HCPCS Level II codes?

   ____

2. How many diagnostic codes may be submitted on the CMS-1500 form?

   ____

3. Which coding system(s) is (are) used for claims submitted by physicians?

   ____

4. Dr. Smith saw a Medicare patient with a diagnosis of rectal abscess in Central Hospital. She performed an incision and drainage in the outpatient surgery department.

   a. Which coding system(s) would Dr. Smith use to bill for her services?

      Diagnosis: ______________________________

      Procedure: ______________________________

   b. Which coding system(s) would Central Hospital use to bill for its services?

      Diagnosis: ______________________________

      Procedure: ______________________________

   c. Which form would Central Hospital use to submit a paper-based claim to Medicare for payment?

      ____

5. Which coding system describes the reason for the patient visit or encounter?

   ____

6. A patient was seen in a physician's office for excision of a 0.5-cm facial nevus (CPT [HCPCS Level I] code 11440). The ICD-9-CM diagnostic code for the benign lesion is 216.3. During this encounter, the physician also evaluated the patient's hyperglycemia (ICD-9-CM code 790.29) and chronic simple anemia (ICD-9-CM code 281.9). A three-specimen glucose tolerance test (HCPCS Level I code 82951) was performed. Using the excerpt from the CMS-1500 form provided in figure 1.3, link the appropriate ICD-9-CM codes found in block 21 with HCPCS Level I codes found in block 24D. In column 24E, select the appropriate number (1, 2, or 3) to indicate which diagnostic code is related to the procedure.

   ____

Figure 1.3. Information for question 6 of exercise 1.1

21. DIAGNOSIS OR NATURE OF ILLNESS OR INJURY (Relate Items 1, 2, 3 or 4 to Item 24E by Line)		22. MEDICAID RESUBMISSION CODE	ORIGINAL REF. NO.
1. ____ . ____	3. ____ . ____	23. PRIOR AUTHORIZATION NUMBER	
2. ____ . ____	4. ____ . ____		

	24. A. DATE(S) OF SERVICE From MM DD YY	To MM DD YY	B. PLACE OF SERVICE	C. EMG	D. PROCEDURES, SERVICES, OR SUPPLIES (Explain Unusual Circumstances) CPT/HCPCS	MODIFIER	E. DIAGNOSIS POINTER	F. $ CHARGES	G. DAYS OR UNITS	H. EPSDT Family Plan	I. ID. QUAL.	J. RENDERING PROVIDER ID. #
1											NPI	
2											NPI	
3											NPI	
4											NPI	
5											NPI	
6											NPI	

Chapter 2
Application of the CPT System

The American Medical Association (AMA) developed *Current Procedural Terminology* (CPT) to provide a uniform language that could be used to accurately designate medical, surgical, and diagnostic services. The CPT coding system is an effective means of facilitating communication among physicians, patients, and third-party payers nationwide. Published in 1966, the first edition of the CPT codebook consisted primarily of surgical procedures and limited codes for medicine, radiology, and laboratory procedures and services. The second edition, published in 1970, expanded the four-digit codes to five digits. And the last two editions, published in the late 1970s, reflected advances in medical technology and introduced a mechanism for updating the CPT codebook annually to keep it in step with changes in the medical field.

The AMA's CPT Editorial Panel, consisting of physicians and representatives from the Health Insurance Association of America, CMS, Blue Cross and Blue Shield, AHIMA, and AHA, is responsible for the annual revision and modification of the codebook. The panel is assisted in this task by the CPT Advisory Committee, which is composed of physicians nominated by the National Medical Specialty Societies, and by the AMA Health Care Professionals Advisory Committee, which is composed of other healthcare professionals. (Links to the AMA and CMS Web sites pertinent to the discussion in this chapter are listed in the Web resources in appendix A of this workbook.)

Organization of CPT

To be included in the CPT codebook, a procedure or service must meet the following conditions: (1) It must be commonly performed by many physicians across the country, and (2) it must be consistent with contemporary medical practice. Consequently, a procedure's inclusion in, or exclusion from, the CPT codebook does not imply that the AMA does or does not endorse it. Nor does it mean that the procedure is or is not covered for reimbursement by insurance plans. For example, although codes exist in CPT to describe cosmetic surgery, most insurance carriers do not provide reimbursement for such procedures. Thus, patients would pay for such services out of pocket. Reimbursement rules and guidelines are not always consistent with CPT coding rules and guidelines. Just as insurance policies for healthcare services vary, so do the reporting requirements involving codes.

The listing of procedures or services and their codes by subsections does not restrict use of these codes to certain specialty groups. For example, when describing a service that has been rendered, a surgeon may use codes from any section, not just those from the surgery section. Similarly, a family practice physician may use a code from the surgery section to describe office procedures or maternity care.

Each main section in the CPT codebook is divided into subsections, subcategories, headings, and procedures/services, as follows:

Surgery	Section
Integumentary system	Subsection
Skin, subcutaneous, and accessory structures	Subcategory
Incision and drainage	Heading
Incision and drainage of pilonidal cyst, simple	Procedure

The subsections, subcategories, and headings may identify any of the following:

- Services
- Procedures or therapies
- Examinations or tests
- Body systems
- Anatomic sites

Table 2.1 provides an example of each subdivision (when applicable) by section.

Exercise 2.1 Organization of CPT

Unless otherwise noted, all answers can be found in appendix D of this book. Answers to selected exercises are located in the Instructor's Guide and available only to faculty of educational programs.

Identify the CPT section and/or Category (I, II, or III) in which the following codes are located.

1. 21310 __________
2. 99232 __________
3. 81000 __________
4. 0503F __________
5. 97001 __________
6. 70486 __________
7. 00918 __________
8. 0085T __________

Identify the CPT subsection in which the following codes are located.

9. 59510 __________
10. 99360 __________
11. 77261 __________
12. 88307 __________

Table 2.1. Examples of CPT subdivisions

Section	Category/Subsection	Subcategory	Heading	Procedure/Service
E/M Services	Hospital Inpatient Services (99221–99239)	Initial Hospital Care (99221–99223)	New or Established Patient (99221–99223)	99223 Initial hospital care
Anesthesia	Head (00100–00222)	—	—	00104 Anesthesia for electroconvulsive therapy
Surgery	Respiratory System (30000–32999)	Nose (30000–30999)	Incision (30000–30020)	30020 Drainage abscess or hematoma, nasal septum
Radiology	Diagnostic Radiology (Diagnostic Imaging) (70010–76499)	Vascular Procedures (75600–75989)	Aorta and Arteries (75600–75791)	75600 Aortography, thoracic, without serialography, radiological supervision, and interpretation
Pathology and Laboratory	Anatomic Pathology (88000–88099)	Postmortem Examination (88000–88099)	—	88020 Necropsy (autopsy), gross and microscopic; without CNS
Medicine	Psychiatry (90801–90899)	Psychiatric Therapeutic Procedures (90804–90899)	Other Psychotherapy (90845–90857)	90845 Psychoanalysis
Category II Codes	Patient Management (0500F–0575F)	—	—	2000F Blood pressure, measured
Category III Codes	—	—	—	0249T Ligation, hemorrhoidal vascular bundle(s), including ultrasound guidance

Conventions and Characteristics of CPT

The CPT codebook follows several conventions, including the use of the following symbols:

- Semicolon ;
- Bullet •
- Triangle ▲
- Facing triangles ▶◀
- Plus symbol +
- Circled bullet ⊙
- Null symbol ⊘
- Pending symbol ⩘
- Out-of-numerical sequence code #
- Recycled/Reinstated code ○

The meanings of these symbols are explained in an introduction section at the beginning of the CPT book.

Semicolons

The format of the CPT codebook is designed to provide descriptions of procedures that can stand alone without additional explanation. To conserve space, many descriptions refer to a common portion of the procedure listed in a preceding entry rather than repeating the procedure in its entirety. When this occurs, the incomplete procedural description or descriptions are indented under the main entry, and the common portion of the main entry is followed by a semicolon (;). This signifies that the main entry applies to, and is part of, all indented entries that follow with their codes. The indented entries can yield different kinds of information, as illustrated in the following examples:

- The indented information may provide diagnostic data.

49520	Repair recurrent inguinal hernia, any age; reducible
49521	incarcerated or strangulated

The common portion of the description for code 49520 (the part before the semicolon) should be considered part of code 49521. Therefore, the full description of code 49521 reads: Repair recurrent inguinal hernia, any age; incarcerated or strangulated.

- The indented entries may describe alternate anatomical sites.

27705	Osteotomy; tibia
27707	fibula
27709	tibia and fibula
27712	multiple, with realignment on intramedullary rod (for example, Sofield-type procedure)

The full description of code 27707 reads: Osteotomy; fibula.

- The indented entries may designate specific procedures.

44150	Colectomy, total, abdominal, without proctectomy; with ileostomy or ileoproctostomy
44151	with continent ileostomy

The full description of code 44151 reads: Colectomy, total, abdominal, without proctectomy; with continent ileostomy

- The indented entries also may describe extensive procedures requiring the assignment of two codes. CPT often designates more extensive procedures by using the code for a stand-alone procedure and the code for an indented procedure to fully describe the extent of the surgery. When both codes are appropriate, the code for the indented description is preceded by the plus symbol (+) for add-on code.

15200	Full-thickness graft, free, including direct closure of donor site, trunk; 20 sq cm or less
+15201	each additional 20 sq cm or part thereof (List separately in addition to code for primary procedure)

- When a 40-sq cm graft is performed on a patient, both codes 15200 and 15201 are assigned. The performance of a 60-sq cm graft requires the following codes to be reported: 15200, 15201, and 15201.

Bullets and Triangles

CPT uses bullets (•) and triangles (▲) to identify changes in the current codebook. A bullet before a code identifies that code as a new addition, and a triangle before a code identifies a revision to the narrative description accompanying that code. Appendix B of the CPT codebook contains a comprehensive list of all revisions, including deletions and additions in code order. The following entry is an example of a new code found in CPT 2012:

• 37619	Ligation of inferior vena cava

The next is an example of a code that has been changed in CPT 2012:

▲32480	Removal of lung, other than pneumonectomy, single lobe (lobectomy)

Facing Triangles

The facing triangles symbol (▶◀) is used to indicate the beginning and ending of new or revised text within the guidelines and instruction notes. The coding professional should carefully review the information identified within facing triangles to ensure correct code assignment. An example of new text found in CPT 2012 can be found beneath code 39010:

> ▶ (For VATS pericardial biopsy, use 32604) ◀

Plus Symbols

When a procedure is commonly carried out with another procedure, it may be designated as an add-on code. Therefore, it should not be used alone. CPT identifies add-on codes with plus symbols. For example:

11000	Debridement of extensive eczematous or infected skin; up to 10% of body surface
+11001	each additional 10 percent of body surface, or part thereof (List separately in addition to code for primary procedure)

The plus symbol (+) indicates that 11001 is an add-on code and must be used with code 11000. It may not be reported alone. Notes reinforce the correct use of add-on codes. For example, after code 11001, the following instructional note appears:

> (Use 11001 in conjunction with code 11000)

Appendix D of CPT 2012 contains a complete list of add-on codes.

Circled Bullets

A circled bullet symbol (⊙) before a CPT code indicates that the use of moderate (conscious) sedation is an inherent part of the procedure. Moderate sedation is often used for procedures that do not require general anesthesia, which causes complete unconsciousness. Moderate sedation works by administering pain relievers and sedatives to induce an altered state of consciousness that minimizes pain and discomfort. The patients who receive moderate sedation are usually able to speak and respond to verbal cues throughout the procedure, and so they are able to communicate any discomfort to the provider.

According to CPT coding guidelines, it is not appropriate for the same physician to report both the service codes and moderate sedation codes (99143–99145) when the sedation is included in the service code. In addition, codes (99148–99150) are not reported in conjunction with codes listed in Appendix G (codes that include moderate sedation) when performed in the nonfacility setting. It is important to note that the inclusion of a procedure from the moderate (conscious) sedation list does not prevent separate reporting of an associated anesthesia procedure or service (CPT codes 00100–01999) when the service was performed by a physician other than the healthcare professional performing the diagnostic or therapeutic procedure. Appendix G of CPT 2012 provides a complete list of the codes that include moderate (conscious) sedation and guidelines on the use of these codes.

Null Symbol

The null symbol (⊘) indicates codes that may not be appended with modifier 51, Multiple Procedures. For example, code 17004, Destruction (e.g., laser surgery, electrosurgery, cryosurgery, chemosurgery, surgical curettement), premalignant lesions (e.g., actinic keratoses), 15 or more lesions may not be used with modifier 51. Appendix E of CPT 2012 provides a complete list of codes that are exempt from the use of modifier 51. (For a more detailed discussion of modifiers, see chapter 3 of this workbook.)

Pending Symbol

The pending symbol (⩘) indicates that the CPT code is for a vaccine that is pending approval from the Food and Drug Administration (FDA). For example:

⩘ 90664	Influenza virus vaccine, pandemic formulation, live, for intranasal use

Appendix K of CPT 2012 contains a list of codes identifying products that are pending FDA approval.

Resequenced Symbol

The resequenced symbol (#) emphasizes that the CPT codes do not appear in numeric sequence. Resequencing codes allow for CPT codes to be relocated without unnecessarily deleting codes. Appendix N of the CPT codebook provides a list of codes that are out of numerical sequence. Note that code 46320 (Excision of thrombosed hemorrhoid, external) was relocated to the hemorrhoidectomy section after code 46230).

Reinstated Code Symbol

The reinstated code symbol applies to codes that have been recycled. The hollowed circle (○) appears in front of the code.

Exercise 2.2 CPT Conventions

Unless otherwise noted, all answers can be found in appendix D of this book. Answers to selected exercises are located in the Instructor's Guide and available only to faculty of educational programs.

Review each of the following questions, and write the appropriate answers in the spaces provided.

1. What is the full description of code 35207?

   ____

2. The reporting of CPT codes 28150 and 28150 indicates the removal of how many toes?

   ____

3. Is code 33206 identified as a code with a new descriptor or a revised descriptor?

   ____

4. What is the full description for code 43219?

   ____

5. Is code 15271 identified as a code with a new descriptor or a revised descriptor?

   ____

6. Can code 15003 be used alone?

   ____

7. Can code 31500 be appended with modifier 51?

   ____

8. Review the range of CPT codes 13150 through 13153. What is the correct code assignment for a 7.8-cm complex wound repair of the ear?

   ____

9. Review the range of CPT codes 40810 through 40816. What is the correct code assignment for an excision of a mucosal lesion of the vestibule of the mouth with a complex repair?

   ____

10. Review the range of CPT codes 31575 through 31578. What is the correct code assignment for a flexible fiberoptic laryngoscopy for removal of a lesion and a separate biopsy of inflamed tissue?

    ____

Category I, II, and III Codes

The AMA continues to focus on enhancing the functionality of CPT nomenclature. As part of this initiative, CPT has been expanded to include the needs of data reporting and data collection without significantly changing the current structure and payment focus of CPT. As a result, three categories of CPT codes have been established.

Category I Codes

Category I codes include the traditional, five-digit numeric codes that identify procedures and services. Code 10021—Fine needle aspiration; without imaging guidance—is an example of a Category I CPT code.

Category II Codes

Category II codes include alphanumeric codes that are used for tracking purposes to represent performance measurements. Category II codes are located in a section after the Medicine codes in the CPT codebook. The use of tracking codes for performance measurement facilitates data collection and minimizes administrative burden. The five-digit alphanumeric codes can be identified by adding the letter *F* at the end of the code. Code 4000F—Tobacco use cessation intervention, counseling—is an example of a Category II code.

The use of Category II codes is optional. The tracking codes are reviewed as part of healthcare quality tracking by the AMA, the Joint Commission, and the National Committee for Quality Assurance (NCQA), among others. Appendix H—Alphabetical Clinical Topics Listing of the codebook has been relocated to the AMA Web site at: http://www.ama-assn.org/go/cpt.

Category III Codes

Category III codes are temporary codes used to represent emerging technology services and procedures. These codes were developed to allow researchers to track the use of emerging technology services. Data collection of Category III codes can assist with the following:

- Clinical efficacy
- Utilization
- Outcomes
- A means to avoid the use of unlisted CPT codes

The codes are included in a section of the codebook that falls after the Category II codes and the Medicine section.

Category III codes are assigned an alphanumeric identifier (for example, 0019T). After they have been approved by the CPT Editorial Panel, new Category III codes are added on a semi-annual (twice-yearly) basis and made available through the AMA Web site. Category III codes are archived when they have not been moved to the Category I section after five years unless it can be demonstrated that the codes are still useful. For example, 0137T appeared in the 2010 edition of CPT, but the procedure (transperineal stereotactic template guided saturation prostate biopsies) was assigned code 55706 in 2011. Therefore, 0130T was deleted from the list of Category III codes. Payment for Category III services and procedures depends on the reimbursement policies of individual payers.

Unlisted Procedures

Because of rapid advances in medical research and technology, new services or procedures may be performed before codes have been added to the CPT system to represent them. In these rare instances, an unlisted code should be reported along with a written report describing the procedure or service. The operative report is usually sufficient when reporting an unlisted surgical code. The introduction to each section of the CPT codebook includes a complete list of the unlisted service or procedure codes available for that section. Unlisted codes for various subsections can be found in the alphabetic index of the CPT codebook under the main heading Unlisted Services and Procedures. Before any unlisted code is assigned, the coding professional should review HCPCS Level II (National) codes to confirm that CMS has not developed a specific code for the procedure or service in question. CPT Category III codes, which are developed specifically for reporting new technology, should also be reviewed. CPT guidelines support the use of a Category III code instead of a Category I unlisted code.

Appendixes

The following is a summary of each of the 14 appendices located after the Category III codes in CPT.

Appendix A—Modifiers

Appendix A provides a complete list of modifiers for use with CPT Level I and HCPCS Level II (National) codes. Chapter 3 of this book will highlight the use of modifiers

Appendix B—Summary of Additions, Deletions, and Revisions

Every year, CPT undergoes a revision process. The summary of this work is provided in Appendix B.

Appendix C—Clinical Examples

In this appendix, CPT provides explanatory paragraphs to assist with guiding the selection of Evaluation and Management (E/M) codes. Chapter 7 of this book will focus on E/M codes.

Appendix D—Summary of CPT Add-on Codes

A complete list of CPT add-on codes is contained in Appendix D. As described earlier in this chapter, these codes appear with a plus sign.

Appendix E—Summary of CPT Codes Exempt from Modifier 51

Codes in Appendix E are not to be appended with the modifier 51. Modifier 51 is assigned when multiple procedures (other than E/M services, physical medicine and rehabilitation services, or provision of supplies) are performed at the same session by the same provider. The primary procedure or service may be reported as listed. The additional procedure or service may be identified by appending modifier 51. The null symbol appears before these codes. Chapter 3 of this book will focus on use of modifiers.

Appendix F—Summary of CPT Codes Exempt from Modifier 63

Codes that appear in this appendix are exempt from being appended with modifier 63 (Procedure Performed on Infants Less than 4 kg).

Appendix G—Summary of CPT Codes That Include Moderate (Conscious) Sedation

The procedure codes listed in this appendix include conscious sedation as an inherent part of the procedure. A circled bullet symbol (⨀) appears before these CPT codes.

Appendix H—Alphabetical Clinical Topics Listing

This listing is no longer in the CPT book but is provided on the AMA's Web site. This appendix contains an alphabetic listing of the diseases with which the measures and codes are associated. This crosswalk to the Category II codes provides an overview of performance measures and reporting instructions.

Appendix I—Genetic Testing Code Modifiers

Genetic testing modifiers are appended to CPT and HCPCS codes to provide diagnostic granularity of service to enable providers to submit complete and precise genetic testing information without altering the testing code descriptors.

Appendix J—Electrodiagnostic Medicine Listing of Sensory, Motor, and Mixed Nerves

To assist with the accurate selection of CPT codes 95900, 95903, and 95904 (nerve conduction study codes), this appendix designates the specific nerve to the corresponding CPT code.

Appendix K—Product Pending FDA Approval

This appendix provides a list of vaccine product codes pending approval from the Federal Drug Administration (FDA). The pending symbol (✗) appears before these CPT codes.

Appendix L—Vascular Families

To assist with CPT coding selection, this appendix contains a diagram of first, second, and third order branches in a vascular family. The diagram assumes that the starting point is catheterization of the aorta. Before using any of the reference material in the appendices, it is important to read the introductory information.

Appendix M—Deleted CPT Codes

Appendix M provides a table that links deleted and renumbered codes from the years 2007 through 2009 to the current 2012 codes. In addition, the appendix provides citations to *CPT Assistant* and *CPT Changes: An Insider's View.*

Appendix N—Summary of Resequenced CPT Codes

Appendix N lists the codes that are not in numerical order.

Notes

Coding professionals using the CPT codebook should pay special attention to the notes located at various levels within the text. Notes may appear at the beginning of a heading, within parentheses before or after a code, or within parentheses in the code description.

Notes placed at the beginning of a heading provide additional information about the services or procedures that follow. For example:

- Integral components of a service or procedure

Example: A note under the heading Endoscopy (31231–31297) states that a surgical sinus endoscopy always includes a sinusotomy (when appropriate) and a diagnostic endoscopy.

- Definitions of terms and codes

  Example: Under the heading Shaving of Epidermal or Dermal Lesions (11300–11313), a note defines *shaving* as "the sharp removal by transverse incision or horizontal slicing to remove epidermal and dermal lesions without a full-thickness dermal excision."

- Directions to assign additional codes

  Example: Under the heading Coronary Artery Bypass–Sequential Combined Arterial–Venous Grafting (33517–33530), the note reminds the coding professional that two codes are required to identify coronary artery bypass grafting using both arterial and venous grafts.

Notes that appear before or after individual codes provide additional coding guidelines. For example:

- Alternative codes

  Example: The note appearing after code 11772 directs the coding professional to use 10080 or 10081 for an incision of a pilonidal cyst.

- Deleted codes

  Example: The note appearing after code 0081T advises the coding professional that 0084T has been deleted. To report the procedure previously identified by code 0084T the coding professional should assign code 53855.

- Add-on codes

  Example: The note appearing after code 19001 instructs the coding professional not to assign code 19001 as a single code. It must be used with code 19000.

- Other instructional information

  Example: The note appearing after code 64611 instructs the coding professional to use modifier 52 if fewer than four salivary glands are injected.

Notes also appear within the text of some codes to provide additional explanation. For example:

Example: Within code 10040, the coding professional is provided with the example of acne surgery.

Coding Tips

The Professional Edition of CPT 2012 includes "Coding Tips" to provide guidance in appropriate code selection. For example, preceding code 11000 is the following tip:

> ---------------------------*Coding Tip*---------------------------
>
> Use of Depth and Surface Area for Reporting Debridement of Wounds
>
> When performing debridement of a single wound, report depth using the deepest level of tissue removed. In multiple wounds, sum the surface area of those wounds that are at the same depth, but do not combine sums from different depths.

Alphabetic Index

At the back of the CPT codebook, an index provides a list of specific codes organized by main entries such as:

Replantation
Report Preparation
Reposition
Repositioning
Reproductive tissue
Reprogramming
Resection

The main entries are printed in boldface type and arranged in alphabetic order. The main entries are based on:

- Procedures, services, or examinations such as coccygectomy, mastopexy, preventive medicine, physical therapy, nuclear medicine, and organ- or disease-oriented panel
- Organs or other anatomic sites such as bladder, blood vessels, ethmoid, ganglion, muscle, and sweat glands
- Conditions or diagnoses such as abrasion, hematoma, heel spur, meningioma, mumps, omphalocele, and septal defect
- Synonyms, eponyms, or abbreviations such as Ewart procedure, FAST, LHR, Pereyra procedure, Pomeroy's operation, TLC screen, and HLA typing

Some of the main entries include subterms that provide additional information that must be reviewed before a code can be selected. For example:

Laryngoscopy
Diagnostic 31505
Direct. 31515–31571
Exploration 31505, 31520–31526, 31575
Fiberoptic 31575–31579
with Stroboscopy 31579
Indirect 31505–31513
Newborn 31520
Operative. 31530–31561

The CPT alphabetic index also uses cross-references to help coding professionals identify the most appropriate code. *See* cross-references appear most frequently with eponyms, synonyms, and abbreviations and refer coding professionals to other main terms. For example, the entry for AHG includes a cross-reference that refers the coding professional to the main entry for clotting factor.

See cross-references can also direct the coding professional to another main term, but only when the information sought did not follow the first main term. For example:

> Sweat Test. 82435
> *See* Chloride, Blood

These examples illustrate the importance of referring to the additional main entries as directed by the cross-references to ensure the highest level of specificity in code selection.

The alphabetic index offers at least one code under each entry, although in some cases more than one code or a range of codes is provided. Every code and its description must be reviewed carefully to ensure accurate code assignment and appropriate payment.

Consider the following example:

> **Mastectomy**
> Gynecomastia 19300
> Modified Radical .19307
> Partial 19301–19302
> Radical 19303–19306
> Simple, Complete .19303
> Subcutaneous 19304

When coding a partial mastectomy, the coding professional must review the descriptions for both 19301 and 19302 before assigning a final code.

The first step in locating a code in the alphabetic index is to find the procedure or service performed, such as jejunostomy or peritoneocentesis. If the service or procedure is not listed, the coding professional should locate the organ or anatomic site involved; the condition or diagnosis; or the synonym or eponym, such as phalanx, Epstein-Barr virus, or Dandy operation. The subterms should be reviewed and any cross-references followed. Each code listed in the index should be noted and each description reviewed until a match is established.

Becoming familiar with the CPT codebook will expedite the coding process. For example, a comprehensive knowledge of the codebook would show that correct codes often are found under several main terms.

Consider these procedures: hallux valgus correction and Mayo bunionectomy. Review of the alphabetic index will yield the following entries and codes:

> **Bunion Repair** 28296–28299
> Mayo Procedure. 28292
>
> **Mayo Procedure**. 28292
>
> **Repair**
> Hallux Valgus. 28290–28299
>
> **Repair**
> Toe
> Bunion 28290–28299
>
> **Repair**
> Bunion 28290–28299

Note: The terms *Hallux valgus* and *Correction, hallux valgus* do not appear in the alphabetic index.

General Rules for CPT Coding

Here are some general rules to consider when applying CPT codes:

- Analyze the note or procedural statement provided by the physician or other healthcare provider and/or included in the health record.
- Determine the procedure, test, or service to be coded.
- Locate the main term in the index by checking under the procedure, anatomic site, condition, synonym, eponym, service, or abbreviation as necessary.
- Review and select the subterms indented below the main term.
- Note the code number(s) found opposite the selected main term or subterm:

  —If a single code number is provided, locate the code in the body of the CPT codebook. Verify the code and its description against the procedural statement to make sure they match.

  —If two or more codes separated by a comma are shown, locate each code in the body of the CPT codebook. Read the description of each code before selecting the appropriate one to match the procedural statement.

  —If a range of codes is shown, locate that range in the body of the CPT codebook. Review the description of each entry before selecting a code. The code description should always match the procedural statement.
- If applicable, follow cross-references.
- Never code directly from the index.
- Read all notes that apply to the code selected. They can appear at the beginning of a section or subsection, directly under, or within the code description.
- Select the appropriate modifier, when applicable, to complete the code description. Modifiers may not always apply to hospital reporting of outpatient hospital procedures. Individual health plans may have specific guidelines for the use of modifiers and for the acceptance of Level II modifiers. For accurate reporting, the coding professional must be familiar with the specific reporting requirements for the circumstances.
- Continue coding all components of the procedure or service according to the directions in the CPT codebook.

Exercise 2.3 Use of the Alphabetical Index

Unless otherwise noted, all answers can be found in appendix D of this book. Answers to selected exercises are located in the Instructor's Guide and available only to faculty of educational programs.

Assign the appropriate CPT codes and provide the corresponding index entries for the following terms.

1. Green operation

   Code: ______________________________

   Index entry: ______________________________

2. Fine needle aspiration of cyst of thyroid, without imaging guidance

   Code: ______________________________

   Index entry: ______________________________

3. Femoropopliteal bypass graft with vein

   Code: ______________________________

   Index entry: ______________________________

4. Repair of reducible recurrent femoral hernia

   Code: ______________________________

   Index entry: ______________________________

5. Incision and drainage of infected bursa, left hip

   Code: ______________________________

   Index entry: ______________________________

6. Anesthesia provided for application of shoulder cast (assign only the code for the anesthesia services)

   Code: ______________________________

   Index entry:

7. Direct diagnostic laryngoscopy for 45-year-old patient

   Code: ______________________________

   Index entry: ______________________________

8. MRI of lumbar spine with contrast material

   Code: ______________________________

   Index entry: ______________________________

9. Paring of a single corn of the right foot

   Code: ______________________________

   Index entry: ______________________________

10. HIV-1 antibody testing

    Code: ______________________________

    Index entry: ______________________________

Exercise 2.3 (Continued)

Note: Answers to exercises 11 through 20 do not appear in appendix D of this text. They are located in the Instructor's Guide and available to faculty of educational programs.

11. Biopsy of posterior third of tongue

    Code: ______________________________

    Index entry: ______________________________

12. Esophagogastroduodenoscopy (EGD) with biopsy

    Code: ______________________________

    Index entry: ______________________________

13. Arthroscopic medial meniscectomy

    Code: ______________________________

    Index entry: ______________________________

14. All-night recording EEG

    Code: ______________________________

    Index entry: ______________________________

15. Removal of metal shaving from cornea without use of slit lamp

    Code: ______________________________

    Index entry: ______________________________

16. Endometrial cryoablation with ultrasound guidance

    Code: ______________________________

    Index entry: ______________________________

17. Beta-blocker therapy prescribed

    Code: ______________________________

    Index entry: ______________________________

18. Excision of rectal tumor, TEMS (transanal endoscopic microsurgery) approach

    Code: ______________________________

    Index entry: ______________________________

19. DXA, vertebral fracture assessment

    Code: ______________________________

    Index entry: ______________________________

20. Excision of recurrent ganglion of wrist

    Code: ______________________________

    Index entry: ______________________________

Abstracting Documentation

This book provides two types of exercises: one-line procedure coding and operative narratives. The one-line procedures offer students the opportunity to use the index to locate the coding selection and apply the guidelines introduced in the chapter. Coding from operative notes found in office records, operative reports, and emergency department notes allows students to practice the skill of abstracting needed information to assign a code successfully. When reviewing the documentation in an operative report, students are encouraged to scan the report for procedures performed (action types of words: excision, incision, aspiration, endoscopy, and so forth) and associated diagnoses.

For example, note the contents of an operative report below with the highlighted action words.

Operative Report

Preoperative Diagnosis: Bladder tumor → [Reason for procedure]

Postoperative Diagnosis: Bladder tumor

Operation: Transurethral resection of a 3-cm bladder tumor → [Procedure performed]

Anesthesia: General

Specimens: Sessile bladder tumor and tumor base → [Tissue sent to laboratory]

Findings: A 3-cm high-grade appearing tumor, thought to be transitional cell carcinoma, right posterior bladder wall.

Indication: A 62-year-old patient with hematuria with bladder tumor identified on CT of the pelvis.

[Describes the beginning of the operative session—preparing the patient for the procedure.] ← Description of procedure: The patient was brought to the operating room. General anesthesia was induced. The patient was placed in lithotomy and genitalia was prepped and draped in the usual manner. The patient was identified and the procedure was confirmed. Resectoscope passed. → [This is the operative approach.] Tumor visualized, right posterior bladder wall, approximately 3 cm in greatest dimension. It is very sessile in nature, quite red and angry-appearing. There were some papillary areas. Overall the tumor had a very high-grade appearance to it. It was near, but did not involve the right ureteral orifice.

[Action word: resected] ← The tumor was resected and the biopsy specimen sent for permanent section.

[Action word: biopsies] ← Separate biopsies were taken of the tumor base to rule out deep muscle invasion. The area was thoroughly cauterized with loop electrode. No bleeding was seen with the bladder decompressed. No other abnormalities were noted. Scope removed. The patient tolerated the procedure well.

[The end of the operative report describes the closure of the operative session.]

After looking in the index and, subsequently, in the main body portion of the CPT codebook to locate coding selections, it will be necessary to note the types of information that may influence the choice of codes and then to read the operative report again for information that will help determine the correct answer.

Exercise 2.4 CPT Coding Process

Unless otherwise noted, all answers can be found in appendix D of this book. Answers to selected exercises are located in the Instructor's Guide and available only to faculty of educational programs.

Operative Report

Preoperative Diagnosis:	History of colon cancer	→ Reason for encounter
Postoperative Diagnosis:	Rectosigmoid polyp	
Procedure:	Colonoscopy and polypectomy	→ Procedure performed
Indications:	The patient has had three previous resections of three different primary carcinomas of the colon. His last resection of carcinoma was in 2000. He has been doing well in general.	
Premedications:	Demerol 50 mg IV and Versed 2.5 mg IV	
Procedure:	The CF100-L video colonoscope was passed without difficulty from the anus up through the anastomosis, which appears to be in the distal transverse colon. The instrument was advanced into the distal small bowel and then slowly withdrawn with good view obtained throughout. A small, 3-mm polyp near the rectosigmoid junction was removed with hot biopsy forceps and retrieved. Otherwise, the patient has a satisfactory postoperative appearance of the colon. It is shortened due to previous resections, but there is no other evidence of neoplasm. The instrument was completely withdrawn without other findings.	

Read the preceding operative report. Then perform the steps in the coding process as listed below. Show your results in the spaces provided.

1. Scan the documentation to identify the procedure performed.

   ____

2. Search the index for Colonoscopy, Removal, Polyp, and identify the code range for the procedure.

   ____

3. Review the coding descriptions to determine what additional documentation is needed before you can accurately select a code.

   ____

4. Read the operative report again to determine the method of removal used.

   ____

5. Choose the code that reflects this documentation.

   ____

Exercise 2.5 CPT Coding Process

Unless otherwise noted, all answers can be found in appendix D of this book. Answers to selected exercises are located in the Instructor's Guide and available only to faculty of educational programs.

Operative Report

Preoperative Diagnosis:	Subepidermal nodular lesion of the forearm ——► Reason for encounter
Operation:	Excision of 2.0-cm lesion of the forearm
Procedure:	Under local anesthesia, the 2.0-cm lesion was removed with 0.5-cm margins. The lesion was submitted to pathology. Bleeding was controlled with electrocautery, and the wound was closed with five vertical mattress sutures of 5-0 nylon. Polysporin and dressing were applied to the wound.
Pathological Diagnosis:	Well-organized basal cell carcinoma

Review the preceding operative report and note the pathological diagnosis. Then perform the steps in the coding process as listed below. Record your results in the spaces provided. (Hint: Be sure to abstract the following information from the operative report: size of lesion and margins; morphology, benign or malignant; location; and method of removal.)

1. Scan the documentation and record the main procedure to be located in the alphabetic index.

   ____

2. Search the index for the main terms/subterms and record the code selections.

   ____

3. Review the code descriptions to determine what additional documentation is needed before you can accurately select a code.

   ____

4. Read the operative report and pathological diagnosis again to determine the additional documentation to clarify the selection.

   ____

5. Choose the code that reflects this documentation.

   ____

Exercise 2.6 CPT Coding Process

Unless otherwise noted, all answers can be found in appendix D of this book. Answers to selected exercises are located in the Instructor's Guide and available only to faculty of educational programs.

Operative Report

Preoperative Diagnosis: Umbilical hernia

Postoperative Diagnosis: Same

This is a 38-year-old man who presents with an umbilical hernia. He has been experiencing influenza-like symptoms, which he describes as crampy abdominal pain. Risks versus benefits including bleeding, infection, and the high recurrence rate because of his obesity were discussed. The patient states he understands and elects to proceed with surgery.

After adequate general endotracheal anesthesia had been induced, the patient was placed in the supine position, and prepped and draped in the usual sterile manner. A curvilinear incision was made just inferior to the umbilicus. This was extended down through adipose tissue to the level of the rectus fascia. The herniosac was amputated and sent to pathology. The fascia was then reapproximated transversely using interrupted 0 prolene sutures. The skin was reapproximated using 4-0 nylon. Sponge and needle counts were accurate. The patient tolerated the procedure well and left the operating room in stable condition.

Review the preceding operative report and abstract the information that is needed for a correct code assignment. Answer the following questions in the spaces provided.

1. What procedure was performed?

   ____

2. What code selections were listed in the index entry for the main terms describing the procedure?

   ____

3. What additional documentation is needed before an accurate code can be assigned?

   ____

4. What is the correct code for the procedure?

   ____

5. Should a CPT code also be assigned for the suturing of the wound at the conclusion of the procedure?

   ____

Identification of Operative Procedures for Coding

New coding professionals often have difficulty determining whether a procedure is an integral part of the main operative procedure or a separately identifiable procedure. For example, when a patient has a breast mass removed, a code for the wound closure would not be assigned because it is an integral part of the main procedure. The ability to discriminate between reportable and non-reportable procedures is a skill that must be developed and one that significantly affects accurate code selection. Coding professionals need to have surgical references to help them understand procedures and techniques. The references section of this book provides a list of helpful resources. In addition to understanding surgical techniques, coding professionals must know when to assign additional codes and will find instructions on doing so in the CPT guidelines. Various types of notes and descriptions located throughout CPT guidelines are illustrated below.

52601	Transurethral electrosurgical resection of prostate, including control of postoperative bleeding, complete (Vasectomy, meatotomy, cystourethroscopy, urethral calibration and/or dilation, and internal urethrotomy are included)

Many CPT codes combine the main procedure with minor procedures that do not warrant additional codes. In these cases, the code description contains a note specifying the secondary procedures that are to be included in the primary code. In the preceding example, if the surgeon performs a transurethral electrosurgical resection of prostate (TURP) with vasectomy, the correct code assignment is 52601. Because the code description states that vasectomy is included in the code for the TURP procedure, the vasectomy is not assigned a separate code.

58150	Total abdominal hysterectomy (corpus and cervix), with or without removal of tube(s), with or without removal of ovary(s)

If the surgeon performs a total abdominal hysterectomy with salpingo-oophorectomy, the only code submitted would be 58150. The code description explains that no additional code would be submitted for the salpingo-oophorectomy.

Some notes in the CPT codebook offer guidance on multiple code assignment for an entire section. For example, look at the note before code 14000 in the Adjacent Tissue Transfer or Rearrangement portion of the integumentary system subsection of the surgery section. The second paragraph includes the following clause: "Excision (including lesion) and/or repair by adjacent tissue transfer or rearrangement." According to this note, when a surgeon removes a skin lesion and the defect is repaired with an adjacent tissue transfer, only the tissue transfer should be coded. The excision of lesion is not identified with an additional code.

Some notes provide instructions for use of add-on codes. For example, code 69990, Operating microscope, is reported only as an additional code. In some procedures, physicians utilize an operating microscope during the surgical episode. CPT provides specific instructions in the note before code 69990 to help the coding professional determine whether this add-on code is to be used with a particular primary procedure code.

Instruction is often given in the form of a note under a specific code, for example, the note under CPT code 63078 that instructs the coding professional not to report code 69990 in addition to codes 63075 through 63078.

Coding References

Both the American Medical Association (AMA) and the Centers for Medicare and Medicaid Services (CMS) are resources for CPT coding guidelines.

American Medical Association

The AMA is the primary, authoritative reference for CPT guidelines and changes. The AMA publishes *CPT Assistant,* a monthly newsletter that provides information on the correct application of CPT codes. The newsletter includes a question-and-answer section that provides answers to coding professionals' questions. The AMA also offers a subscription service for assistance with coding questions. Most large healthcare facilities subscribe to an online version of *CPT Assistant.* Exercises 2.7 and 2.8 require access to *CPT Assistant.*

Exercise 2.7 Coding References

Unless otherwise noted, all answers can be found in appendix D of this book. Answers to selected exercises are located in the Instructor's Guide and available only to faculty of educational programs.

Exercise 2.4 asked you to analyze documentation and assign the correct code for a colonoscopy with a polypectomy procedure. For correct CPT assignment, you needed to know what method was used to remove the polyp. In the operative report for that exercise, the surgeon used hot biopsy forceps. For this exercise, assume that a surgeon removed the tiny polyp by using a cold biopsy forceps. The polyp was so small that it was completely removed during the biopsy.

1. What is the correct coding assignment for this procedure?

   ____

2. What volume of *CPT Assistant* provided the information needed to arrive at this code assignment?

   ____

Centers for Medicare and Medicaid Services

The federal government provides some interpretative guidance on the use of CPT codes and modifiers as an element of HCPCS. The HCPCS guidelines are published in the form of transmittals, manuals, and other documents. Most of the Medicare and Medicaid manuals are available for downloading from the CMS Web site (http://www.cms.gov/transmittals).

Exercise 2.8 Coding References

Unless otherwise noted, all answers can be found in appendix D of this book. Answers to selected exercises are located in the Instructor's Guide and available only to faculty of educational programs.

In exercise 2.5, the surgeon excised a lesion of the forearm. Suppose that the surgeon took a biopsy of the lesion before removing it. (The following exercise requires reference to *CPT Assistant.*)

1. Should both the biopsy and the excision be coded or just the excision?

   ____

2. Which volume of *CPT Assistant* provided the information needed to answer this question?

   ____

Exercise 2.9 Chapter 2 Review

Unless otherwise noted, all answers can be found in appendix D of this book. Answers to selected exercises are located in the Instructor's Guide and available only to faculty of educational programs.

Answer the following questions in the spaces provided.

1. Which symbol indicates that a procedure code is new in CPT?

   ____

2. Refer to CPT codes 11100 and 11101. Assume that a surgeon performed a biopsy of two different skin lesions during the same procedure. Which code should be assigned?

   ____

3. Which category of CPT codes is reserved for emerging technology?

   ____

4. Refer to CPT codes 42310 and 42320. Assume that a surgeon drained an external submaxillary abscess. Which code should be assigned?

   ____

5. Refer to CPT codes 40840 through 40844. Assume that a surgeon performed a bilateral, posterior vestibuloplasty. Which code should be assigned?

   ____

Note: Answers to exercises 6 through 10 do not appear in appendix D of this text. They are located in the Instructor's Guide and available to faculty of educational programs.

6. Refer to CPT code 56630. What documentation in the operative report would be needed to support the use of this code?

   ____

7. Refer to CPT codes 54050 through 54060. Assume a surgeon removed condylomas of the penis. What medical record documentation would be needed to assign one of the codes accurately?

   ____

8. Assume that a gastroenterologist performed an EGD (CPT code 43235) and administered Versed during the procedure. Would the physician submit codes to reflect both the procedure (43235) and the administration of anesthesia?

   ____

9. Refer to CPT codes 76856 through 76857. Documentation indicates that a radiologist examined the fallopian tubes and ovaries to compare the abnormal surgical findings to an ultrasound performed the preceding month. What would be the correct code assignment?

   ____

10. Refer to CPT codes 11730 through 11732. Assume that a physician performed a complete avulsion of the nail plate of the thumb and index and ring fingers. What would be the correct code assignment?

    ____

Chapter 3

Modifiers

(Please note that for purposes of instruction and for ease in reading, this book uses a dash to separate each five-character CPT code from its two-character modifier. However, dashes are not used in actual code assignments and reimbursement claims, which report seven-character codes with no spaces between the characters when the assignment of modifiers is appropriate.)

Modifiers may be reported along with a CPT code to indicate that a particular event modified the service/procedure, but with no change to its basic definition. Modifiers may indicate any of the following situations:

- A service/procedure has both a professional component and a technical component.
- A service/procedure was performed by more than one physician or in more than one location.
- A service/procedure has been increased or reduced in scope.
- A service was performed only partially.
- An adjunctive service was performed.
- A bilateral procedure was performed.
- A service/procedure was performed more than once.
- An unusual event occurred during the service/procedure.

Example of Modifier:

> 50 Bilateral Procedure: Unless otherwise identified in listings, bilateral procedures that are performed at the same operative session should be identified by adding modifier 50 to the appropriate five-digit code.
>
> Code assignment for *bilateral* repair of recurrent inguinal hernia
>
> 49520–50
>
> CPT code ← → Modifier 50

There is a distinct advantage to conveying as much information as possible to the third-party payer to ensure appropriate payment when billing for professional physician services or services provided by an ambulatory surgery or service center. Use of a modifier, in selected cases, allows the healthcare provider to explain special circumstances that surround the charge for the service and may affect claim payment. Use of an appropriate modifier also can prevent a claim from being denied.

Appendix A of the CPT codebook includes a complete list of currently accepted modifiers and their descriptions. Coding professionals should examine modifier descriptions carefully for conditions that may limit use of a modifier to a specific section of CPT. For example, modifier 25 is limited by definition to evaluation and management codes and would not be appended to a code from the surgery section. Modifier 78 (Return to Operating Room for a Related Procedure During the Postoperative Period) would only be appended to a CPT surgical code. (Links to the CMS Web site pertinent to the discussion in this chapter are in the Web resources at the back of this book.)

Use of Modifiers

The CPT and HCPCS systems for describing and reporting medical procedures and services include the use of special supplementary codes called modifiers. Modifiers are two-character codes that can be appended to some of the CPT Level I codes and the HCPCS Level II codes to provide additional information.

Different sets of modifiers apply to different services and settings. For example, two-digit numerical modifiers can be appended to CPT codes for reporting additional information relevant to physician and outpatient hospital services. In addition, two-digit alphabetic or alphanumeric modifiers permit more concise reporting of services in Level II (National) HCPCS codes.

Several specific CPT modifiers are required for reporting hospital outpatient services and are designated for hospital use only.

Use of Modifiers for Physician Services

In most cases, modifiers applicable to the codes for physician services are simply appended to the appropriate CPT code, as in the following example:

Example: 35840–78

Postoperatively, a patient is taken to the operative room for exploration of postoperative hemorrhage.

Some third-party payers have special reporting requirements that affect the assignment of modifiers. For example, they may ask that claims for surgical procedures performed bilaterally include the appropriate surgical code twice, with modifier 50 assigned only on the second listing of the code to indicate that the same procedure was performed twice. This practice does not follow the AMA's guidelines for reporting bilateral procedures, and CMS requires a one-line method of reporting bilateral procedures for Medicare claims.

Example: 49500
49500–50 Required reporting by some payers

49500–50 AMA and CMS method of reporting

In addition to the CPT modifiers, HCPCS Level II National Codes include many modifiers for more concise reporting of procedures performed by physicians. A complete list of HCPCS Level II Modifiers can be located on the CMS web page (http://www.cms.gov). Use the CMS site's search engine to locate HCPCS Release & Code Sets. These two-digit alphanumeric modifiers can be used to identify:

- The specific finger or toe involved (for example, F3 for left hand, fourth digit)
- A visit for a second or third opinion (for example, SM for second opinion)
- A service provided by someone other than a physician (for example, GN for outpatient speech language services)
- Right- or left-side involvement (for example, RT for right side)

Use of Modifiers for Ambulatory Surgery Center (ASC) Hospital Outpatient Use

CPT Level I Modifiers

The following CPT modifiers are available for use by hospitals for outpatient Medicare services. The modifiers should be reported as two digits appended to the appropriate CPT code in field location 44 of the CMS-1450 form (UB-04). (See figure 1.2)

25 Significant, separately identifiable evaluation and management service by the same physician on the same day of a procedure or other service
27 Multiple outpatient hospital E/M encounters on the same date
50 Bilateral procedure
52 Reduced services
58 Staged or related procedure or service by the same physician during the postoperative period
59 Distinct procedural service
73 Discontinued outpatient procedure prior to the administration of anesthesia
74 Discontinued outpatient procedure after anesthesia administration
76 Repeat procedure or service by same physician or other qualified health care professional
77 Repeat procedure or service by another physician or other qualified health care professional
78 Unplanned return to operating/procedure room by the same physician or other qualified health care professional following initial procedure for a related procedure during the postoperative period
79 Unrelated procedure or service by the same physician during the postoperative period
91 Repeat clinical diagnostic laboratory test

Level II (HCPCS/National) Modifiers

In addition, the following Level II modifiers are acceptable for hospital use:

LT Left side (used to identify procedures performed on the left side of the body)
RT Right side (used to identify procedures performed on the right side of the body)
BL Special acquisition of blood and blood products
CA Procedure payable only in the inpatient setting when performed emergently on an outpatient who expires prior to admission

CR	Catastrophe/disaster related
E1	Upper left, eyelid
E2	Lower left, eyelid
E3	Upper right, eyelid
E4	Lower right, eyelid
FA	Left hand, thumb
F1	Left hand, second digit
F2	Left hand, third digit
F3	Left hand, fourth digit
F4	Left hand, fifth digit
F5	Right hand, thumb
F6	Right hand, second digit
F7	Right hand, third digit
F8	Right hand, fourth digit
F9	Right hand, fifth digit
TA	Left foot, great toe
T1	Left foot, second digit
T2	Left foot, third digit
T3	Left foot, fourth digit
T4	Left foot, fifth digit
T5	Right foot, great toe
T6	Right foot, second digit
T7	Right foot, third digit
T8	Right foot, fourth digit
T9	Right foot, fifth digit
LC	Left circumflex coronary artery
LD	Left anterior descending coronary artery
RC	Right coronary artery
FB	Item provided without cost to provider, supplier, or practitioner, or full credit received for replaced device (examples, but not limited to covered under warranty, replaced due to defect, free samples)
FC	Partial credit received for replaced device
GA	Waiver of liability statement on file
GG	Performance and payment of a screening mammogram and diagnostic mammogram on the same patient, same day
GH	Diagnostic mammogram converted from screening mammogram on same day
Q0	Investigational clinical service provided in a clinical research study that is in an approved clinical research study
Q1	Routine clinical service provided in a clinical research study that is in an approved clinical research study
QM	Ambulance service provided under arrangement by a provider of services
QN	Ambulance service furnished directly by a provider of services

Example of use of Level II Modifier:

Surgical procedure: exploratory arthrotomy of left elbow	
24000–LT	Arthrotomy, elbow, including exploration, drainage, or removal of foreign body
Level II modifier LT is appended to indicate the procedure was performed on the left	

A complete list of modifiers is located in appendix A in CPT 2012. Application of modifiers for use with surgical codes is provided in figure 3.1 of this book.

Figure 3.1. Modifiers for use with surgical codes

22 Increased Procedural Services

Modifier 22 is intended only for use by physicians. The modifier is assigned to indicate that the work required was substantially greater than typically required. Carriers may or may not increase the fee as a result. It may be necessary to submit supportive documentation to justify the use of this modifier.

Example: Because of the patient's extreme obesity, a physician required an additional 30 minutes to perform a cholecystectomy. He should report 47600–22.

47 Anesthesia by Surgeon

Modifier 47, also for physician use only, may be reported to indicate that the surgeon provided regional or general (not local) anesthesia for a surgical procedure. This modifier should not be reported with the anesthesia codes (00100–01999).

Example: Obstetrician performs emergency cesarean delivery for an out-of-town patient visiting relatives. He also administers a pudendal block (regional anesthesia). Moreover, he will provide postpartum care for the patient until she is able to return home. The physician should report 59515–47 and 64430.

50 Bilateral Procedure

Modifier 50 may be reported by both physicians and hospitals to identify bilateral procedures that are performed during the same operative episode. However, if the code describes the procedure as bilateral, modifier 50 should not be reported.

Example: Physician performs a complex anterior packing of both nares for a nosebleed. Both physicians and hospitals providing this service for Medicare patients should report 30903–50.

51 Multiple Procedures

Modifier 51 may be reported to identify that multiple procedures (other than E/M services, physical medicine or rehabilitation services, or provision of supplies) were performed at the same session by the same provider. The procedure listed first should identify the major or most resource-intensive procedure, which usually is paid at 100 percent of the allowed reimbursement. Subsequent or secondary procedures should be appended by modifier 51, and payment may be reduced according to the terms of the health plan. Policies on payment of multiple procedures vary depending on the payer, so a complete understanding of the individual payer's policies is required to ensure appropriate reimbursement. It is not appropriate to append modifier 51 to CPT codes listed in appendix D of the book. This is a physician-only modifier and is not used in the hospital setting.

Example: Physician performed an excision of a chalazion and a dacryolith from the lacrimal passage. She should report 67800 and 68530–51.

Some procedures in the CPT codebook are not intended to stand alone, so they are reported as add-on codes to describe a more extensive procedure. Modifier 51 should not be appended to these codes.

Example: Percutaneous transluminal coronary angioplasty is performed on two coronary arteries. The physician should report 92982 and 92984. Modifier 51 should not be reported in this situation because code 92984 is considered an add-on code and thus must be reported with code 92982.

(Continued on next page)

Figure 3.1. (Continued)

52 Reduced Services

Modifier 52 may be reported by physicians and hospitals to indicate that a service or procedure is partially reduced in scope or eliminated at the discretion of the physician.

Although this modifier serves the purpose of identifying a reduction in the procedure or service, many physicians also use it to report a reduction in the charge for a particular procedure because the complete procedure was not performed. However, CMS directs hospitals to use modifier 73 instead of 52 when a procedure is partially reduced or eliminated at the physician's election before anesthesia is induced. This would apply when the patient has been prepared and taken to the room for surgery, but the surgery is not carried out due to specified circumstances. Modifier 73 was added to differentiate the definitions between physicians and hospitals for this situation.

Example: Patient was taken to the operating room (OR) for excisional débridement of a decubitus ulcer. However, before anesthesia was administered, the physician was called for emergency surgery of a trauma patient, and the ulcer surgery was postponed until a later date. In this case, the hospital would report the appropriate code for the excisional débridement, along with modifier 73 to indicate that, at the discretion of the physician, the surgery was not performed. The physician would not report a procedure code because no professional services were rendered.

53 Discontinued Procedure

Modifier 53 is appropriate in circumstances where the physician elects to terminate or discontinue a surgical or diagnostic procedure, usually because of a risk to the patient's well-being. However, this modifier should not be used to report the elective cancellation of a procedure prior to the patient's surgical preparation or prior to the induction of anesthesia. Also, the appropriate ICD-9-CM code should be assigned to identify the reason for the procedure's termination or discontinuation. For hospital reporting, the CMS guidelines state that modifier 74, not 53, should be used when a procedure must be discontinued at the physician's election after the induction of anesthesia or after the procedure is underway. Elective cancellation of a procedure by the patient is not reported in this way.

Example: Patient was admitted for a cystourethroscopy with bladder biopsy. Twenty minutes into the procedure, the patient developed some arrhythmia and the surgery was stopped. The physician should report 52204–53. The hospital should report 52204–74.

54 Surgical Care Only

Modifier 54 may be reported by physicians only to indicate that one physician performed the surgical procedure and another provided the preoperative and postoperative care.

Example: Dr. Reynolds is asked to perform an extracapsular cataract extraction for his partner, Dr. Owens, who is detained out of town. Dr. Owens provided the preoperative care and will provide postoperative care for his patient. Dr. Reynolds should report 66940–54.

55 Postoperative Management Only ***(for physician use only)***

Modifier 55 may be reported to identify that the physician provided only postoperative care services for a particular procedure.

Example: Patient sustains a fracture of the distal femur while skiing in Colorado. The physician in Colorado performed a closed treatment of the fracture with manipulation. However, the patient's postoperative care will be provided by his hometown physician, Dr. Rogers. Dr. Rogers should report 27510–55.

56 Preoperative Management Only

Modifier 56 may be reported by physicians to indicate that the physician provided only preoperative care services for particular procedure.

Example: Dr. Smith provides preoperative care services for his patient, who will be transferred later the same day to another hospital to undergo a lower lobectomy of the right lung. The physician should report 32480–56.

Figure 3.1. (Continued)

58 Staged or Related Procedure or Service by the Same Physician During the Postoperative Period

Both hospitals and physicians may report modifier 58 to indicate that a staged or related procedure performed by the same physician is provided during the postoperative period. This procedure may have been planned (staged) prospectively at the time of the original procedure, it may be more extensive than the original procedure, or it may be for therapy following a diagnostic surgical procedure.

Example: Physician performed the first stage of a hypospadias repair 1 month ago. The patient now returns for the second-stage repair, which includes a urethroplasty with a free skin graft obtained from a site other than genitalia. The physician should report the following for the second-stage procedure: 54316–58.

59 Distinct Procedural Service

Modifier 59 may be used by physicians and hospitals to identify that a procedure/service was distinct or independent from other services provided on the same day. Furthermore, modifier 59 is useful when circumstances require that certain procedures/services be reported together, even though they usually are not. Use of this modifier often signifies a different session or patient encounter, a different procedure or surgery, a different site or organ system, a separate incision/excision, or a separate lesion or injury not ordinarily encountered or performed on the same day by the same physician. Modifier 59 should not be reported if another modifier can more appropriately describe the circumstance.

Example: Procedures 23030 (Incision and drainage of shoulder area; deep abscess or hematoma) and 20103 (Exploration of penetrating wound; extremity) are performed on the same patient during the same operative session. Ordinarily, if these codes were reported together without a modifier, code 20103 would be denied as integral to code 23030. Because incision and drainage of the shoulder is the definitive procedure, any exploration of the area (code 20103) preceding this would be considered an inherent part of the more comprehensive service. If the exploration procedure were performed on the other limb, modifier 59 explains that the codes are distinct from each other and both services are eligible for reimbursement from the health plan.

62 Two Surgeons

Physicians may report modifier 62 to identify that two surgeons were required to perform a particular procedure. Each surgeon should report his or her distinct operative work by adding the modifier to the procedure code and any associated add-on code(s) for that procedure as long as both surgeons continue to work together as primary surgeons. To expedite payment, the operative note dictated by each physician should be sent to the third-party payer.

63 Procedure Performed on Infants Less than 4 kg

Modifier 63 may be appended to codes in the 20000 through 69999 series when a procedure or service is performed on a neonate or infant with a body weight of up to 4 kg. Use of this modifier indicates that the procedure involved significantly increased complexity of physician work, which is commonly associated with these patients. Modifier 63 should only be assigned by physicians and should not be appended to any CPT code listed in the evaluation and management services, anesthesia, radiology, pathology and laboratory, or medicine sections.

66 Surgical Team

Modifier 66 may be reported by physicians only to identify a complex procedure performed by a team of physicians and other highly skilled personnel.

Example: Patient is admitted for a liver transplant. All the physicians involved in performing this complex procedure should report 47135–66.

(Continued on next page)

Figure 3.1. (Continued)

73 Discontinued Outpatient Procedure Prior to Anesthesia Administration

Modifier 73 is approved for hospital use only. If a surgical patient is taken to the operating room (or cystoscopy suite, gastrointestinal laboratory, and so on) and is prepared for surgery, but the surgery is cancelled before anesthesia is administered, the intended procedure code, along with modifier 73, is assigned. This modifier is not to be reported for an elective cancellation of a procedure. The medical record documentation should reflect the circumstances surrounding the cancellation.

Example: Patient is scheduled for a knee arthroscopy for a lateral meniscus repair. The patient is taken to the OR and prepped, but it was noted that before anesthesia was administered, the patient was experiencing severe hypotension. The procedure was cancelled. The correct code assignment would be 29882–73.

74 Discontinued Outpatient Procedure After Anesthesia Administration

Modifier 74 is reported by hospitals only when a patient's surgery is cancelled after administration of anesthesia or after the procedure was begun (for example, after an incision was made or after an endoscope was inserted). The procedure in progress at the time of cancellation should be reported, not all intended procedures.

Example: Patient is scheduled for a knee arthroscopy for a lateral meniscus repair. The patient is taken to OR, prepared for surgery, and anesthesia is administered. Ten minutes into the procedure, the patient develops cardiac arrhythmia and the surgery is cancelled. The correct code assignment would be 29882–74.

76 Repeat Procedure or Service by Same Physician

Modifier 76 may be reported by hospitals and physicians to identify a procedure or service that was repeated by the physician who performed the original procedure/service. Use of this modifier will help to clarify that the provider is not submitting a duplicate claim. Some third-party payers may require supportive documentation. Hospitals also may report this modifier.

Example: Patient is admitted with significant pleural effusion and congestive heart failure, and the physician performs a thoracentesis. Later in the day, the lungs again fill up with fluid and the same physician performs a second thoracentesis. The physician or hospital should report the following: 32421 (first thoracentesis); 32421–76 (second thoracentesis identified as a repeat procedure with modifier 76).

77 Repeat Procedure by Another Physician

Modifier 77 may be reported by hospitals and physicians to identify a procedure that was repeated by a physician other than the one who performed the original procedure. As with modifier 76, some third-party payers may require supportive documentation. Hospitals also may report this modifier as appropriate.

Example: Dr. Reynolds performs a percutaneous transluminal balloon angioplasty of the renal artery. Later in the day, a diagnostic evaluation determines that the artery has occluded again. Because Dr. Reynolds cannot be reached, Dr. Smith repeats the earlier procedure. Dr. Reynolds should report 35471 to identify the first angioplasty performed, and Dr. Smith should report 35471–77 to identify the repeat angioplasty.

78 Unplanned Return to the Operating/Procedure Room by the Same Physician Following Initial Procedure for a Related Procedure During the Postoperative Period (approved for physician and facility use)

This modifier reflects circumstances when it is necessary for a patient to return to the operating room (unplanned) during the postoperative period. The procedure performed for the subsequent surgery is related to the initial procedure. It is important to note that the modifier specifically states that the subsequent surgery is performed by the ***same*** physician.

Example: Dr. Bailey performs an excision of a hydrocele (55040). Two days later, the patient develops a postoperative wound abscess. Dr. Bailey takes the patient to the operating room and performs an incision and drainage of the abscess (10180). Modifier 78 would be reported with CPT code 10180.

Figure 3.1. (Continued)

79 Unrelated Procedure or Service by the Same Physician During the Postoperative Period (approved for physician and facility use)

Modifier 79 is applicable to situations when a procedure is performed during the postoperative period that was unrelated to the original procedure (by the same physician).

Example: Patient is seen for an excision of a 2.0-cm soft-tissue tumor of the back (21930). Three days later, the same general surgeon performs an emergency cholecystectomy (47562). Modifier 79 would be appended to code 47562. The modifier conveys to the payer that the two procedures are not related and the cholecystectomy was not part of the global surgical period.

80 Assistant Surgeon

Modifier 80 may be reported by physicians only to indicate that the physician provided surgical assistant services for a particular procedure. The surgeon who assists another physician reports the code for the procedure that was performed along with modifier 80. The operating surgeon should not report modifier 80. (Assistant surgeons are usually assumed to have been present throughout the entire surgical procedure.)

Example: Dr. Reynolds performs a total abdominal hysterectomy with removal of fallopian tubes and ovaries. Dr. Jones provides surgical assistance. Dr. Reynolds should report 58150, and Dr. Jones should report 58150–80

81 Minimum Assistant Surgeon

Modifier 81 may be reported by physicians only to indicate that a physician provided minimal surgical assistance when another surgeon's presence typically is not required throughout the entire procedure. The physician who provided minimal assistance reports the code for the procedure performed, along with modifier 81. As in the case of modifier 80, the operating surgeon should not report modifier 81

82 Assistant Surgeon (when qualified resident surgeon not available)

Modifier 82 may be reported by physicians only when a physician provides surgical assistance to another surgeon and a resident surgeon is unavailable. This situation occurs primarily in teaching facilities where resident surgeons typically assume the role of assistant surgeon. When a qualified resident surgeon is unavailable, another physician may serve as an assistant surgeon and report the appropriate procedure code along with modifier 82. As in the case of modifiers 80 and 81, the operating surgeon should not report modifier 82.

99 Multiple Modifiers

Modifier 99 may be reported by physicians only to alert third-party payers that more than one modifier is being submitted on a claim. Many health plans have limitations on the number of modifiers recognized.

Other Uses of Modifiers

New in 2012

A new modifier was added to CPT 2012: -33 Preventive Services.

Modifier -33 (Preventive Service) is to be appended to a service when the primary purpose is the delivery of an evidence based service in accordance with a U.S. Preventive Services Task Force (USPSTF) A or B rating. The entire list of services is available on the website of the task force. The following is an excerpt from the list:

Topic	Description	Grade	Date in Effect
Syphilis screening: pregnant women	The USPSTF recommends that clinicians screen all pregnant women for a syphilis infection	A	May 2009

Category II Modifiers

Category II performance measurement modifiers indicate that a service specified in the measure(s) was considered but, due to either medical or patient circumstances(s), was not provided. The new modifiers are as follows:

1P Performance Measure Exclusion Modifier due to Medical Reasons

2P Performance Measure Exclusion Modifier due to Patient Reasons

3P Performance Measure Exclusion Modifier due to System Reasons

8P Performance Measure Reporting Modifier—Action Not Performed, Reason Not Otherwise Specified

Category II modifiers should only be reported with Category II codes and the circumstances must be documented in the medical record.

Use of Modifiers for Genetic Testing Code Modifiers

CPT/HCPCS also includes a list of alphanumeric modifiers to be used for reporting the molecular laboratory procedures performed for the purpose of genetic testing. (The list is provided in appendix I of CPT 2012.) The modifiers report additional information without altering the CPT/HCPCS code descriptions for the laboratory procedures. Coding guidelines for applying these modifiers are provided in the molecular diagnostic and molecular cytogenetic code sections in CPT.

The first character of these modifiers is numeric, and it indicates the disease category, and the second (alphabetic) character identifies the gene type. The modifiers for genetic testing are categorized according to the type of genetic mutation being tested for, specifically:

- Neoplasia (solid tumors or lymphoid/hematopoietic conditions)
- Nonneoplastic hematology/coagulation
- Histocompatibility/blood typing
- Neurologic, nonneoplastic
- Muscular, nonneoplastic
- Metabolic, other

- Metabolic, transport
- Metabolic, pharmacogenetics
- Dysmorphology

Example of Genetic Testing Code Modifier:

Neoplasia (solid tumor, excluding sarcoma and lymphoma)		
OA	BRCA1	(hereditary breast/ovarian cancer)

Use of Physical Status Modifiers

The Anesthesia section of CPT contains a list of six levels for ranking the physical status of patients. The codes are alphanumeric and appended to the appropriate CPT code. The following is a list of the physical status modifiers:

P1 A normal healthy patient
P2 A patient with mild systemic disease
P3 A patient with severe systemic disease
P4 A patient with severe systemic disease that is a constant threat to life
P5 A moribund patient who is not expected to survive without the operation
P6 A declared brain-dead patient whose organs are being removed for donor purposes

These modifiers provide additional information about the condition of the patient and the complexity of the case.

Medicare Transmittals

Periodically, CMS issues its own guidelines or clarification memos pertaining to coding issues. Whenever CMS sees the need to alter or provide additional clarification on the correct usage of CPT codes or modifiers for Medicare reimbursement, it issues one of these memorandums. These guidelines are published as transmittals and an archive of these documents can be found at the following Web site: http://www.cms.hhs.gov/Transmittals/01_overview.asp.

Exercise 3.1 Chapter 3 Review

Unless otherwise noted, all answers can be found in appendix D of this book. Answers to selected exercises are located in the Instructor's Guide and available only to faculty of educational programs.

Refer to appendix A of the CPT 2012 codebook to identify the appropriate modifiers to be reported for the procedures in items 1 through 5.

1. The modifier that is to be assigned to indicate that a physician provided only postoperative care.

 ____

2. The modifier that is to be used when a different physician repeated a procedure on the same date.

 ____

3. The modifier that is to be used when a surgical procedure took a great deal of extra work and time due to the complexity of the case.

 ____

4. The modifier that can be appended to a code to indicate that two surgeons were required to perform the procedure.

 ____

5. The modifier that is to be used when a procedure was begun but had to be discontinued because of deterioration in the patient's condition (coding is for physician services, not hospital).

 ____

For items 6 through 11, assign the correct CPT code(s) and the appropriate modifiers (CPT and HCPCS National).

Note: Answers to exercises 6 through 11 do not appear in appendix D of this text. They are located in the Instructor's Guide and available to faculty of educational programs.

6. A patient undergoes carpal tunnel releases on both the left and right wrists.

 ____

7. The physician performed a partial avulsion of the nail plate of the left thumb.

 ____

8. A patient was taken to the outpatient surgery suite for an excisional debridement of the skin that extended into the muscle. The patient was prepared for surgery, but before anesthesia was administered, the physician was called for an emergency surgery of a trauma patient and the outpatient surgery was cancelled. (Assign code[s] to be reported by the hospital.)

 ____

9. Bilateral chemodenervation of salivary glands (two glands injected).

 ____

10. The patient underwent a percutaneous core needle biopsy of the left breast with the use of imaging.

 ____

11. The surgeon performed an open reduction with internal fixation for a right, fifth metatarsal fracture.

 ____

Chapter 4

Surgery

To assign codes accurately from the surgery section, physicians and coding professionals must work together to ensure that the documentation in the health record supports the code(s) selected. In the hospital setting, as in the office setting, the operative or procedure report serves as the source document when identifying the type of procedure that has been performed.

Introduction to Surgery Section

The Surgery section provides codes for procedures performed by physicians of any specialty type (general surgeons, ophthalmologists, cardiovascular surgeons, neurosurgeons, and so on). It is further divided into the following subsections:

Subsection	**Code Range**
General	10021–10022
Integumentary System	10040–19499
Musculoskeletal System	20005–29999
Respiratory System	30000–32999
Cardiovascular System	33010–37799
Hemic and Lymphatic Systems	38100–38999
Mediastinum and Diaphragm	39000–39599
Digestive System	40490–49999
Urinary System	50010–53899
Male Genital System	54000–55899
Reproductive System Procedures	55920
Intersex Surgery	55970–55980
Female Genital System	56405–58999
Maternity Care and Delivery	59000–59899
Endocrine System	60000–60699
Nervous System	61000–64999
Eye and Ocular Adnexa	65091–68899
Auditory System	69000–69979
Operating Microscope	69990

This chapter reviews the guidelines and conventions specific to surgical coding and introduces specific subsections. (Links to various Web sites pertinent to the discussion in this chapter are located in the Web resources at the back of this book.)

Surgical Packages

The term *surgical procedure* refers to any single, separate, systemic process upon or within the body that is complete in itself. Surgical procedures are performed for a number of purposes, including:

- To restore disunited or deficient parts
- To remove diseased or injured tissues
- To extract foreign matter from the body
- To assist in obstetrical delivery
- To provide diagnostic information

Each individual *surgical operation* includes one or more surgical procedures performed at one time for one patient via a common approach or for a common purpose. For example, consider a patient who has had an initial, incisional hernia repair with implantation of mesh. The surgical operation is the herniorrhaphy, which includes several surgical procedures such as incision, removal of hernia and implantation of the mesh, and closing of the wound. In this surgical case, the CPT code 49560 would be assigned for the repair of the hernia, and an additional code of 49568 is assigned for implantation of mesh. The incision, closure of the wound, and other minor intraoperative procedures are not assigned a code, because they are considered an integral part of the operation.

CPT Definition of Surgical Package

The term *surgical package* refers to a combination of individual *services* provided during one surgical operation. A surgical package is treated as one single service for purposes of reimbursement, and a single payment is issued for each package of related surgical services. The services covered in each surgical package include the following:

- The actual surgical procedure(s)
- Local infiltration, metacarpal/metatarsal/digital block, or topical anesthesia
- After the decision to perform surgery has been made, one related evaluation and management (E/M) encounter on the date of, or immediately prior to, the date of the procedure (including history and physical)
- Immediate postoperative care, including dictation of operative notes and talking with the family and other physicians
- Preparation of orders
- Evaluation of the patient in the postanesthesia recovery area
- Typical postoperative follow-up care

This reimbursement concept is sometimes referred to as global surgery payment. For example, if a physician performed a surgical operation and a few days later saw the patient in her office for standard follow-up care (for example, removal of sutures), the follow-up visit provided by the physician would not be reported separately. It would be included under the code(s) for the surgical procedure(s) performed during the first encounter, and both encounters would be submitted as a single reimbursement claim. In some cases, however, the code for the postoperative follow-up visit (99024) might also be reported for documentation purposes.

Example: Four weeks ago, Dr. Smith repaired a closed tibial shaft fracture without manipulation. Today, the patient has returned to Dr. Smith's office to have his cast removed. Dr. Smith may bill only for the repair of the fracture, which includes the normal, uncomplicated follow-up care, including cast removal. Thus, only code 27750 is reported on his claim. The subsequent visit for removal of the cast is not billed separately; however, for tracking purposes only, code 99024 may be assigned for that encounter.

Services other than standard postoperative care, however, would not be included in the same surgical package. Follow-up visits for the treatment of complications resulting from the surgical procedure (for example, wound infection at operative site) would be reported with codes for the appropriate E/M level of service, along with the appropriate ICD-9-CM code, to describe the complication.

Example: Two weeks ago, Dr. Smith performed a cholecystectomy. Today, the patient returns with complaints of redness, inflammation, and oozing from the wound site. Dr. Smith determines that the patient has developed an infection at the operative wound site and treats it appropriately. For the second office visit, Dr. Smith should report the appropriate E/M level of service code and assign ICD-9-CM code 998.59 to describe the wound infection.

Medicare guidelines for reimbursement for services involving complications are slightly different from CPT. These guidelines can be referenced in the manuals published by the Centers for Medicare and Medicaid Services (CMS). A complete list of manuals, including the Medicare Claims Processing Manual, can be located at the following Web site: http://www.cms.hhs.gov/Manuals/IOM/list.asp.

The surgical package or global surgery concept does not apply in the hospital outpatient setting. Hospitals may report postoperative visits that occur on subsequent days by using standard billing procedures, such as assigning the appropriate ICD-9-CM diagnosis code to describe the reason for the visit.

Example: Patient returns to the outpatient department of Central Hospital for a change of surgical dressing. The hospital assigns ICD-9-CM code V58.3 (Attention to surgical dressings) to identify the reason for the visit. The E/M code appropriate to the circumstance (new or established) reflects the service rendered.

Medicare Definition of a Surgical Package

The services included in a surgical package may vary depending on individual third-party payer requirements. Unlike CPT, the postoperative period for Medicare claims is not open-ended. Medicare assigns postoperative global periods of 90 days for major surgeries and 0 to 10 days for minor surgeries and endoscopies. The Medicare global surgery definition for major surgeries includes the following types of services:

- The actual surgical procedure
- Preoperative services provided 1 day prior to surgery or the day of surgery, except when modifier 57 or modifier 25 applies
- Follow-up visits during the postoperative period of the surgery that are related to recovery from the surgery
- Complications following surgery: All additional medical or surgical services required of the surgeon during the postoperative period of the surgery because of complications that do not require additional trips to the operating room
- Postsurgical pain management provided by the surgeon
- Insignificant surgical procedures not performed in the operating room, including dressing changes, removal of operative packs, and care of the operative incision site; removal of sutures, staples, wires, lines, tubes, drains, casts, and splints; insertion, irrigation, and removal of urinary catheters; routine peripheral intravenous lines; removal of nasogastric tubes and rectal tubes; care of tracheostomy tubes

The Medicare global surgery definition for minor and endoscopic surgeries includes the following types of services:

- The actual surgical procedure
- Preoperative services provided 1 day prior to surgery or the day of surgery, except when modifier 57 or modifier 25 applies
- Postoperative services provided within 0 to 10 days of the surgical procedure, except when modifier 24 applies

Follow-up Care for Diagnostic and Therapeutic Procedures

Follow-up care for diagnostic or therapeutic procedures includes only that care related to recovery from the diagnostic procedure itself or care that is usually part of the surgical service. When follow-up care involves the initiation of treatment for the condition that has been diagnosed or for a complication, the treatment should be coded and reported separately. Complication, exacerbation, or recurrence, or the presence of other diseases or injuries requiring additional services should be reported with the appropriate code for that procedure.

Separate Procedures

The CPT codebook defines a separate procedure as one that, when performed in conjunction with another service, is considered an integral part of the major service; therefore, it should not be coded separately. In normal circumstances, it is fraudulent to report the codes separately and charge separate fees for each procedure.

However, the separate procedure may be coded when it is performed independently and not in conjunction with the so-called larger or major procedure. A modifier, such as modifier 59 (Distinct Services), may be added to explain special circumstances where the separate procedure was not performed integral to the larger procedure. For example, assume that the following procedures were performed on a patient:

Example: 58720 Salpingo-oophorectomy, complete or partial, unilateral or bilateral (separate procedure)

58150 Total abdominal hysterectomy (corpus and cervix), with or without removal of tube(s), with or without removal of ovary(s)

Assignment of code 58720 would be appropriate in circumstances where *only* a salpingo-oophorectomy was performed. If the salpingo-oophorectomy was done as part of a larger procedure, as described in code 58150, an additional code of 58720 is inappropriate and would be considered unbundling of services. Unbundling is the practice of using multiple codes that describe individual components of a procedure rather than an appropriate single code that describes all steps in the procedure performed.

In another example, assume the physician performed a flexible bronchoscopy with cell washings (CPT code 31622) and a transbronchial lung biopsy (CPT code 31628). In this example, only CPT code 31628 is reported. CPT code 31622 is a separate procedure code and would not be assigned with 31628.

National Correct Coding Initiative

A list of coding edits has been developed by CMS in an effort to promote correct coding nationwide and to prevent the inappropriate unbundling of related services. The National Correct Coding Initiative (NCCI) edits help CMS to detect inappropriate codes submitted on claims and are based on CPT coding guidelines, current standards of medical/surgical coding practice, and advice from specialty societies. There are two major types of coding edits: the comprehensive/component edit and the mutually exclusive edit.

Comprehensive/Component Edit

The comprehensive/component edit pertains to HCPCS codes that should not be used together. Note the following table as an example of a NCCI listing. Under the NCCI, if bills contain a procedure in both the comprehensive code column and the component code column for the same patient on the same date of service, only the code in the comprehensive code column is covered (provided that code is on the list as an approved procedure for reimbursement). For example:

Comprehensive Code	Component Code(s)
20912	12014, 13152

In the preceding example, code 20912 describes a cartilage graft of nasal septum. During the procedure, the surgeon may mention that a wound repair (12014, 13152) was performed, but it is considered part of the more involved procedure (20912) and should not be coded. If the coding professional assigned the additional wound repair codes, it would be considered unbundling.

Mutually Exclusive Edit

The mutually exclusive edit applies to improbable or impossible combinations of codes. For example, code 69601, Revision mastoidectomy; resulting in complete mastoidectomy, would never be performed with code 69604, Revision mastoidectomy; resulting in tympanoplasty.

NCCI edits are included in most encoding software packages. The software vendors are responsible for maintaining up-to-date edits to support the coding/billing function. More information about NCCI edits can be found on the CMS Web site.

Medical Unlikely Edits

For Part B claims, CMS has developed "medical unlikely edits" to reduce error rates for items on the claim form that reference units of service. For each HCPCS/CPT code, the edits list the maximum units of service that a provider would report under most circumstances for a single beneficiary on a single date of service.

Integumentary System

The integumentary system subsection includes codes for procedures performed on the following body parts:

- Skin and subcutaneous structures, including excision of skin lesions, wound closure, skin grafting, burn treatment, Mohs' chemosurgery, incision and drainage, and debridement
- Nails, including debridement, excision, and reconstruction of nail bed
- Breast, including needle, incisional, and excisional biopsies, and all types of mastectomies

Figure 4.1 shows the skin and its components.

The integumentary system subsection includes many definitions that are located at various levels within the subsection. A careful review of each definition is necessary before codes are assigned.

Figure 4.1. The skin and its components

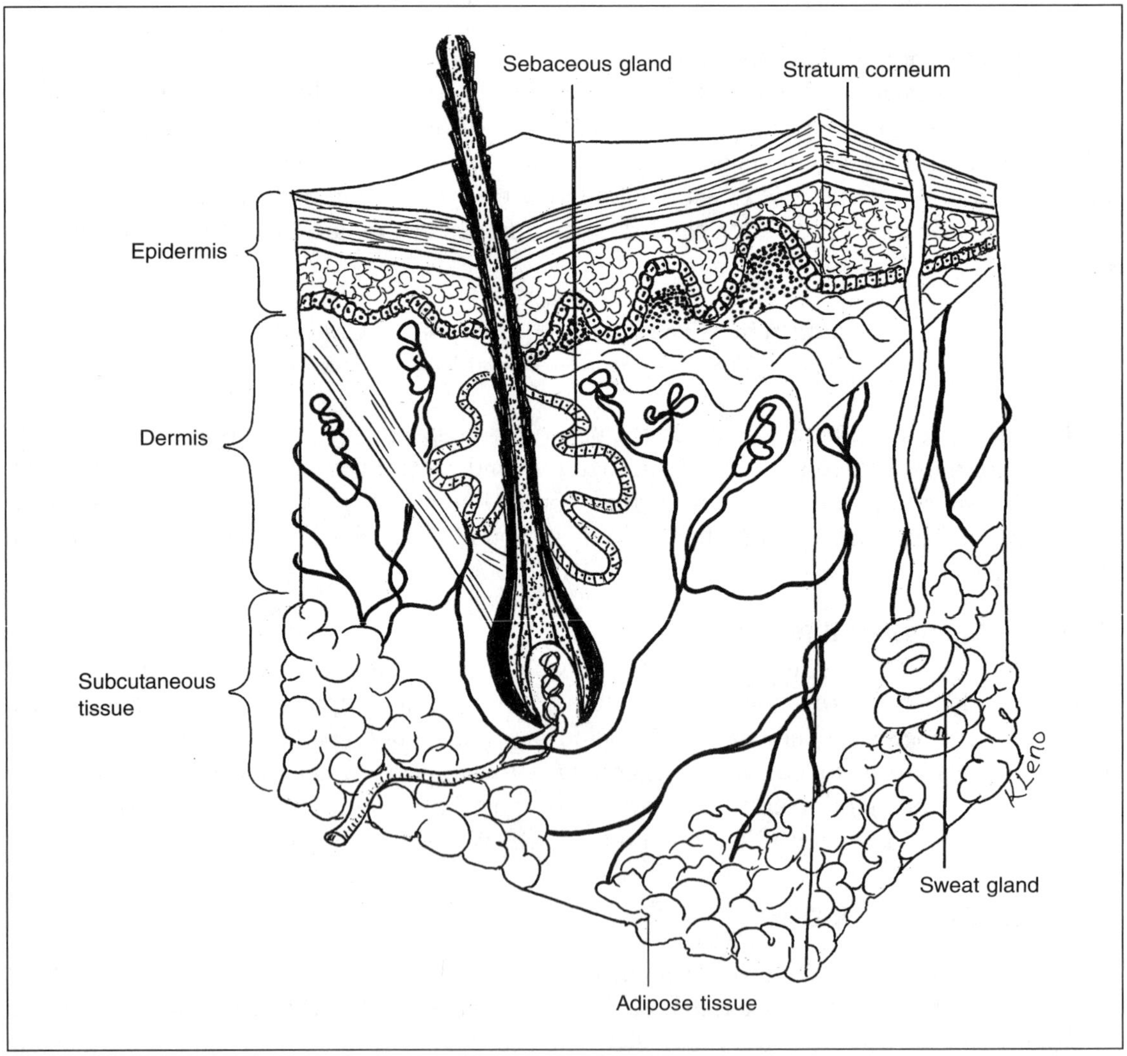

Debridement

CPT provides a variety of codes to reflect the treatment of damaged or infected tissue. A good coding practice is to review a selection of codes and identify the unique characteristics. For example, scan the codes in the following list and differentiate each.

- 11000: This code reflects the treatment via debridement for infected skin and eczema. The wound size is dependent on the percent of body surface.
- 11004–11006: Code 11004 starts a family of codes used to identify a more serious type of infection (necrotic soft tissue infection) that can extend to the depth of bone. Site includes external genitalia, perineum, and abdominal wall.
- 11008: This code involves removal of prosthetic material associated with an abdominal wall infection. A plus sign (+) in front of this code indicates that it is an "add-on code" and should not be reported separately.
- 11010–11012: This family of codes is reserved for debridement associated with open fractures. The hierarchy of codes is related to the depth (11011 extends to the muscle, while 11012 extends to the bone).
- Note the series of entries under code 11012 that refers a coder to different sections of CPT if the debridement is associated with burns (16020–16030) or active wound care.

Wound debridement (11042–11047) is a surgical method in which a patient's dead, damaged, or infected tissue is removed to assist the healing process. The coding selection is differentiated by depth (subcutaneous, bone, muscle) and size. CPT provides the following guidelines to support an accurate code assignment:

- For a single wound, report the depth using the deepest level of tissue removed.
- For multiple wounds, sum the surface areas that are at the *same depth* (do not combine sums from different depths).

Example #1: The physician debrided a 3.0-sq cm wound of the buttocks (in the muscle) and another 4.0-sq cm wound (in the muscle) of the heel.

Coding rationale: Both wounds were at the same depth (*in the muscle*), so a sum of the wounds would be reported (3.0 sq cm + 4.0 sq cm = 7.0 sq cm). Code 11043

Example #2: The physician debrided a 3.0-sq cm wound of the buttocks (*in the muscle*) and another 4.0-sq cm wound (*in the bone*) of the heel.

Coding rationale: The wounds are *not* at the same depth. The wound of the buttocks was debrided in the muscle, but the wound of the heel extended down to the bone. The correct coding assignment would be 11043 (wound of buttocks) and 11044 (wound of heel).

Note: The sequencing of these codes, for reporting on a claim form, would require knowledge of reimbursement amounts and payer guidelines offered by current software programs. Typically, the more resource-intensive code (in this case 11044) is sequenced first on the claim form.

Exercise 4.1 Integumentary System—Debridement

Unless otherwise noted, all answers can be found in appendix D of this book. Answers to selected exercises are located in the Instructor's Guide and available only to faculty of educational programs.

Assign appropriate CPT code(s) to the following debridement procedures and indicate the index entries that were used to identify the codes. Assign only CPT surgical codes (no E/M codes) and append any applicable modifiers.

1. Patient has a Grade III ulcer of the left heel. The physician debrided the 5.0-sq cm ulcer to the subcutaneous tissue. The #15 blade removed the fibrinous tissue.

   Code(s): ____________________

   Index entries: ____________________

   ____

2. Patient was involved in a motorcycle accident and sustained a fractured fibula. The wound was debrided down to the subcutaneous tissue for removal of contaminating material (gravel and glass). *(Only assign CPT code for the debridement in this case.)*

   Code(s): ____________________

   Index entries: ____________________

   ____

3. The patient had a mesh inserted during an inguinal hernia repair a couple of years ago. The patient presents for removal of the infected mesh and debridement of the necrotic tissue. The physician performed a debridement of the wound, including the fascia, and removed the mesh.

   Code(s): ____________________

   Index entries: ____________________

   ____

Lesions

A lesion is tissue that has suffered damage through injury or disease. Skin lesions can include moles, cysts, keloids, warts, or skin tags. Most are benign; however, they are sometimes removed if they are painful, unsightly, or restrictive of movement. Surgical removal is the most common treatment for most skin lesions. Warts are also removed by the use of liquid gas to freeze them off, or they may be treated with chemical paint. If the lesion is suspected of being malignant, a biopsy is taken and analyzed in a laboratory for any signs of cancerous cells.

Removal of Skin Lesions

There are a variety of methods used to remove skin lesions. The physician may elect to remove the lesion by any of the following techniques: shaving, paring, excising, or with the use of laser. Coding professionals should read the documentation to determine the method used to remove the lesion. Depending on the method of removal and the CPT code description, other documentation is also necessary. Table 4.1 displays the supportive documentation required for different methods of removing different types of skin lesions.

Table 4.1. Necessary documentation for removal of skin lesions

Method of Removal	Necessary Documentation	CPT Code Range
Paring of lesions	• Diagnosis of benign hyperkeratotic lesion • Number of lesions removed	11055–11057
Removal of skin tags	• Diagnosis of skin tag(s) • Number of skin tags removed	11200–11201
Shaving of epidermal or dermal lesions	• Diagnosis of epidermal or dermal lesion • Diameter of lesion • Location of lesion	11300–11313
Excision of benign lesion(s)	• Diagnosis of benign skin lesion • Excised diameter • Location of lesions	11400–11471
Excision of malignant lesion(s)	• Diagnosis of malignant skin lesion • Excised diameter • Location of lesions	11600–11646
Destruction of benign or premalignant lesions	• Diagnosis of benign or premalignant skin lesion • Lesion removed by methods such as electrosurgery, cryosurgery, laser, or chemical treatment • Number of lesions removed	17000–17004 17110–17250
Destruction of malignant lesions	• Diagnosis of malignant skin lesion • Lesion removed by destruction • Diameter of lesion • Location of lesion	17260–17286

Excision of Lesions

Two separate code ranges can be found in this subsection to describe the excised site of benign (11400–11471) and malignant (11600–11646) lesions. Both series of codes are further subdivided, first by body part and then by lesion size. To accurately code excision of lesions, the coding professional must be able to answer the following questions:

- *Is the lesion malignant or benign?* Careful review of the operative report and, more important, the pathology report is required to determine the lesion type. Coding from superbills or encounter forms, which do not reveal pathology results, often leads to inappropriate code assignment.
- *What site or body part is involved with the lesion?* The operative report should be reviewed for this information.
- *How large is the excised area (in centimeters, including margins, if applicable)?* During surgery, physicians may take some normal-looking skin around the growth. Removal of the normal-looking skin is known as taking margins. This is done to be sure no cancer cells are left behind. The total size of the excised area, including margins, is needed for accurate coding. (See figure 4.2.) Usually, this information is provided in the operative report. It is very important that surgeons be educated and trained to provide accurate lesion size information. The pathology report typically provides the specimen size

Figure 4.2. Melanoma excision

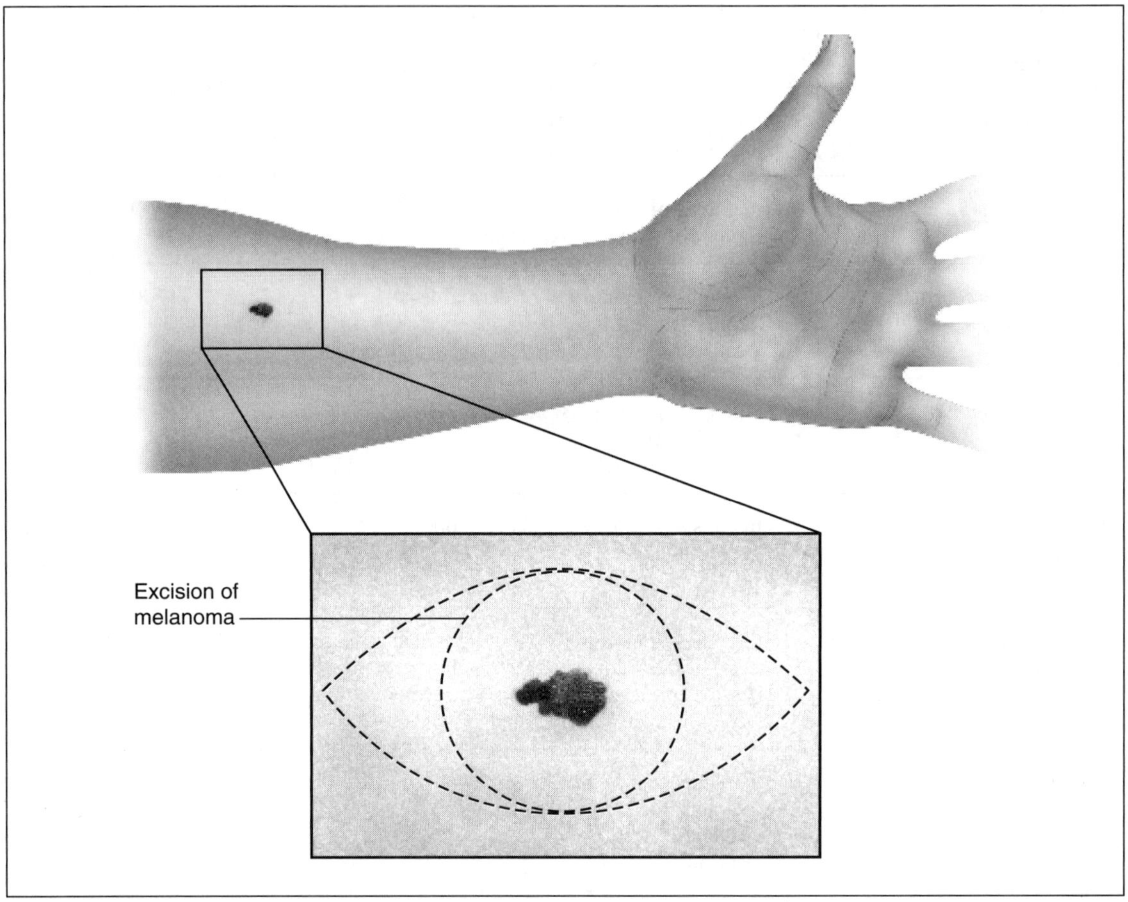

rather than the lesion or excised size. Because the specimen tends to shrink, this is not an accurate measurement according to the intent of the code assignment. Inches should be converted to centimeters, when necessary.

1 mm	=	0.1 cm
10 mm	=	1.0 cm
1 inch	=	approximately 2.54 cm
1 cm	=	0.4 inch

- *What type of wound closure was performed?* Both series of codes (11400–11471 and 11600–11646) include simple closure. Separate codes should be reported when the excision requires more than simple closure, such as an intermediate repair.

When more than one dimension for an excised area is provided, the size is equal to the largest dimension of the excision, including margins.

Example: The physician excised a malignant melanoma of the hand that was reported as 3.0 cm × 2.0 cm. Documentation in the operative report states that 0.5-cm margins were excised around the lesion. For coding purposes, the size of the excision was 3.0 cm + 0.5 cm + 0.5 cm = 4.0 cm in total. The correct code assignment would be 11624.

Excision of Lesion Followed by Adjacent Tissue Transfer

When excision of a malignant or benign lesion involves repair by adjacent tissue transfer—such as Z-plasty, W-plasty, V-Y plasty, rotation, advancement, or double pedicle flap—codes 14000–14350 should be reported. It should be noted that these codes include both the excision and the tissue transfer or rearrangement. A separate code should not be reported for the lesion excision. A more detailed discussion of adjacent tissue transfer techniques follows in the section on skin grafts later in this chapter.

Every excised lesion should be reported individually with the correct CPT code. Multiple lesion excisions are not treated as a single excision.

Excision of Lipomas

Lipomas are usually benign fatty tumors commonly found in superficial tissue, although they can also be present in subfascial and submuscular locations. Whether the lipoma is confined to the skin or extends into the deeper tissues will be the deciding factor for accurate code assignment. For example, if the patient has a lipoma of the back that extends into the dermis, then a code for excision of skin lesion is appropriate. However, if the lipoma extends into the soft tissue of the back, including the muscle, then the code would be selected from the musculoskeletal section. For example, looking at code 21930 for Excision, tumor, soft tissue of back or flank, *soft tissue* refers to tissues that connect, support, or surround other structures and organs of the body. Soft tissue includes muscles, tendons (bands of fiber that connect muscles to bones), fibrous tissues, fat, blood vessels, nerves, and synovial tissues (tissues around joints). In addition, codes for removal of soft-tissue tumors are differentiated by site and size.

Examples:	21555	Excision, tumor, soft tissue of neck or anterior thorax, subcutaneous; less than 3 cm
	#21552	3 cm or greater

Note that the symbol (#) indicates that the codes are out of numerical sequence.

Exercise 4.2 Integumentary System—Lesions

Unless otherwise noted, all answers can be found in appendix D of this book. Answers to selected exercises are located in the Instructor's Guide and available only to faculty of educational programs.

Assign appropriate CPT code(s) to the following procedures and indicate the index entries that were used to identify the codes. Assign only CPT surgical codes (no E/M codes) and append any applicable modifiers.

1. Physician excises two benign skin lesions. The excised areas are 2.0 cm from arm and 1.0 cm from neck.

   Code(s): ______________________________

   Index entries: ______________________________

   ____

2. Laser removal of four benign skin lesions from the back.

   Code(s): ______________________________

   Index entries: ______________________________

   ____

(Continued on next page)

Exercise 4.2 (Continued)

3. Physician excises a lesion from the chin. The excised dimension is 1.5 cm. Pathology report reveals malignant melanoma.

   Code(s): ______________________________

   Index entries: ______________________________

   ____

4. In the physician's office, the patient has seven skin tags removed.

   Code(s): ______________________________

   Index entries: ______________________________

   ____

Note: Answers to exercises 5 through 7 do not appear in appendix D of this text. They are located in the Instructor's Guide and available to faculty of educational programs.

5. Physician excised an area 3.0 cm × 2.0 cm × 1.5 cm from the patient's back. The pathology report shows a lipoma in the subcutaneous layer of skin.

   Code(s): ______________________________

   Index entries: ______________________________

   ____

6. Physician excised a 2.0-cm squamous cell carcinoma from the forehead. The total excision, including margins, was 3.5 cm in diameter.

   Code(s): ______________________________

   Index entries: ______________________________

   ____

7. Excision of malignant melanoma of the forehead (1.0 cm) and nose (0.5 cm).

   Code(s): ______________________________

   Index entries: ______________________________

   ____

Exercise 4.3 Integumentary System

Unless otherwise noted, all answers can be found in appendix D of this book. Answers to selected exercises are located in the Instructor's Guide and available only to faculty of educational programs.

Operative Report

Preoperative Diagnosis:	Sebaceous cyst, left face
Postoperative Diagnosis:	Same
Procedure:	Excision of left-face sebaceous cyst
Anesthesia:	Local with IV sedation

The patient is a 69-year-old woman who has a sebaceous cyst, which has started to grow larger, on the left side of her face. She presents now for excision of the cyst.

The patient was brought to the OR and placed on the operating table in the supine position. She was given 50 mg of Demerol and 1 mg of Versed IV. The left face was prepped and draped in the usual sterile fashion. The area overlying the cyst was anesthetized with 1% lidocaine with epinephrine. An elliptical incision was made of the cyst in the direction of the facial wrinkles. The cyst itself was 1 cm in diameter. The underlying cyst was dissected away from the surrounding tissues, taking care to remove the entire cyst, with an excised area of 2.0 cm × 0.5 cm. Hemostasis was obtained using electrocautery. The wound was then closed with 3-0 Vicryl. It was then dressed with Masticel and Steri-Strips. The patient tolerated the procedure well and was taken to the recovery room in stable condition.

Pathology Report

Clinical Diagnosis:	Cyst of the face
Specimen:	Ellipse of skin measuring 2.0 × 0.5 × 0.2 cm
Pathological Diagnosis:	Epidermal inclusion cyst with rupture, marked acute and chronic inflammation

Assign appropriate CPT code(s) for the preceding procedure and indicate the index entries that were used to identify the code(s). Assign only CPT surgical codes (no E/M codes) and append any applicable modifiers.

1. Code(s): ______________________________

   Index entries: ______________________________

   ____

Exercise 4.4 Integumentary System

Unless otherwise noted, all answers can be found in appendix D of this book. Answers to selected exercises are located in the Instructor's Guide and available only to faculty of educational programs.

Operative Report

Preoperative Diagnosis: Epidermoid nevus of scalp

Postoperative Diagnosis: Same

Procedure: Shave excision of 4.0-cm benign scalp lesion

This patient is on chronic anticoagulation. A subgaleal lipoma has previously been removed. At that time he was not interested in having his seborrheic keratosis removed from his scalp, although the offer was made to do so. He has had a very nice result from his original surgery and is now willing and wishing to undergo removal of what I believe is a seborrheic keratosis. Although, according to the history, it has been there as long as he can remember, it may be an epidermal nevus. A small portion is sent for biopsy to create the definitive diagnosis. The patient understands the risks of bleeding.

The patient was brought to the operating room and made comfortable in a supine position on the table. The area to be worked up was infiltrated with 1% lidocaine with 1:100,000 parts epinephrine. The area was then prepared and draped in the usual sterile fashion. A #15 blade was used to remove a small portion of the lesion, which was carefully labeled and sent to pathology for examination. The rest was then shaved off at the level of the dermis, where there was punctate bleeding. Hemostasis was achieved with cautery. A dressing of Gelfoam soaked in thrombin was placed over this, and the patient was allowed to return to the recovery room with stable vital signs. The estimated blood loss was less than 15 cc, which was replaced with crystalloid solution only. Sponge, needle, and instrument counts were reported as correct.

Assign appropriate CPT code(s) for the preceding procedure and indicate the index entries that were used to identify the code(s). Assign only CPT surgical codes (no E/M codes) and append any applicable modifiers.

1. Code(s): ____________________

   Index entries: ____________________

   ____

Wound Repair/Closure

The CPT codebook describes three types of wound repair/closure: simple, intermediate, and complex.

Simple Wound Repair

A simple repair is a superficial repair that primarily involves the epidermis, dermis, or subcutaneous tissues without involvement of deeper structures. This repair usually requires simple suturing of only one layer of skin.

Intermediate Wound Repair

An intermediate repair, like a simple wound repair, is considered a superficial repair, requiring that one or more of the deeper layers of the subcutaneous tissue and superficial (non-muscle) fascia, as well as the skin (epidermal and dermal), be closed in layers. In other words, wounds that require closure of subcutaneous tissue or more than one layer of tissue beneath the dermis should be coded as intermediate, unless the criteria for a complex closure are met. Wounds that are closed with only one layer, but which are so heavily contaminated that they require extensive cleaning or removal of foreign material, such as gravel or glass, also may be classified as an intermediate repair.

Example: Surgeon documents the defect is to the epidermis, dermis, and subcutaneous tissue. Procedure description includes that the absorbable sutures were placed within the subcutaneous tissue and deep dermis. In order to close the defect, epidermal sutures were placed in interrupted or running fashion (intermediate closure).

Complex Wound Repair

A complex repair of a wound goes beyond a layer closure and requires scar revision, debridement, extensive undermining, stents, or retention sutures. Wounds described as angular, jagged, irregular, or stellate may require complex repair. Layered closure is part of this wound repair.

Example: Wound edges were undermined extensively. Buried absorbable sutures were used to close the subcutaneous and dermal components of the defect. Simple interrupted sutures were used to approximate the epidermal edges.

Coding of Wound Repairs/Closures

To accurately code wound closures, the following questions must be answered:

- *What type of repair is being performed: simple, intermediate, or complex?*
- *What site or body part is involved, and what is the extent of the wound?* The operative report should be reviewed for mention of blood vessel, tendon, or nerve involvement. The wound repair codes include simple ligation of blood vessels and simple exploration of the nerves, vessels, or tendons, so they should not be reported separately. However, a separate code is warranted if the extent of the laceration requires repair of the nerves, vessels, or tendons.
- *What is the length of the repair (in centimeters)?*

When multiple wounds are repaired, the coding professional should add together the lengths of those in the same classification and from all anatomic sites that are grouped together into the same code descriptor. For example, add together the lengths of intermediate repairs to the trunk and extremities. Do not add lengths of repairs from different groupings of anatomic sites (for example, face and extremities). Also, do not add together the lengths of different classifications (for example, intermediate and complex repairs).

Example #1: Simple wound repair of two lacerations of the arm measuring 2.5 cm and 1.5 cm. The sum of the two lacerations is 4.0 cm, and the code reported is 12002.

Example #2: Emergency department physician documents a simple repair of the following lacerations: 2.0 cm of arm, 3.0 cm of leg, and 1.5 cm of cheek. In addition, the physician documented the following layered wound closures: 2.0 cm of foot, 1.5 cm of leg, and 3.0 cm of knee. Note the correct code assignment:

Simple Repairs	Intermediate Repairs
2.0 cm arm	2.0 cm foot
3.0 cm leg	1.5 cm leg
1.5 cm cheek	3.0 cm knee
Add 2.0 cm of arm and 3.0 of leg and assign CPT code 12002 (5.0-cm repair). An additional code, 12011, would be assigned for the repair of the cheek.	*Add 1.5 cm of leg and 3.0 cm of knee to assign CPT code 12032 (4.5-cm repair). An additional code, 12041, would be assigned for the 2.0-cm repair of the foot.*

When more than one classification of wounds is repaired, the most complicated repair is listed first, followed by the less complicated repairs. Modifier 51 (for physician billing) also should be reported to identify the performance of more than one procedure. Debridement may be reported separately only when gross contamination requires prolonged cleansing, considerable amounts of devitalized or contaminated tissue are removed, or debridement is carried out separately without immediate primary closure.

A note under the wound repair subheading refers the coding professional to codes 20100 through 20103 if the wound required any of the following:

- Enlargement
- Extension of dissection
- Debridement
- Removal of one or more foreign bodies
- Ligation or coagulation of minor subcutaneous and/or muscular blood vessel(s)

Superficial wound repairs requiring only Steri-Strips or bandages are reported with the appropriate E/M services code. Surgical codes are inappropriate because no surgical repair was performed. Repairs with tissue adhesive, such as 2-cyanoacrylate (Dermabond), are reported using the appropriate code from the repair category.

Tissue Adhesives

It is important to note that Medicare requires a Level II HCPCS code to identify a wound closed with tissue adhesives. Instead of assigning the CPT code for wound repair, the following code should be assigned: G0168, Wound closure utilizing tissue adhesive(s) only. (HCPCS Level II codes are discussed further in chapter 10.)

Exercise 4.5 Integumentary System—Wound Repairs

Unless otherwise noted, all answers can be found in appendix D of this book. Answers to selected exercises are located in the Instructor's Guide and available only to faculty of educational programs.

Assign appropriate CPT code(s) for the following procedures and indicate the index entries that were used to identify the codes. Assign only CPT surgical codes (no E/M codes) and append any applicable modifiers.

1. A child is seen in the physician's office for a superficial laceration of the right knee. The physician repairs the 3.0-cm laceration with simple suturing.

   Code(s): ____________________

   Index entries: ____________________

   ____

2. The patient is treated in the emergency department for a deep 3.5-cm wound of the right arm. A routine cleansing and deep non-muscle layer closure was required.

   Code(s): ____________________

   Index entries: ____________________

   ____

3. A patient is treated for multiple wounds of the right forearm, hand, and knee. The physician sutured the following: simple repair, 2.5 cm forearm; intermediate repair, 1.5 cm hand; 2.0 cm simple repair, knee.

   Code(s): ____________________

   Index entries: ____________________

   ____

Exercise 4.6 Integumentary System

Unless otherwise noted, all answers can be found in appendix D of this book. Answers to selected exercises are located in the Instructor's Guide and available only to faculty of educational programs.

Emergency Department Record

Chief Complaint:	Laceration, left hand
History of Present Illness:	Patient is a 67-year-old woman who tripped over a brick. As she tried to break her fall, she somehow cut her left hand. She has a laceration at the base of her fifth finger on the palm side, but no other injuries.
Past Medical History:	Unremarkable
Medications:	None
Allergies:	None
Physical Examination:	
General:	Alert female in no acute distress
Extremities:	Left upper extremity examination reveals a 2.5-cm full-skin-thickness laceration on the palm side of the left hand just at the base of the finger over the volar metacarpal phalangeal joints. She has full active and passive range of motion.
Procedure:	Anesthesia local injection 2 cc 1% lidocaine plain; prepped and routine exploration revealed no foreign body. No neurovascular tendon injury noted. Repaired with six 5-0 nylon sutures. Polysporin ointment and dressing placed on the wound.
Diagnosis:	2.5-cm simple laceration, left hand
Disposition and Plan:	Wound care instructions given and advised to have sutures taken out in 10 to 12 days

Assign appropriate CPT code(s) for the preceding procedure and indicate the index entries that were used to identify the code(s). Assign only CPT surgical codes (no E/M codes) and append any applicable modifiers.

1. Code(s): ______________________________

   Index entries: ______________________________

   ____

Exercise 4.7 Integumentary System

Unless otherwise noted, all answers can be found in appendix D of this book. Answers to selected exercises are located in the Instructor's Guide and available only to faculty of educational programs.

Emergency Department Record

Chief Complaint:	Right arm laceration
History of Present Illness:	This 24-year-old man presents here after attempting to punch out a window in his garage door with his elbow in an attempt to enter his own house.
Medications:	None
Allergies:	Keflex
Last Known Tetanus:	Unknown
Review of Systems:	No shoulder pain, no wrist pain. Complains of multiple lacerations of the forearm.

Exercise 4.7 (Continued)

Extremities:	Right elbow and right forearm reveal multiple lacerations in various lengths from proximal and working distally. Over the area of the olecranon, there is noted to be a 3-cm superficial laceration. There is also noted to be several simple lacerations distally: approximately four measuring 1 cm and three others measuring 2 cm each. There is noted to be a 5-cm laceration involving deeper layers of skin.
Procedure:	After adequate anesthesia was obtained with local infiltration of all lacerations with 1% lidocaine with epinephrine, the wounds were explored. No foreign bodies were appreciated. Each wound was vigorously irrigated and draped individually in a sterile fashion. Initially, the 3-cm laceration along the area of the olecranon was closed with two interrupted sutures of 4-0 Ethilon. The remaining smaller wounds were closed with simple sutures. The 5-cm laceration required closing with 3-0 Vicryl for the subcutaneous layer and 4-0 Vicryl to close the skin. Wound edges were painted with Benzoin and Steri-Strips applied. The patient tolerated the procedure well.

Assign appropriate CPT code(s) for the preceding procedure and indicate the index entries that were used to identify the code(s). Assign only CPT surgical codes (no E/M codes) and append any applicable modifiers.

1. Code(s): ____________________

   Index entries: ____________________

   ____

Exercise 4.8 Integumentary System

Unless otherwise noted, all answers can be found in appendix D of this book. Answers to selected exercises are located in the Instructor's Guide and available only to faculty of educational programs.

Emergency Department Operative Note

Chief Complaint:	Head laceration
History of Present Illness:	This 85-year-old man was found in his basement with a bleeding head laceration. Examination revealed a scalp laceration, which is at the superior occiput. The laceration was approximately 8 cm and required a complex repair. The wound was irrigated as well as possible with normal saline. Subsequently, using 4-0 Vicryl suturing, some of the deeper structures were reapproximated with some hemostasis. Approximately three Vicryl sutures were placed deep in these structures. Multiple 4-0 nylon interrupted suturing were placed, with eventual control of the hemostasis. Several other staples were placed as well for further cosmetic closure of the skin. The procedure did provide complete resolution of the symptoms. There was a very complex and deep wound with active hemorrhage. Subsequent to this, it was cleansed and Neosporin was placed. Please note that multiple areas of hair were trimmed with scissors prior to this procedure.

Assign appropriate CPT code(s) for the preceding procedure and indicate the index entries that were used to identify the code(s). Assign only CPT surgical codes (no E/M codes) and append any applicable modifiers.

1. Code(s): ____________________

   Index entries: ____________________

   ____

Exercise 4.9 Integumentary System

Unless otherwise noted, all answers can be found in appendix D of this book. Answers to selected exercises are located in the Instructor's Guide and available only to faculty of educational programs.

Operative Report

Preoperative Diagnosis:	Pigmented nevus, arm
Postoperative Diagnosis:	Melanoma
Operation:	Excision 1.5-cm nevus of arm

The patient was brought into the surgery center and prepped and draped in the usual manner. Local anesthesia was injected under the lesion. The lesion with 0.5-cm margins was excised taking full-thickness skin, transversely oblique. Hemostasis was obtained with cautery. The skin was closed in layers of 3-0 Vicryl in fascia, 5-0 Vicryl subcuticular, and 6-0 nylon in the skin. Dressing was applied.

Assign appropriate CPT code(s) for the preceding procedure and indicate the index entries that were used to identify the code(s). Assign only CPT surgical codes (no E/M codes) and append any applicable modifiers.

1. Code(s): ______________________

   Index entries: ______________________

   ____

Skin Grafting

Skin grafting is a method of treating damaged or lost skin in which a piece of skin is taken from another area of the body and transplanted to the area of the damaged or missing section. There are several code ranges to identify skin graft procedures.

Adjacent Skin Grafts

The first series of codes (14000–14350) identify grafts that maintain their own blood supply. If a lesion is removed and it results in an adjacent skin graft to cover the defect, the excision of the lesion is included in the skin graft procedure. Examples of tissue transfer or rearrangement (also known as local skin flaps) are: Z-plasty, W-plasty, V-Y plasty, rotation, advancement, or double pedicle flap. These codes are categorized first by body part involved and then by size of defect in square centimeters.

An additional code may be reported to describe any skin grafting required to close the secondary defect.

The following definitions are helpful when coding adjacent tissue transfer or arrangement procedures:

- *Advancement:* The sliding of a pedicle graft into its new position.
- *Pedicle graft:* Grafted tissue that remains connected to its vascular bed.
- *Z-plasty:* A tissue transfer that surgically releases tension in the skin caused by a laceration, contracted scar, or a wound along the flexion crease of a joint. It is characterized by a Z-shaped incision that is above, through, and below the scar or defect. This type of technique is used to reposition a scar so that it more closely conforms to the natural lines and creases of the skin, where it will be less noticeable.

- *W-plasty:* A tissue transfer performed to release tension along a straight scar. A W-shaped incision creates a series of triangular flaps of skin. The triangle flaps on both sides of the scar are removed, and the remaining skin triangles are moved together and sutured into place.
- *V-Y plasty:* A tissue transfer that begins with a V-shaped skin incision and with advancement and stretching of the skin and tissue. The defect is covered and forms a Y when sutured together.
- *Rotational flap:* These flaps are curved or semicircular and include the skin and subcutaneous tissues. A base is left, and the remaining portion of the flap is freed and rotated to cover the defect and then sutured into place.

Skin Replacement Surgery

The next range of skin graft codes are categorized into two groupings: Autograft (or tissue cultured autograft) and Skin Substitute Grafts. The subsection begins with surgical preparation codes (15002–15005).

Surgical Preparation

Codes 15002–15005 include surgical preparation of a site by excision of open wounds, eschar, or scar, including subcutaneous tissue. The code selection also includes incisional/excisional release of scar contracture. Code differentiation is made by the site and size of the area. A percentage of body surface for adults (and children age 10 years and older) is measured in increments of 100 square centimeters. The measure of infants and children (younger than 10 years) is in percentages of body surface area.

Autograft (or Tissue Cultured Autograft) Grafts

The next series of codes describes autograft skin grafts. Skin transplanted from one location to another on the same individual is termed an autograft. (See figure 4.3 for an illustration of a skin graft.)

These codes are categorized by type of graft (for example, pinch graft, split-thickness graft, or full-thickness graft), body part involved, and size of defect in square centimeters (except for pinch grafts, which are measured in centimeters). If the donor site requires skin grafting or local flaps, an additional code should be reported. CPT code 15040 is to be assigned for harvesting of skin for tissue-cultured skin autograft.

The following definitions are helpful when coding skin grafts:

- *Pinch graft:* This is a piece of skin graft about 0.25 inch in diameter that is obtained by elevating the skin with a needle and slicing it off with a knife.
- *Split-thickness graft:* This graft consists of only the superficial layers of the dermis.
- *Full-thickness graft:* This graft is composed of skin and subcutaneous tissues. (See figure 4.4 for an illustration of depth of split-thickness and full-thickness grafts.)
- *Allograft:* This graft is obtained from a genetically dissimilar individual of the same species (one individual to another). It is also known as allogenic graft and homograft.
- *Autograft:* A graft transferred from one part of the patient's body to another part.
- *Dermal autograft:* An autograph from which epidermis and subcutaneous fat has been removed; can be used in place of fascia.
- *Epidermal autograft:* An autograft consisting primarily of epidermal tissue including keratinocytes cells but with little dermal tissue.

- *Skin substitute:* Biomaterial engineered tissue or a combination of material and cells or tissues that can be substituted for skin autograft or allograft in a clinical procedure
- *Xenograft:* This graft is obtained from a species different from the recipient (for example, animal to human). It is also called xenogenic graft, heterograft, and heterotransplant. Currently, pig skin is the most popular xenograft.

Figure 4.3. Skin graft harvest

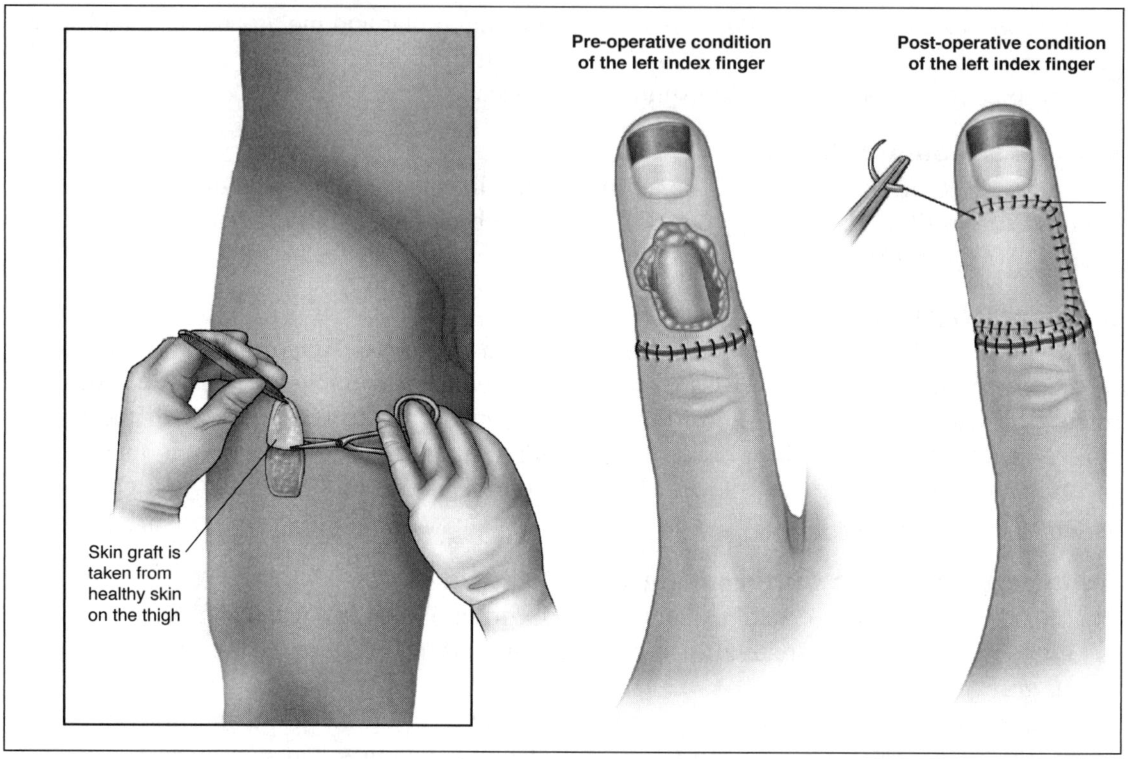

Figure 4.4. Depth of split-thickness and full-thickness grafts

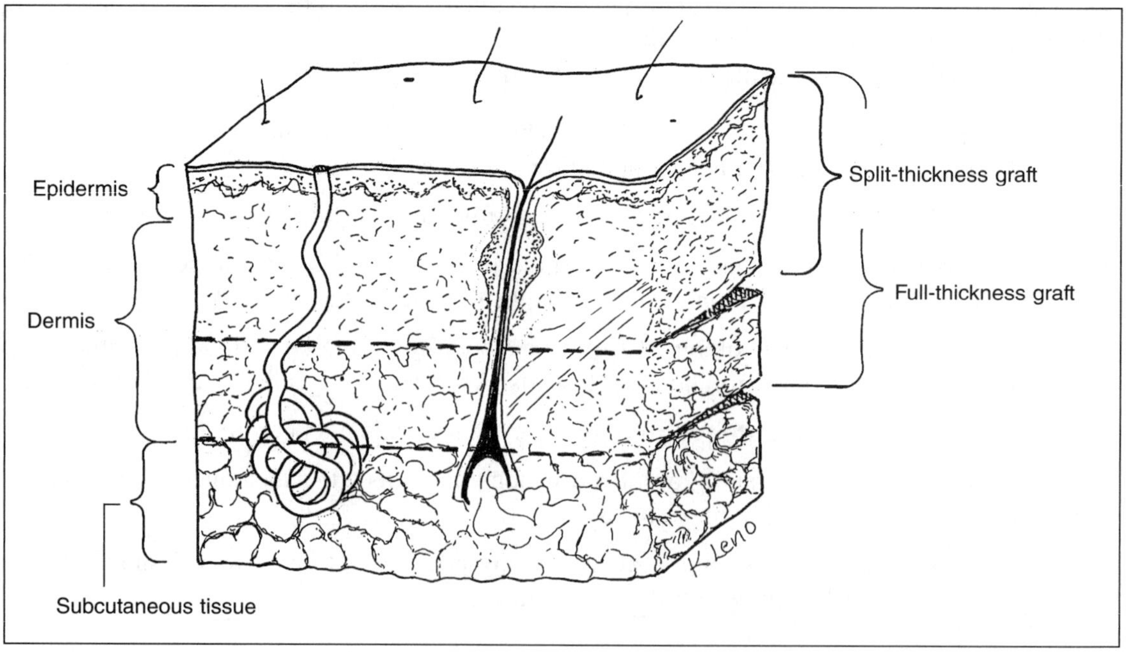

Tissue-Cultured Autograft

CPT codes 15150–15157 are assigned for tissue-cultured autograft procedures. Studies have supported the fact that these grafts are not rejected by the patient's immune system because they are recognized by the immune system as being part of the person's own body. Codes are differentiated by the size and location of the recipient site.

Epicel® is an example of a tissue-cultured autograft process. Living, unburned skin cells are removed from a burn patient and used to grow thin sheets of new cells in a laboratory. Cells are harvested and then placed in a cultured medium, co-cultured with mouse cells, where the tissue is nutritionally supported and grown to the size of a playing card. This method is often used to treat deep dermal or full-thickness burns comprising a total body surface area of greater than or equal to 30 percent.

Skin Substitute Grafts

Codes 15271–15278 are used to identify application of skin substitute grafts that are not autologous. Common skin substitute grafts include:

- Biobrane®—consists of a nylon mesh which acts as a "dermis" and a silicon membrane which acts as an "epidermis"
- Integra®—a silicone membrane is used as an epidermal layer
- Alloderm®—a skin substitute derived from a cadaveric dermis

Free Skin Grafts

Included in the Autograft subsection is a range of codes to identify full-thickness free skin grafts (15200–15261). If the dermis is included in its entirety, the appropriate term is full-thickness skin graft. Mirroring the other skin graft codes, the coding selection is based on site and size.

Removal of Skin Lesion with Skin Replacement/Substitute Graft

When an excision of a lesion requires a skin replacement/substitute graft for repair of the defect, the coding professional is directed to also assign a code to identify the excision of the lesion, using a code from the range 11400 through 11471 or 11600 through 11646.

Flaps (Skin and/or Deep Tissues)

This series of codes (15570–15738) includes procedures describing pedicle flaps, muscle, myocutaneous or fasciocutaneous flaps, and delayed flap transfers. The codes are categorized first by type of flap (for example, pedicle) and then by recipient body part.

Codes 15600 through 15630, which describe delayed transfer, identify the donor site, not the recipient site. An additional code should be reported when repair of the donor site requires skin grafting or local flaps.

The following definitions are helpful when coding flaps:

- *Pedicle flap:* This flap consists of detached skin and subcutaneous tissue in which the attached end or base contains an adequate blood supply. It is partially transferred to the recipient site with the base still attached to the donor site. After the recipient site has established a good blood supply, the base or pedicle is cut off and the graft completed.

- *Myocutaneous flap:* This flap involves the transfer of intact muscle, subcutaneous tissue, and skin as a single unit rotated on a relatively narrow blood supply of the muscle.

Other Flaps and Grafts

The last range of codes for skin grafts (15740–15776) identifies specialty procedures such as punch graft for hair transplants and neurovascular pedicle procedures. Add-on code 15777 is used for implantation of biologic implant. For example, use of acellular dermal matrix for breast reconstruction would include both the reconstruction code and 15777.

Exercise 4.10 Integumentary System—Skin Grafts

Unless otherwise noted, all answers can be found in appendix D of this book. Answers to selected exercises are located in the Instructor's Guide and available only to faculty of educational programs.

Assign appropriate CPT code(s) for the following procedure and indicate the index entries that were used to identify the code(s). Assign only CPT surgical codes (no E/M codes) and append any applicable modifiers.

1. Physician performs a wide resection of a 3.0-cm malignant skin lesion of the left leg. The defect required an adjacent tissue transfer measuring 15 sq cm.

   Code(s): ______________________________

   Index entries: ______________________________

   ____

2. A 35-year-old patient sustained third-degree burns three weeks ago. A small skin graft was harvested at the time and submitted for tissue culturing. The patient is now admitted for grafting of the cultured tissue. A total of 72 sq cm is grafted onto the patient's lower abdomen during this encounter.

   Code(s): ______________________________

   Index entries: ______________________________

   ____

3. Surgeon performs a full-thickness skin graft from the buttocks to the arm covering the 2 cm × 4 cm defect.

   Code(s): ______________________________

   Index entries: ______________________________

   ____

Exercise 4.11 Integumentary System

Unless otherwise noted, all answers can be found in appendix D of this book. Answers to selected exercises are located in the Instructor's Guide and available only to faculty of educational programs.

Operative Report

Preoperative Diagnosis:	Basal cell carcinoma of the forehead
Postoperative Diagnosis:	Same
Procedure:	Excision of basal cell carcinoma with split-thickness skin graft

The patient was given a local IV sedation and taken to the OR suite. The face and left thigh were prepped with Phisohex soap. The cancer was outlined for excision and measured 5 × 4 cm. The forehead was infiltrated with 1% Xylocaine with 1:100,000 epinephrine.

The cancer was excised and carried down to the frontalis muscle. A suture was placed at the 12 o'clock position. The specimen was sent to pathology for frozen section.

Attention was then turned to the skin graft. A pattern of the defect was transferred to the left anterior thigh using a new needle. A local infiltration was performed on the thigh. Using a freehand knife, a split-thickness skin graft was harvested. The thigh was treated with Tegaderm and a wraparound Kerliz and Ace wrap. The skin graft was applied and sutured to the forehead defect with running 5-0 plain catgut.

Xeroform with cotton soaked in glycerin was sutured with 4-0 silk. A sterile dressing was applied. The patient tolerated the procedure well, with no complications or blood loss.

Assign appropriate CPT code(s) for the preceding procedure and indicate the index entries that were used to identify the code(s). Assign only CPT surgical codes (no E/M codes) and append any applicable modifiers.

1. Code(s): ____________________

   Index entries: ____________________

   ____

Exercise 4.12 Integumentary System

Unless otherwise noted, all answers can be found in appendix D of this book. Answers to selected exercises are located in the Instructor's Guide and available only to faculty of educational programs.

Operative Report

Preoperative Diagnosis:	Open wound, left thigh, status post fasciotomy
Postoperative Diagnosis:	Same
Procedure:	Split-thickness skin graft, left thigh, donor site from left thigh. Graft was approximately 12 × 5 cm.

The patient is status post trauma. A tree fell on him and he sustained a significant injury to his thigh. He had compartment syndrome of his thigh, requiring a fasciotomy. He presents today for a skin graft to the fasciotomy site.

The patient was brought to the operating room and placed supine on the operating table. Following the adequate induction of general anesthesia, his left thigh and fasciotomy site were prepped and draped in the standard surgical fashion. Attention was first directed to the patient's anterior thigh. The Betadine prep was gently removed with normal saline. We then applied mineral oil to the anterior thigh. We then used a dermatome to harvest an approximately 12 × 5-cm split-thickness skin graft in the depth of 0.015. Following removal of our donor site, an epinephrine-soaked sponge was applied to the donor site. We then went in to the back table and meshed our graft 1:1. Following this, we prepared our graft bed for graft placement. The excellent granulation tissue bed was roughed up using a gauze sponge, and the skin graft was applied and secured in place using surgical staples. The edge of the skin was then trimmed accordingly. Following adequate placement and securing our graft, we then fashioned the dressing. A Bacitracin-coated Adaptic was then applied over the graft and Reston foam was applied over that. Fine mesh gauze was then used to secure it in place, and the Reston and mesh gauze were secured also using surgical staples. There was an excellent compression against the graft. Following this, we turned our attention to the donor site. Epinephrine-soaked gauze was removed, and Calgiswab dressing was applied. There was excellent hemostasis from the donor site. Following this, a Kerlix roll was placed around the left thigh and secured with paper tape. The patient tolerated the procedure without complications. The patient was then taken to the PACU for recovery.

Assign appropriate CPT code(s) for the preceding procedure and indicate the index entries that were used to identify the code(s). Assign only CPT surgical codes (no E/M codes) and append any applicable modifiers.

1. Code(s): ______________________________

   Index entries: ______________________________

   ____

Mohs Micrographic Surgery

Mohs surgery (17311–17315) is a specialized treatment for skin cancer cases that usually involves several stages with histologic examination of 100 percent of the surgical margins. The selective removal of skin cancer allows for preservation of as much of the surrounding normal tissue as possible. After the removal of the visible portion of the tumor, the surgeon excises a thin layer of tissue that is processed and examined under the microscope. This process includes dividing the tumor specimen into pieces, and each individual piece is embedded into an individual tissue block that is histopathologically examined. If any tumor is seen during the microscopic examination, its location is established, and a thin layer of additional tissue is excised from the involved area. The microscopic examination is then repeated. The entire process is repeated until no tumor is found. The Mohs surgery codes are differentiated by the stage of the procedure, site, and number of tissue blocks.

Surgical Procedures of the Breast

Codes 19000 through 19499 describe procedures performed on the breast, such as biopsy, mastectomy, and reconstruction. These codes are categorized first by general type of procedure (incision, excision, reconstruction/repair) and then by specific procedure.

The codes describing breast procedures refer to unilateral procedures, and modifiers LT or RT should be appended. If a bilateral procedure is performed, modifier 50 should be reported.

Breast Biopsy

In coding breast biopsies, the coding professional must determine the type of biopsy performed: percutaneous, excisional, or incisional:

- *Percutaneous biopsy:* A biopsy that involves the insertion of a hollow needle to remove a biopsy specimen of breast tissue. This procedure is reported with code 19100. See figure 4.5.
- *Excisional biopsy:* A biopsy that involves total removal of the lesion, whether malignant or benign, from the breast. To make this determination, the coding professional should review both the operative report and the pathology report. The operative report may indicate that the lesion was removed completely. In the case of malignant lesions, the pathology report may indicate that the margins of the specimen are negative for malignancy or free of tumor. If the excisional biopsy was performed with identification by preoperative placement of radiologic marker, codes 19125 through 19126 should be reported. When appropriate, an additional code(s) to describe placement of the needle localization wire (19290–19291) or metallic localization clip (19295) should be reported.
- *Incisional biopsy:* A biopsy of the breast (19101) that typically involves removal of only a portion of the lesion for pathologic examination.

Mastectomy

Codes 19300 through 19307 describe the various types of mastectomy:

- Code 19301, Partial mastectomy, refers to the partial removal of part of the breast tissue, leaving the breast almost intact. This also may be referred to as a lobectomy or lumpectomy. If an axillary lymphectomy is also performed, the correct coding assignment would be 19302.

Figure 4.5. Needle breast biopsy

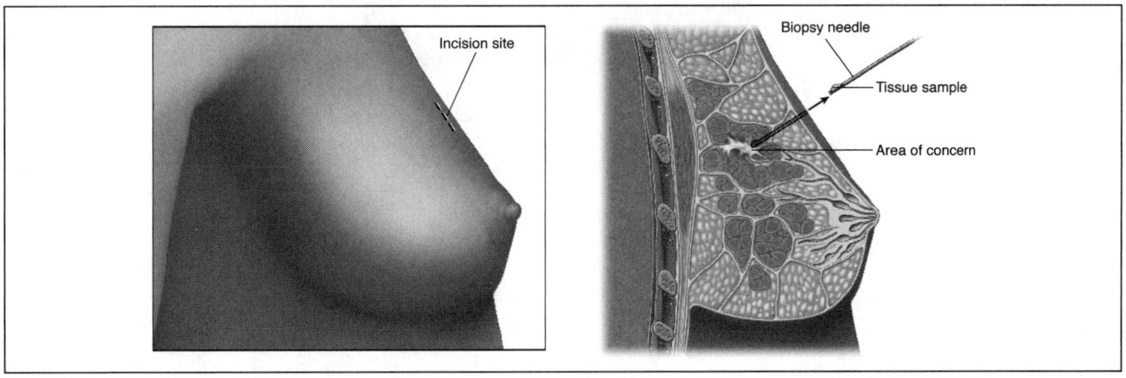

- Code 19303, Simple, complete mastectomy, is assigned for the excision of all the breast tissue, with the lymph nodes and muscle left intact.
- Code 19304, Subcutaneous mastectomy, is used for excision of breast tissue with the skin and nipple intact.
- Code 19305, Radical mastectomy, refers to the excision of breast tissue including the pectoral muscles and the axillary lymph nodes.
- Code 19306, Radical mastectomy, is assigned for the excision of breast tissue including the pectoral muscles and axillary lymph nodes (see code 19305 above), and also includes the internal mammary lymph nodes.
- Code 19307, Modified radical mastectomy, is used for the excision of breast tissue including the axillary lymph nodes. The pectoralis minor muscles may or may not be removed, but the pectoralis major muscles are left intact. Figure 4.6 illustrates a modified radical mastectomy.

Insertion of breast prosthesis may be reported as an additional code when performed at the same time as the mastectomy (19340) or when performed at a later date (19342).

Figure 4.6. Modified radical mastectomy

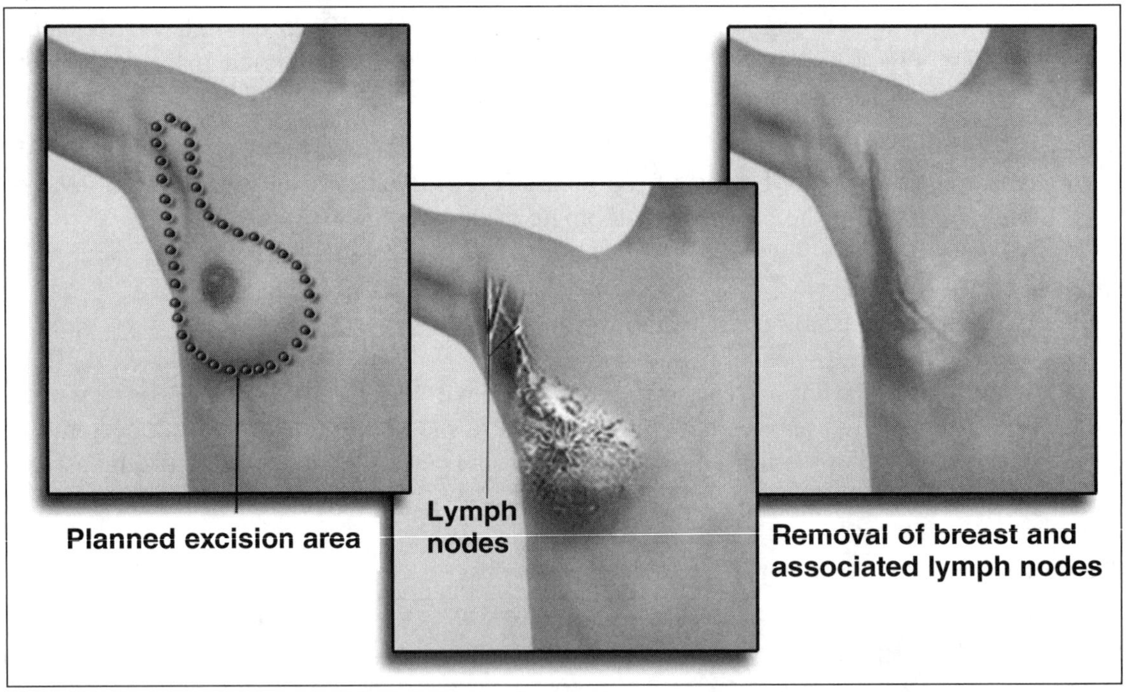

Exercise 4.13 Integumentary System

Unless otherwise noted, all answers can be found in appendix D of this book. Answers to selected exercises are located in the Instructor's Guide and available only to faculty of educational programs.

Physician Office Operative Note

This patient has come to see me for follow-up for a cyst present in the left breast area. I did a needle aspiration biopsy, and fluid was sent out for cytology. If the biopsy is negative, I can see her back in the office in four months, or earlier if there are any problems.

The right breast feels benign. There is no axillary adenopathy. No cervical adenopathy.

Hospital pathology of a sample from a left breast aspiration revealed only a few benign lipocytes.

Assign appropriate CPT code(s) for the preceding procedure and indicate the index entries that were used to identify the code(s). Assign only CPT surgical codes (no E/M codes) and append any applicable modifiers.

1. Code(s): ____________________

   Index entries: ____________________

   ____

Exercise 4.14 Integumentary System

Unless otherwise noted, all answers can be found in appendix D of this book. Answers to selected exercises are located in the Instructor's Guide and available only to faculty of educational programs.

Operative Report

Preoperative Diagnosis: Abnormal mammogram, left breast

Postoperative Diagnosis: Same

The patient is a 61-year-old G3, P3 female with a family history of positive carcinoma of the breast. She underwent a screening mammogram in the spring of this year that demonstrated a localized density in the subareolar tissue of the left breast. Physical examination demonstrated no palpable abnormality in the area.

The patient was brought to the OR after undergoing placement of a hook wire localizing needle in the mammography suite by the radiologist. She was placed on the OR table in a supine position. After ensuring an adequate level of conscious sedation, her left breast and chest wall were prepped and draped in a sterile fashion. A needle/wire complex was protruding from the left breast approximately 2 centimeters above the nipple. The skin surrounding the needle in the breast tissue in the subareolar area was infiltrated with 1% Xylocaine to achieve local anesthesia. A 5-cm incision was made around the localizing wire. Small superior and inferior skin flaps were elevated, exposing the underlying subcutaneous fat. Dissection with electrocautery was begun into the breast about the wire. The needle wire complex was grasped using Allis clamps and drawn into the operative wound. The breast tissue and subcutaneous fat surrounding the needle were excised in this fashion until all the tissue surrounding the needle/wire complex was excised. The specimen was then forwarded to the radiology suite for specimen mammography.

As the specimen mammogram was being obtained, the wound was examined for hemostasis, which was thought to be complete. The deeper breast tissues were closed using interrupted 3-0 Vicryl figure-of-8 sutures. Subcutaneous tissues were approximated in a similar fashion. The wound was irrigated and again examined for hemostasis, which was thought to be complete. The skin was closed using a running 5-0 Maxon subcuticular suture. The wound was washed and dried and sterile dressings applied. The operative field was not disturbed until a call was received from the radiology suite indicating that the specimen contained the area of interest identified on the patient's original mammogram. At this point, the patient was transferred to the recovery area in stable condition.

Assign appropriate CPT code(s) for the preceding procedure and indicate the index entries that were used to identify the code(s). Assign only CPT surgical codes (no E/M codes) and append any applicable modifiers.

1. Code(s): ____________________

   Index entries: ____________________

   ____

Exercise 4.15 Integumentary System

Unless otherwise noted, all answers can be found in appendix D of this book. Answers to selected exercises are located in the Instructor's Guide and available only to faculty of educational programs.

Operative Report

Preoperative Diagnosis:	Probable carcinoma of the right breast
Postoperative Diagnosis:	Carcinoma of the right breast
Operation:	Excisional biopsy

The patient was brought to the OR. Under satisfactory general endotracheal anesthesia, the right breast was prepped and draped in the usual manner. Through an elliptical incision in the upper outer quadrant, a small nodule was excised. Bleeders were electrocoagulated. The deep layer was closed with interrupted 3-0 Vicryl. The skin was closed with clips. A dry sterile dressing was applied, and the patient returned to the recovery room in good condition.

Pathology Report

Clinical Diagnosis:	Right breast mass
Specimen:	Mass, right breast, frozen section
Pathological Diagnosis:	Breast mass, right: infiltrating ductal carcinoma, Grade 2/3, 0.7 cm; resected margins negative for carcinoma

Assign appropriate CPT code(s) for the preceding procedure and indicate the index entries that were used to identify the code(s). Assign only CPT surgical codes (no E/M codes) and append any applicable modifiers.

1. Code(s): ____________________

   Index entries: ____________________

   ____

Exercise 4.16 Integumentary System Review

Unless otherwise noted, all answers can be found in appendix D of this book. Answers to selected exercises are located in the Instructor's Guide and available only to faculty of educational programs.

Assign appropriate CPT code(s) for the following procedures and indicate the index entries that were used to identify the code(s). Assign only CPT surgical codes (no E/M codes) and append any applicable modifiers.

1. Debridement and dressing of first-degree (partial-thickness) burn of the index finger

   Code(s): ____________________

   Index entries: ____________________

   ____

2. Wide excision of a malignant lesion of arm (3.0 × 2.0 cm) with adjacent skin graft

   Code(s): ____________________

   Index entries: ____________________

   ____

Exercise 4.16 (Continued)

3. Layered closure of 2.0-cm laceration of right forearm and 2.5-cm laceration of left elbow

   Code(s): ______________________

   Index entries: ______________________

   ____

4. With the use of imaging, the surgeon placed a metallic clip to identify the suspicious tissue in the left breast. A percutaneous core needle biopsy was performed.

   Code(s): ______________________

   Index entries: ______________________

   ____

5. Excision of malignant melanoma of left arm (3.0 × 1.5 cm, with 1.0-cm margins surrounding the lesion)

   Code(s): ______________________

   Index entries: ______________________

   ____

Note: Answers to exercises 6 through 10 do not appear in appendix D of this text. They are located in the Instructor's Guide and available to faculty of educational programs.

6. Excision of pilonidal cyst requiring single-layer suture

   Code(s): ______________________

   Index entries: ______________________

   ____

7. Complete excision of nail and matrix, left great toe

   Code(s): ______________________

   Index entries: ______________________

   ____

8. Dermabrasion of cheek for severe acne

   Code(s): ______________________

   Index entries: ______________________

   ____

9. Electrosurgical removal of 3.0-cm squamous cell carcinoma of the hand

   Code(s): ______________________

   Index entries: ______________________

   ____

10. Debridement of below-knee amputation stump. The necrotic wounds were sharply excised down to and including the fascia with a 10-blade scalpel (15 sq cm).

    Code(s): ______________________

    Index entries: ______________________

    ____

Musculoskeletal System

The musculoskeletal subsection is categorized first by body part and then by general type of procedure, with the individual codes describing the specific procedure performed. The first series of codes (20005–20999) describes general musculoskeletal procedures such as bone biopsy, application of fixation device, bone graft, replantation of body part, wound exploration, and arthrocentesis. A lengthy note at the beginning of this subsection defines terms related to the treatment of fractures.

The codes listed in this subsection include the application and removal of the first cast and/or traction device. Subsequent replacement of the cast and/or traction device may be reported with codes 29000 through 29799 and codes located at the beginning of the general subsection.

Integumentary vs. Musculoskeletal Codes

In the integumentary system section, it was noted that procedure codes associated with skin abscesses/cysts (tumors) may be found in the Musculoskeletal system section. Fascia is a layer of fibrous connective tissue that surrounds muscles. Soft tissue tumors may extend beyond the skin into the subcutaneous fascia (located beneath the dermis) or in the subfascia (below [deep] fascia but not involving the bone). Coding professionals must read the documentation to determine the location and size of the soft tissue tumors. If the physician documents an incision of an abscess that extends beyond the skin into the soft tissues (muscle, fascia, or tendon), then the musculoskeletal code would be appropriate. Note the following examples:

Example #1: Patient is seen in the physician's office for an infected epidermal inclusion cyst of the arm that requires an incision and drainage. (Integumentary code 10060)

Example #2: Physician removes a 1.5-cm lipoma located in the subcutaneous layer of the scalp. (Musculoskeletal code 21011)

Example #3: Physician excises a 1.5-cm lipoma located in the subfascial tissue of the scalp. (Musculoskeletal code 21013)

Fractures and Dislocations

To report the diagnosis and treatment of fractures and dislocations accurately, coding professionals must answer the following questions:

- *What body site is involved?* The operative report and/or any diagnostic tests performed, such as x-rays or computed tomography (CT) scans, should be reviewed.
- *Was the fracture/dislocation treatment open or closed or with percutaneous skeletal fixation?* **Closed treatment** refers to treatment of the fracture/dislocation without a surgical incision into the site. **Open treatment** refers to the treatment of a fracture or dislocation that includes exposing the site via a surgical incision or when a fractured bone is opened remote from the fracture site in order to insert an intramedullary nail across the fracture site (fracture site is not opened and visualized). **Percutaneous skeletal fixation** involves treatment of a fracture by placing fixation devices such as pins across the fracture site, usually under x-ray imaging.

- *Was the fracture/dislocation manipulated?* Manipulation refers to the attempted reduction or restoration of a dislocated joint or fracture. CPT codes are available for reporting nondisplaced fractures treated without manipulation.

  Example: Code 27238 is used for reporting closed treatment of an intertrochanteric fracture, without manipulation.

- *Did the procedure include internal or external fixation?*

Application of Casts and Strapping

The series of codes (29000–29750) describing the application of casts and strapping can be reported in the following scenarios:

- To identify replacement of a cast or strapping during or after the period of normal follow-up care (global postoperative period)
- To identify an initial service performed without any restorative treatment or stabilization of the fracture, injury, or dislocation and/or to afford pain relief to the patient
- To identify an initial cast or strapping when the same physician does not perform, or is not expected to perform, any other treatment or procedure
- To identify an initial cast or strapping when another physician provided or will provide restorative treatment

CPT guidelines for hospital outpatient reporting of casting/strapping/splinting can be found in *CPT Assistant* (Vol. 12, Issue 4, April 2002).

Exercise 4.17 Musculoskeletal System—Fractures

Unless otherwise noted, all answers can be found in appendix D of this book. Answers to selected exercises are located in the Instructor's Guide and available only to faculty of educational programs.

Assign appropriate CPT code(s) for the following procedures and indicate the index entries that were used to identify the codes. Assign only CPT surgical codes (no E/M codes) and append any applicable modifiers.

1. Diagnosis: Closed fracture of ulnar shaft, left
   Procedure: Open reduction of ulnar shaft fracture

   Code(s): ______________________________

   Index entries: ______________________________

   ____

2. Closed treatment of two uncomplicated rib fractures

   Code(s): ______________________________

   Index entries: ______________________________

   ____

(Continued on next page)

Exercise 4.17 (Continued)

3. Closed reduction of proximal humerus fracture, right

   Code(s): ____________________

   Index entries: ____________________

   ____

4. The orthopedic surgeon reduces a fracture of the right proximal tibia. After closed treatment and skeletal traction, the physician applies a short leg cast.

   Code(s): ____________________

   Index entries: ____________________

   ____

Note: Answers to exercises 5 through 7 do not appear in appendix D of this text. They are located in the Instructor's Guide and available to faculty of educational programs.

5. The patient was diagnosed with a dislocated right patella. The surgeon performed a closed reduction with the patient under anesthesia.

   Code(s): ____________________

   Index entries: ____________________

   ____

6. Open reduction with internal fixation, fracture of distal end (medial condyle) of left femur

   Code(s): ____________________

   Index entries: ____________________

   ____

7. Patient is diagnosed with right humeral shaft fracture. The orthopedic surgeon performs an open treatment of the fracture using an intramedullary implant and locking screws.

   Code(s): ____________________

   Index entries: ____________________

   ____

Exercise 4.18 Musculoskeletal System

Unless otherwise noted, all answers can be found in appendix D of this book. Answers to selected exercises are located in the Instructor's Guide and available only to faculty of educational programs.

Emergency Department Record

Chief Complaint:	Right ankle injury
History of Present Illness:	The patient is a 39-year-old woman who injured her right ankle yesterday. While stepping around some puppies to avoid hitting them, she suffered an inversion injury to her ankle. She complains of lateral ankle and foot pain, and has pain on weight bearing.
Past Medical History:	Status post hysterectomy
Medications:	None
Allergies:	Codeine, which causes nausea
Physical Examination:	Alert female in no acute distress. Right lower extremity: proximal mid tibia-fibula are nontender. Ankle shows moderate diffuse swelling over the lateral ankle extending onto the dorsolateral foot with ecchymoses. Good distal neurovascular status. Decreased range of motion secondary to pain and swelling.
Emergency Department	X-ray of right foot and ankle shows an avulsion fragment off the distal fibula,
Course:	Otherwise soft tissue swelling.
Diagnosis:	Acute right ankle sprain with avulsion fracture
Disposition and Plan:	Short leg splint applied. Crutches. No weight bearing. Ice and elevate. Vicodin #30 1–2 q 4–6 h. She tolerates it well. Orthopedic referral.

Assign appropriate CPT code(s) for the preceding procedure and indicate the index entries that were used to identify the code(s). Assign only CPT surgical codes (no E/M codes) and append any applicable modifiers.

1. Code(s): ____________________

   Index entries: ____________________

   ____

Exercise 4.19 Musculoskeletal System

Unless otherwise noted, all answers can be found in appendix D of this book. Answers to selected exercises are located in the Instructor's Guide and available only to faculty of educational programs.

Operative Report

Preoperative Diagnosis:	Fracture of distal fibula, left
Postoperative Diagnosis:	Same
Procedure:	Closed reduction of fibular fracture

This 14-year-old gymnast feels pain in her left leg after vaulting at practice. She is unable to bear any weight on her foot.

Physical examination showed foot and ankle to be normal. The neurovascular status of the foot was normal. The ankle was nontender and not swollen. Findings were confined to the distal fibula, 2 inches proximal to the lateral malleolus. There was point tenderness in this area. An x-ray of the tibia and fibula shows a displaced fracture of the distal fibula.

The fracture was reduced and the patient placed in a short leg splint with extensive padding over the fracture site. She was given Tylenol #3 for pain and instructed to follow up with her physician in 10 days.

Assign appropriate CPT code(s) for the preceding procedure and indicate the index entries that were used to identify the code(s). Assign only CPT surgical codes (no E/M codes) and append any applicable modifiers.

1. Code(s): ______________________________

   Index entries: ______________________________

   ____

Arthroscopy

Procedures describing both diagnostic and therapeutic arthroscopy are reported with codes 29800 through 29909. These codes are categorized first by body part involved and then by type—surgical or diagnostic. The surgical arthroscopic codes are further divided to identify the specific procedure performed, such as synovectomy or debridement. A surgical arthroscopy always includes a diagnostic component that should not be reported separately. Figure 4.7 illustrates an arthroscopy of the knee.

Figure 4.7. Knee surgery—injuries with arthroscopic repair

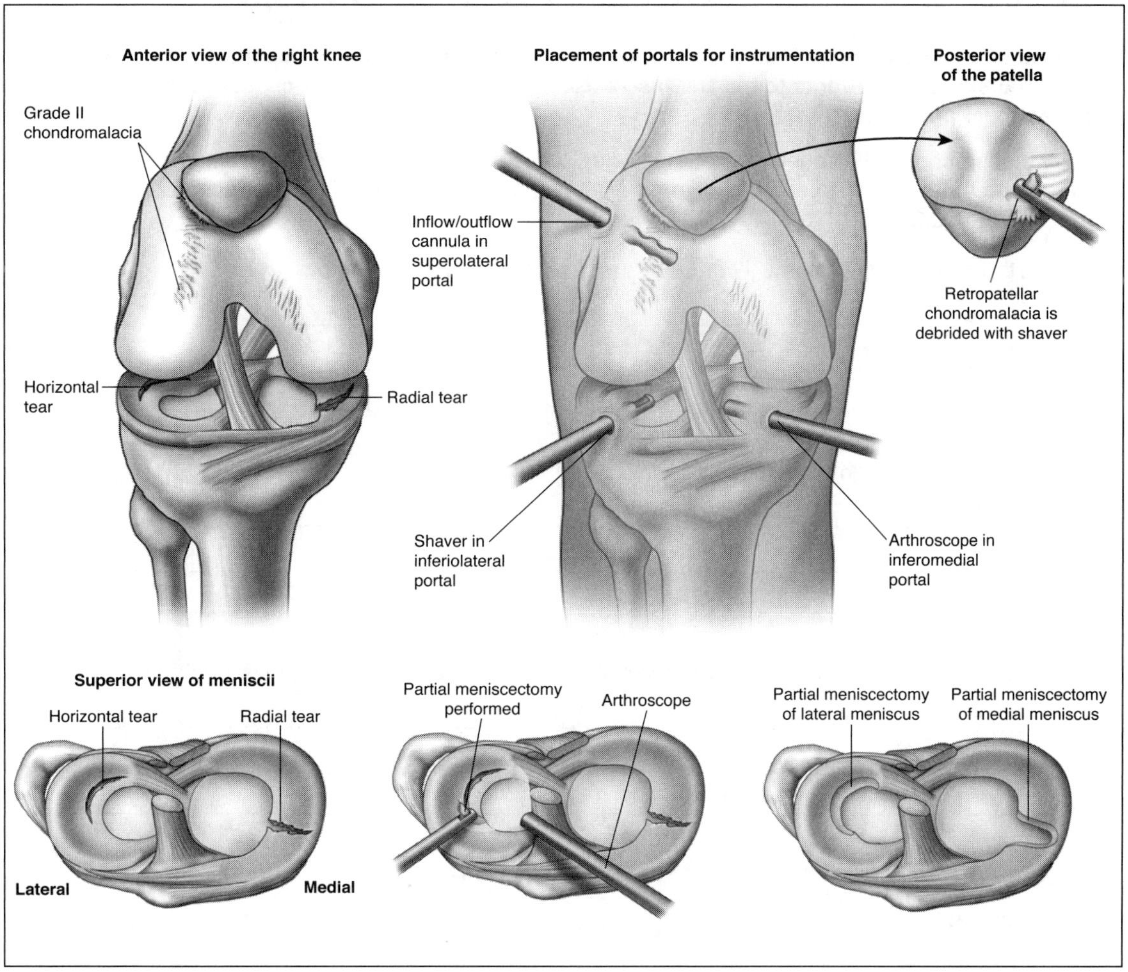

Exercise 4.20 Musculoskeletal System—Arthroscopy

Unless otherwise noted, all answers can be found in appendix D of this book. Answers to selected exercises are located in the Instructor's Guide and available only to faculty of educational programs.

Assign appropriate CPT code(s) for the following procedures and indicate the index entries that were used to identify the codes. Assign only CPT surgical codes (no E/M codes) and append any applicable modifiers.

1. Arthroscopic synovectomy (limited) of the left knee

   Code(s): ______________________________

   Index entries: ______________________________

   ____

2. Arthroscopy of right shoulder with rotator cuff repair

   Code(s): ______________________________

   Index entries: ______________________________

   ____

3. Arthroscopy of the left wrist with repair of triangular fibrocartilage and joint debridement

   Code(s): ______________________________

   Index entries: ______________________________

   ____

4. Arthroscopy of the left elbow with limited debridement

   Code(s): ______________________________

   Index entries: ______________________________

   ____

Exercise 4.21 Musculoskeletal System

Unless otherwise noted, all answers can be found in appendix D of this book. Answers to selected exercises are located in the Instructor's Guide and available only to faculty of educational programs.

Operative Report

Preoperative Diagnosis: Tear of the right medial meniscus

Postoperative Diagnosis: Same

Operation: Meniscus repair

The patient was brought to the OR and anesthetized. An inflatable tourniquet was placed about the proximal thigh, and the operative area was prepared and draped in a sterile fashion with the leg placed in the instrument maker leg holder. Following this, incisions were made for insertion of the arthroscope inflow cannula and probe. Video arthroscopy was then carried out. He was found to have a tear of the posterior horn of the medial meniscus, and this was repaired. The anterior cruciate ligament was examined and found to be intact. The lateral meniscus also appeared to be intact. The patellofemoral joint was within normal limits. While the patient was asleep, the knee was examined and stressed. There was no opening of the medial collateral ligament region and no instability in that area. After completion of the arthroscopy, the instruments were withdrawn from the wound and the incisions closed. The incisions were injected marginally with local anesthetic for postoperative analgesia. After closure of the incisions, Betadine ointment and dressings were placed over the knee, and the patient was returned to the recovery room in stable condition.

Assign appropriate CPT code(s) for the preceding procedure and indicate the index entries that were used to identify the code(s). Assign only CPT surgical codes (no E/M codes) and append any applicable modifiers.

1. Code(s): ____________________

   Index entries: ____________________

   ____

Exercise 4.22 Musculoskeletal System Review

Unless otherwise noted, all answers can be found in appendix D of this book. Answers to selected exercises are located in the Instructor's Guide and available only to faculty of educational programs.

Assign appropriate CPT code(s) for the following procedures and indicate the index entries that were used to identify the codes. Assign only CPT surgical codes (no E/M codes) and append any applicable modifiers.

1. Closed reduction of two metatarsal fractures of left foot

   Code(s): ____________________

   Index entries: ____________________

   ____

2. Repair of hammertoe, second digit of left foot

   Code(s): ____________________

   Index entries: ____________________

   ____

(Continued on next page)

Exercise 4.22 (Continued)

3. Open reduction of fracture of right medial malleolus

   Code(s): ______

   Index entries: ______

4. Surgical exploration of stab wound of chest with included coagulation of blood vessels and enlargement of the wound.

   Code(s): ______

   Index entries: ______

5. Incision and drainage of hematoma of shoulder

   Code(s): ______

   Index entries: ______

Note: Answers to exercises 6 through 10 do not appear in appendix D of this text. They are located in the Instructor's Guide and available to faculty of educational programs.

6. Repair of lateral collateral ligament of right elbow using local tissue

   Code(s): ______

   Index entries: ______

7. Midtarsal arthrodesis, left foot

   Code(s): ______

   Index entries: ______

8. Arthroscopy of the right wrist with partial synovectomy

   Code(s): ______

   Index entries: ______

9. Excision of bone cyst, toe (third digit of left foot)

   Code(s): ______

   Index entries: ______

10. Removal of sliver of metal from deep tissue in the right knee

    Code(s): ______

    Index entries: ______

Respiratory System

The respiratory subsection includes surgical procedures involving the nose and sinuses, larynx, trachea and bronchi, and lungs and pleura. Figures 4.8 and 4.9 illustrate the respiratory system.

Nasal Sinus Endoscopy

Codes 31231 through 31297 describe nasal sinus endoscopic procedures. These procedures allow the physician to visualize the interior of the nasal cavity, the middle and superior meatus, the turbinates, and the sphenoethmoid recess. The purpose of the procedures may be either diagnostic or surgical in nature. A surgical endoscopy may be performed to control a nosebleed or to perform a maxillary antrostomy or sphenoidotomy. The coding professional should always review the documentation carefully to clarify the extent of the procedure. A surgical endoscopy includes the diagnostic component. The diagnostic endoscopy should not be reported separately when performed during the same operative episode. Also, if performed, a sinusotomy is considered part of the endoscopic procedure and not reported separately.

Unless otherwise stated, codes in the 31231 through 31297 range are assumed to be unilateral. When the documentation indicates that a bilateral procedure was performed and the specific code does not state *bilateral,* modifier 50 may be assigned. Key points to remember include:

- Separate codes should not be assigned to identify a diagnostic nasal/sinus endoscopy when it is performed in conjunction with a surgical nasal/sinus endoscopy.
- A surgical endoscopy includes a sinusotomy. Only the code for the surgical endoscopy should be assigned when both are performed during the same operative episode.
- Modifier 50 should be assigned to identify a bilateral procedure only if the code does not specify bilateral.

Figure 4.8. The upper respiratory system

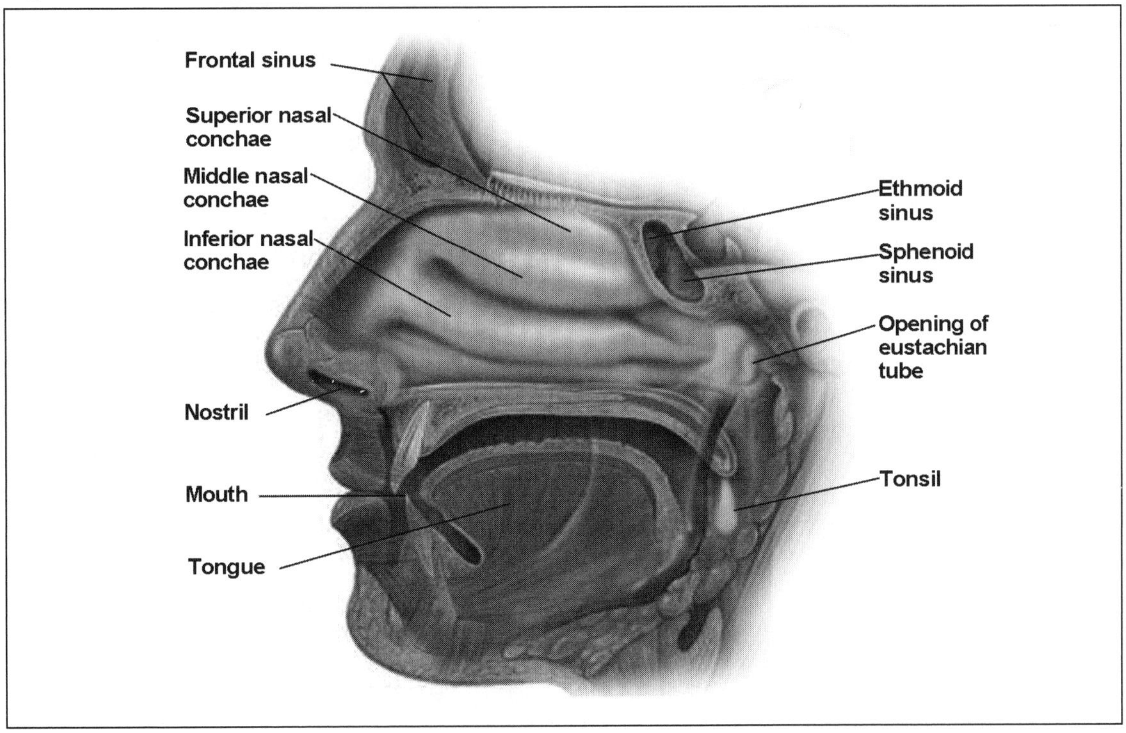

Figure 4.9. The lower respiratory system

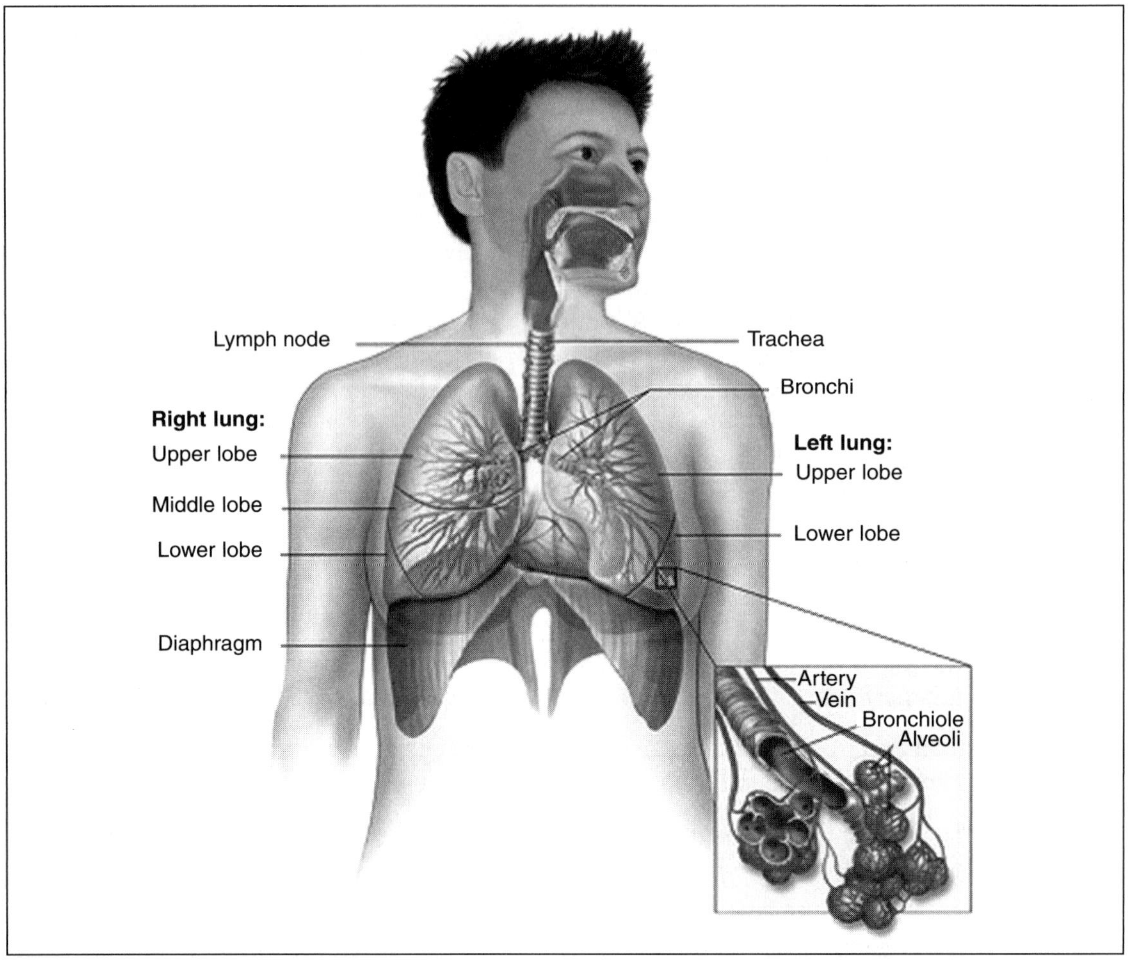

Exercise 4.23 Respiratory System—Endoscopy

Unless otherwise noted, all answers can be found in appendix D of this book. Answers to selected exercises are located in the Instructor's Guide and available only to faculty of educational programs.

Assign appropriate CPT code(s) for the following procedures and indicate the index entries that were used to identify the codes. Assign only CPT surgical codes (no E/M codes) and append any applicable modifiers.

1. Bilateral nasal endoscopy with total ethmoidectomy

   Code(s): ______________________________

   Index entries: ______________________________

   ____

2. Left nasal endoscopy for control of epistaxis

   Code(s): ______________________________

   Index entries: ______________________________

   ____

3. Diagnostic maxillary sinusoscopy, bilateral

   Code(s): ______________________________

   Index entries: ______________________________

   ____

Exercise 4.24 Respiratory System

Unless otherwise noted, all answers can be found in appendix D of this book. Answers to selected exercises are located in the Instructor's Guide and available only to faculty of educational programs.

Operative Report

Preoperative Diagnosis: Deviated nasal septum, chronic maxillary sinusitis, turbinate hypertrophy, nasal obstruction

Postoperative Diagnosis: Same

Procedure Performed:
1. Septoplasty
2. Nasal endoscopy, with bilateral maxillary antroscopy, removal of maxillary polyp
3. Submucous resection of the inferior turbinates, bilaterally

This 26-year-old woman was seen by ENT service for complaints of chronic sinusitis and difficulty breathing through the nose. She was noted to have a severely deviated septum toward the right with turbinate hypertrophy, nasal obstruction (CT scans confirmed this), as well as obstruction of the ostiomeatal complexes with mucosal thickening. A decision for the above-stated procedure was then made after she had failed conservative care.

The patient was brought to the operative suite, given general anesthetic, and properly prepped and draped. 5% cocaine pledgets were placed in each nasal chamber. 1% lidocaine with 1:100,000 epinephrine was injected into the caudal columnar region into the septum, as well as the middle uncinate middle turbinate region. Then, with the #1 scalpel blade, an incision was made along the left caudal columnar region in the septum, down to the mucoperichondrium. The mucoperichondrium was carefully elevated off the nasal septum cartilage, exposing a portion of the deviation. The contralateral portion was also freed up. With a Seiler knife, a portion of the deviation was removed. A large septal spur, touching the lateral wall, was carefully freed up and removed.

After the patient exhibited a much improved nasal septum, a piece of cartilage was morcellized and inserted between the septal mucosa layers, and the submucosa was closed with 4-0 plain suture in interrupted form. Attention was then brought to the middle turbinates, which were found to be lateralized. A decision to medialize them was made by placing 4-0 Vicryl to the left middle turbinate, sent through the right middle turbinate, back to the septum, and tied off on the left side.

Next, with the scope, the left nasal chamber was examined. The natural os was located. With the frontal probe, it was further enlarged with microbiter straight shot and back-biters. There was a moderate amount of mucosal thickening around this opening, just on the inside. After it was widely patent and cleaned out, attention was brought to the right side. The right os was located in a similar fashion and widely enlarged with the microbiter straight shot and back-biters. Again, a moderate amount of mucosal thickening was noted around this opening. When this was completed, attention was brought to the inferior turbinates.

The inferior turbinates were infractured and clamped with a Carmel clamp for five minutes, then submucosal resection was performed in the usual fashion. The rods of the turbinates were then cauterized with suction cautery. This was repeated in a similar fashion bilaterally. Silastic splints were sewn into place along the septum with 3-0 Ethilon, and tampons coated in Bactroban were inserted into both nasal chambers. The oral cavity was suctioned of all serosanguineous debris, and the patient exhibited good hemostasis. She recovered from the anesthetic and was transferred to the recovery room in stable condition.

Assign appropriate CPT code(s) for the preceding procedure and indicate the index entries that were used to identify the code(s). Assign only CPT surgical codes (no E/M codes) and append any applicable modifiers.

1. Code(s) to be submitted for the *hospital* services: ______________________

   ____

   Index entries: ______________________

   ____

Laryngoscopy

A laryngoscopy is an endoscopic procedure that allows the physician to visualize the larynx, or voice box. This examination may be diagnostic only or may be performed for surgical purposes such as for a biopsy or removal of a lesion. Codes 31505–31579 describe these diagnostic and surgical endoscopic procedures.

Indirect Laryngoscopy

Codes 31505 through 31513 refer to an indirect laryngoscopy. An indirect laryngoscopy is the simplest way to examine the larynx. One technique involves the use of a small mirror placed in the back of the throat. With the aid of a light source, the image of the larynx can be visualized in the mirror. The physician may view the image of the oropharynx, posterior third of the tongue, lateral laryngeal walls, posterior pharyngeal wall, epiglottis, valleculae, and piriform sinuses. He or she also may be able to view the aryepiglottic folds, posterior epiglottis, and vocal cords. Although an indirect laryngoscopy is the simplest and least expensive way to examine the larynx, it does require a great deal of skill on the part of the physician. Moreover, this technique may be impossible to perform on a patient who has a strong gag reflex, and it cannot be used on small children.

Direct Laryngoscopy

Codes 31515 through 31571 are used to identify a direct laryngoscopy. This range of codes identifies the performance of procedures such as biopsy, removal of a lesion, arytenoidectomy, and removal of a foreign body. Laryngoscopes that are commonly used include Kleinsasser, Jako, Dedo, Jackson, Lindholm, Nagashima, Holinger, and Benjamin. During this complex procedure, the physician looks directly at the larynx. The patient is usually placed under general anesthesia to avoid the difficulties associated with the gag reflex. A microscope also may be used during the procedure to magnify the image of the larynx. Because the code assignment will be affected, the coding professional should review the operative report carefully for any mention of a microscope or for terms such as "microlaryngoscopy." It is inappropriate to use code 69990, Use of operating microscope, in addition to any laryngoscopy code identified as being done with an operating microscope.

Flexible Fiberoptic Laryngoscopy

Codes 31575 through 31578 are used for a laryngoscopy performed with flexible fiberoptic equipment. After administration of a topical anesthesia and vasoconstrictor, the instrument is passed through the nasal cavity. This type of laryngoscope provides a more comfortable approach to visualizing the larynx, the pharynx, and the nasal cavity.

Code 31579 identifies a laryngoscopy with stroboscopy. A strobe light provides a very bright light in short flashes. Because of the flashing produced by the stroboscopy, the physician is better able to examine moving vocal cords.

The following questions should be answered before assigning codes for laryngoscopies:

- *What was the purpose of the laryngoscopy?*
- *Which type of laryngoscope was used: direct, indirect, or flexible fiberoptic?*
- *Was stroboscopy used?*

In cases during which an operating microscope was used, the combination code should be assigned and not code 69990.

Exercise 4.25 Respiratory System—Laryngoscopy

Unless otherwise noted, all answers can be found in appendix D of this book. Answers to selected exercises are located in the Instructor's Guide and available only to faculty of educational programs.

Assign appropriate CPT code(s) for the following procedures and indicate the index entries that were used to identify the codes. Assign only CPT surgical codes (no E/M codes) and append any applicable modifiers.

1. Direct laryngoscopy with stripping of vocal cords

   Code(s): ______________________________

   Index entries: ______________________________

   ____

2. Flexible fiberoptic laryngoscopy performed for removal of a dime lodged in the patient's larynx

   Code(s): ______________________________

   Index entries: ______________________________

   ____

3. Indirect laryngoscopy with biopsy

   Code(s): ______________________________

   Index entries: ______________________________

   ____

4. Using an operating microscope, the surgeon performs a laryngoscopy with excision of a polyp

   Code(s): ______________________________

   Index entries: ______________________________

   ____

Exercise 4.26 Respiratory System

Unless otherwise noted, all answers can be found in appendix D of this book. Answers to selected exercises are located in the Instructor's Guide and available only to faculty of educational programs.

Operative Report

Preoperative Diagnosis: Laryngeal lesion

Postoperative Diagnosis: Same

Operation: Direct laryngoscopy and biopsy of vocal cord lesion using an operating microscope

The patient was placed on the OR table in the supine position, induced under general anesthesia, and intubated. The Dedo laryngoscope was introduced into the oral cavity, slipped under the tip of the epiglottis, and suspended from the Lewy suspension apparatus. The lesion involved the entire left vocal cord and extended through the ventricle to the false vocal cord and into the anterior commissure area. It also slightly involved the anterior portion of the right vocal cord. In addition, some subglottic extension was present. A biopsy was taken and sent out for frozen section. The laryngoscope was then removed and the procedure terminated. The patient tolerated the procedure well and left the room in good condition.

Assign appropriate CPT code(s) for the preceding procedure and indicate the index entries that were used to identify the code(s). Assign only CPT surgical codes (no E/M codes) and append any applicable modifiers.

1. Code(s): ______________________________

   Index entries: ______________________________

   ____

Bronchoscopy

A bronchoscope is an instrument that can be inserted into either the nose or the mouth and passed through the trachea, past the larynx, and into the bronchial tubes. Indications for this procedure include hemoptysis, a persistent cough that is unresponsive to medication, shortness of breath, an acute upper airway obstruction, or an abnormal chest x-ray or infection.

A physician may elect to use a flexible or rigid bronchoscope. The rigid scope, also referred to as an open-tube bronchoscope, is inserted through the mouth and most often is used to remove foreign objects or to secure a larger-than-normal biopsy sample. The more commonly performed flexible bronchoscopy consists of a flexible tube with many small glass fibers that allow the transmission of light. Codes in the 31622 through 31656 range are used to identify a variety of procedures using either type of bronchoscope.

The note at the beginning of this section advises coding professionals that a surgical bronchoscopy includes a diagnostic bronchoscopy. It is important to note that codes 31622–31646 include fluoroscopic guidance, if performed. Fluoroscopic equipment serves as an image intensifier and is frequently used during bronchoscopies. It is incorrect to use an additional code to identify fluoroscopy.

Frequently, the purpose of the bronchoscopy is to obtain tissue to allow the physician to make an accurate diagnosis. Specimens may be collected in several ways. Cell washings may be obtained by introducing saline solution into the airways, which then is removed and sent to the laboratory for cytological examination. Code 31622 identifies a bronchoscopy *with* or *without* cell washings.

Brushings of tissue is another method of specimen collection. One advantage to this method is that brushings allow the diagnosis to be made on the basis of tissue that could not be obtained normally with biopsy forceps. Either a fixed brush or a protected specimen brush (PSB) may be introduced through the bronchoscope. A PSB is a brush contained in a double catheter. A wax plug at the top prevents contamination of the specimen by upper airway flora. Code 31623 is assigned when a bronchoscopy is performed to collect specimen(s) with either a fixed brush or a PSB.

Code 31624 identifies a bronchoscopy with bronchial alveolar lavage (BAL). This procedure is performed to collect cells from peripheral lung tissue. During a BAL, sterile saline is instilled into the airway in aliquots of 20 mL up to 50 mL. The saline is suctioned out and sent for cytological examination.

CPT provides two codes for placement of fiducial markers during a bronchoscopic procedure. Code 31626 describes a stand-alone code for placement of fiducial markers, which help mark the position of a tumor, especially providing guidance to locate lesions in the distal regions of the lung. Code 31627 (computer assisted image-guided navigation) is an add-on code for the fiducial marker placement.

Code 32997 is assigned for total lung lavage (unilateral).

When a lesion can be visualized with the bronchoscope, the physician may elect to use forceps to obtain a sample of tissue. This procedure allows a more precise sample of tissue to be obtained for pathological diagnosis. Code 31625 is used to identify a bronchoscopy with bronchial or endobronchial biopsy, single or multiple sites.

When the diagnosis of a lung disease requires a sample of lung tissue, a transbronchial lung biopsy may be performed. During the bronchoscopy, forceps are used to puncture the bronchus and take samples of the lung tissue. This procedure is less invasive than an open-lung biopsy and thus carries less risk of morbidity. Code 31628 is assigned to identify a bronchoscopy with a transbronchial lung biopsy of a single lobe. To report transbronchial lung biopsies performed in additional lobes, assign add-on code 31632.

The following questions should be answered before assigning a code for a bronchoscopy:

- *Why was the bronchoscopy performed?*
- *Was a diagnostic bronchoscopy performed in conjunction with a surgical bronchoscopy?* If so, only the code for the surgical procedure should be assigned.
- *Was the procedure one of the bronchoscopies described by a code from the series 31622 through 31646?* If so, a separate code to identify fluoroscopy should not be assigned because fluoroscopic guidance is considered part of the procedures identified by that series of codes.

Lung Procedures

The codes associated with removal of the lung or a portion of the lung (32440–32540) refer to surgical procedures such as resection of segment, pneumonectomy, or wedge resection. Note the following definitions that differentiate between the procedures:

- Pneumonectomy—removal of entire lung
- Lobectomy—removal of one lobe of the lung; removal of two lobes is called bilobectomy
- Wedge resection—removal of small, wedge-shaped portion of the lung
- Segmental resection—removal of a large portion of the lung lobe (larger than a wedge resection)

Figure 4.10 illustrates the following lung procedures: wedge resection, lobectomy, and pneumonectomy.

Figure 4.10. Lung procedures

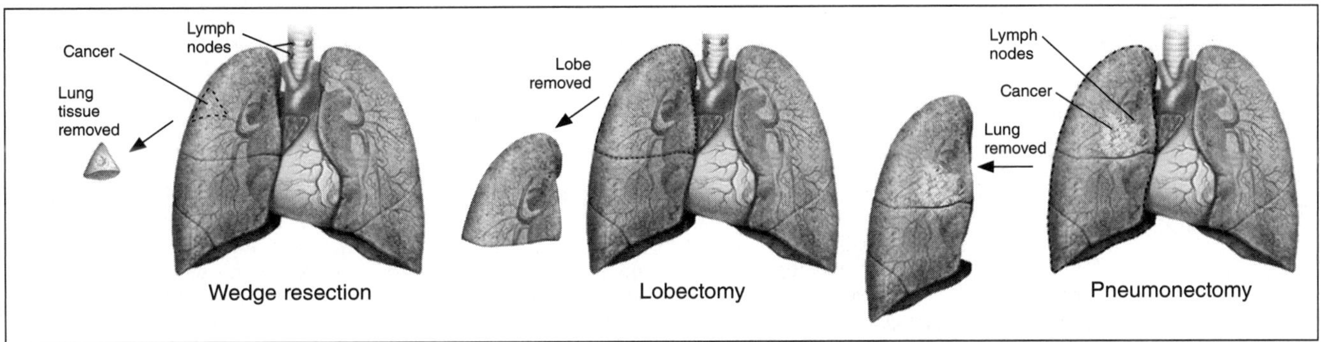

Exercise 4.27 Respiratory System—Bronchoscopy

Unless otherwise noted, all answers can be found in appendix D of this book. Answers to selected exercises are located in the Instructor's Guide and available only to faculty of educational programs.

Assign appropriate CPT code(s) for the following procedures and indicate the index entries that were used to identify the codes. Assign only CPT surgical codes (no E/M codes) and append any applicable modifiers.

1. Bronchoscopy with transbronchial biopsy of lung

   Code(s): ______________________________

   Index entries: ______________________________

   ____

2. Bronchoscopy with laser destruction of a lesion of the bronchus

   Code(s): ______________________________

   Index entries: ______________________________

   ____

3. Flexible bronchoscopy with cell washings, brushings, and biopsy

   Code(s): ______________________________

   Index entries: ______________________________

   ____

Exercise 4.28 Respiratory System

Unless otherwise noted, all answers can be found in appendix D of this book. Answers to selected exercises are located in the Instructor's Guide and available only to faculty of educational programs.

Operative Report

Preoperative Diagnosis:	Persistent cough, dyspnea
Postoperative Diagnosis:	Probable bronchitis
Procedure:	Bronchoscopy
Medications:	Versed 13 mg given just prior to and during the procedure; topical aerosolized lidocaine and atropine 0.4 mg IM and aerosolized albuterol 2.5 mg

The left nares was cannulated. The posterior nasopharynx was normal. The vocal cords, although with exogenous tissue consistent with obesity, were normal and normally apposed. The main carina was normal as was the trachea itself. The left lower lobe anatomy was a variant of normal with two main subsegments, each having three sub-subsegments in the left upper lobe. Very slight erythema is seen in the medial aspect of the left upper lobe subsegment. Brushings were obtained from this area.

The right inside anatomy was entirely normal. No endobronchial lesions were seen throughout.

Pathology

Gross Description:	Received are two prepared slides
Microscopic Description:	The bronchial brushing slides demonstrate benign bronchial epithelial cells and macrophages. The background contains mucus with minimal inflammation. There is no atypia or malignancy.
Diagnosis:	Lung, left upper lobe, bronchial brushings. Negative for malignant cells.

Assign appropriate CPT code(s) for the preceding procedure and indicate the index entries that were used to identify the code(s). Assign only CPT surgical codes (no E/M codes) and append any applicable modifiers.

1. Code(s): ______________________________

   Index entries: ______________________________

   ____

Exercise 4.29 Respiratory System Review

Unless otherwise noted, all answers can be found in appendix D of this book. Answers to selected exercises are located in the Instructor's Guide and available only to faculty of educational programs.

Assign appropriate CPT code(s) for the following procedures and indicate the index entries that were used to identify the codes. Assign only CPT surgical codes (no E/M codes) and append any applicable modifiers.

1. Thoracoscopy with wedge resection of lung that contains a cancerous tumor

   Code(s): ______________________________

   Index entries: ______________________________

   ____

2. Scalpel excision of polyp from inside the nose, performed in the physician's office

   Code(s): ______________________________

   Index entries: ______________________________

   ____

Exercise 4.29 (Continued)

3. Flexible bronchoscopy with bronchial biopsies

   Code(s): ____________________

   Index entries: ____________________

   ____

4. Removal of pebble from child's nasal passage, performed in the physician's office

   Code(s): ____________________

   Index entries: ____________________

   ____

5. Nasal endoscopy with polypectomy

   Code(s): ____________________

   Index entries: ____________________

   ____

Note: Answers to exercises 6 through 10 do not appear in appendix D of this text. They are located in the Instructor's Guide and available to faculty of educational programs.

6. Patient treated in the emergency department for severe epistaxis; physician performs extensive anterior packing, bilateral

   Code(s): ____________________

   Index entries: ____________________

   ____

7. Direct laryngoscopy for removal of lesion

   Code(s): ____________________

   Index entries: ____________________

   ____

8. Puncture aspiration of lung

   Code(s): ____________________

   Index entries: ____________________

   ____

9. Flexible fiberoptic laryngoscopy with biopsy of tissue

   Code(s): ____________________

   Index entries: ____________________

   ____

10. Partial excision of inferior turbinate

    Code(s): ____________________

    Index entries: ____________________

    ____

Cardiovascular System

The cardiovascular subsection includes surgical procedures involving the heart and pericardium, arteries, and veins. (Figure 4.11 illustrates the heart, veins, and arteries.) The codes are categorized first by body part involved and then by procedure performed, such as insertion of pacemaker, coronary artery bypass, embolectomy, and venipuncture. Assignment of codes for many of the cardiac procedures requires advanced knowledge and skill. The reference section of this book provides a list of recommended resources for coding cardiac procedures.

Vascular Injection Procedures

Careful review of the note at the beginning of this subsection will help the coding professional select the appropriate codes.

Intra-Arterial/Intra-Aortic Injections

Selective arterial catheterizations require that the catheter be removed, manipulated, or guided into a part of the arterial system other than the aorta or the vessel punctured. Nonselective arterial catheterizations involve placement of a catheter or needle directly into an artery, or a needle is negotiated only into the thoracic or abdominal aorta from any approach.

Intravenous Injections

Selective venous catheterizations include catheter placement in those veins that rise directly from the vena cava or the vein punctured directly (primary branches) and any subsequent (secondary) branches of the primary venous branches. Nonselective venous catheterizations involve direct puncture of peripheral veins and the vena cavae; or placement of the catheter in the inferior or superior vena cava by any route.

Pacemaker or Pacing Cardioverter-Defibrillator

Cardiac pacemakers are devices that send a small current through a lead (wire) to stimulate the heartbeat. There are two components to a pacemaker: generator (battery) and, attached to the generator, one or two leads. A pacemaker is usually implanted under local anesthesia and sedation. A small incision is made under the collarbone, and the generator is placed under the skin in a pocket created above the muscle. The lead or leads are passed to the heart via a vein and placed in the right atrium and/or right ventricle. Pacemakers may be either single chamber (either atrium or ventricle) or dual chamber (both atrium and ventricle).

An implantable cardioverter defibrillator (ICD) is a device that monitors heart rhythms and delivers shocks if dangerous rhythms are detected.

The CPT coding process involves reviewing documentation (that is, operative reports, physician notes, pathology reports, radiology reports) and applying it to the CPT code selection(s). In this subsection, some of the key documentation elements, or questions, include:

- *Was the electrode inserted into the atrium, ventricle, or both?*
- *Did the procedure involve inserting, replacing, or repositioning the device?*
- *Did the surgeon use the epicardial or transvenous approach?*

Pacemakers, pacing cardioverters, and defibrillator systems are classified with codes from the series 33202 through 33249. Guidelines in this section should be reviewed for descriptions of what comprises the various kinds of pacemaker and defibrillator systems.

Figure 4.12 illustrates a pacemaker insertion.

Figure 4.11. The heart and the veins and arteries that branch from it

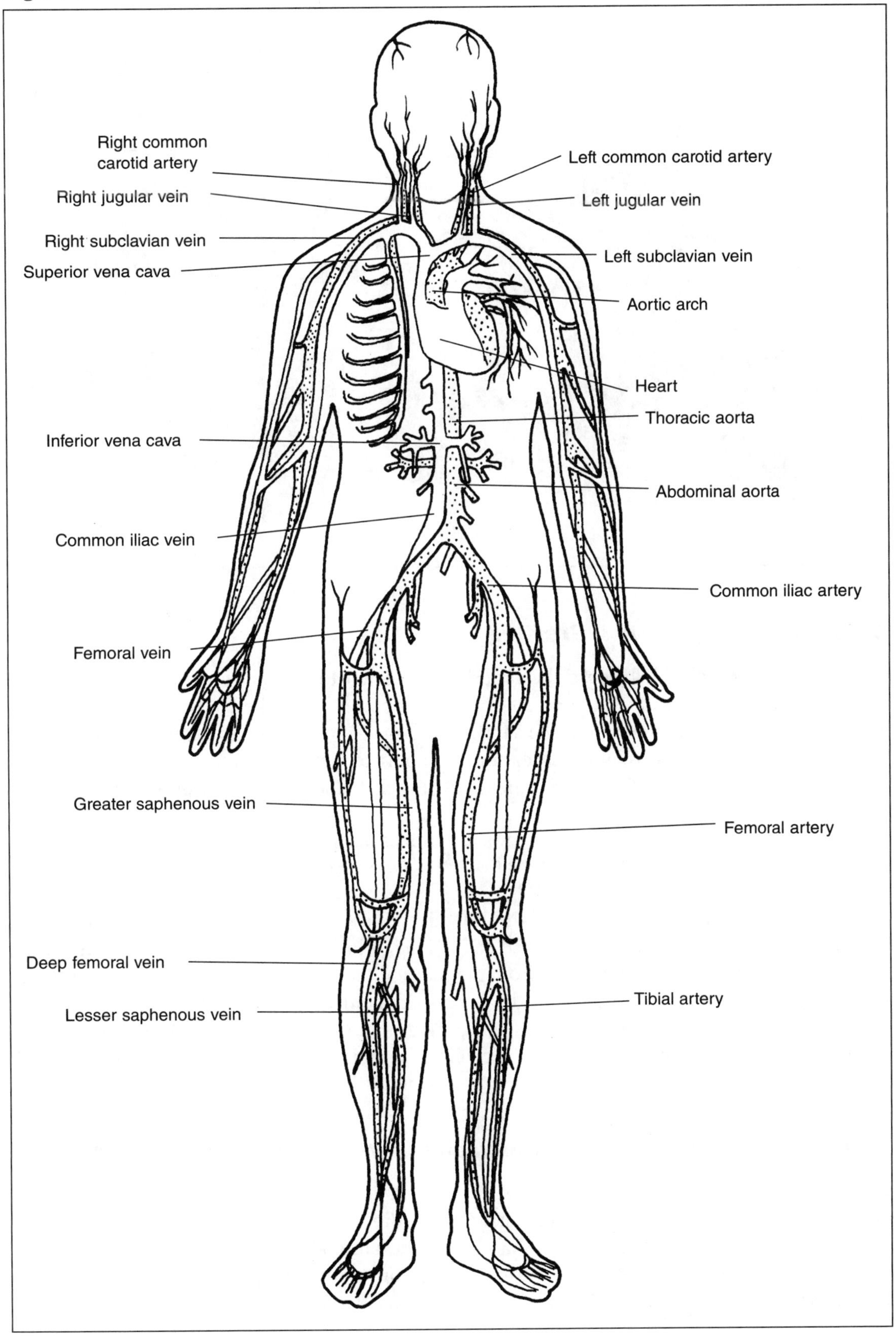

Figure 4.12. Pacemaker insertion

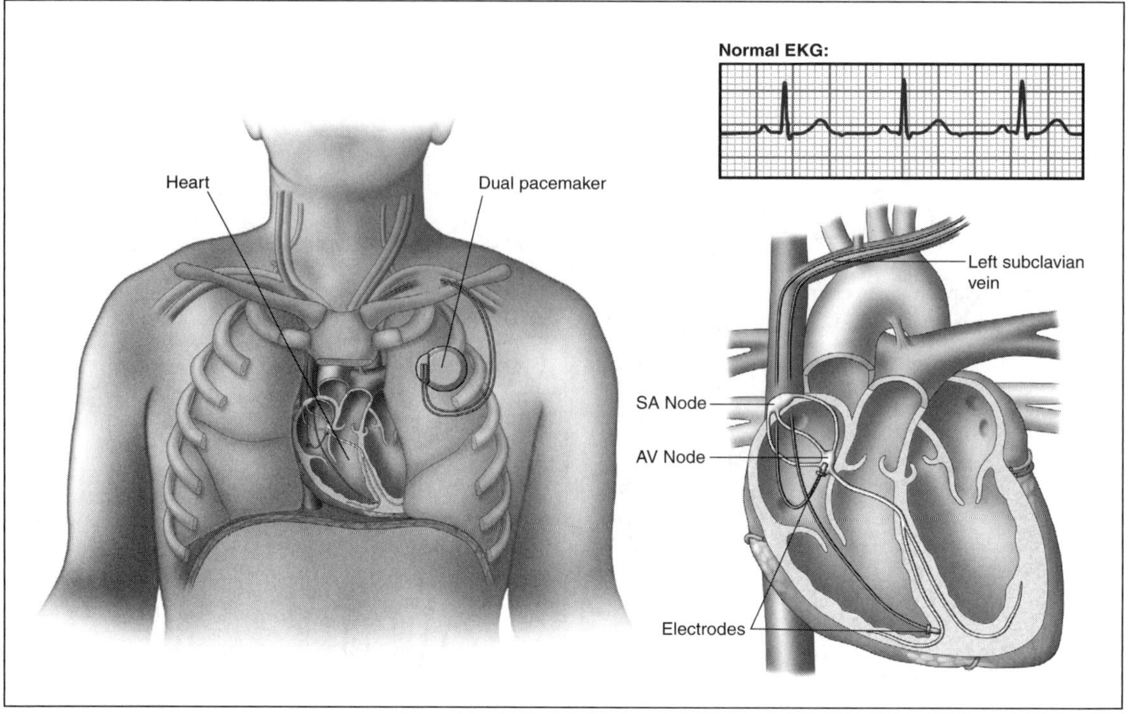

Coronary Artery Bypass Grafting

Codes 33510 through 33548 describe procedures related to coronary artery bypass grafting (CABG). The first series of codes (33510–33516) is reported when the CABG uses only venous grafts, such as those obtained from the saphenous vein. To code this procedure accurately, the coding professional must review the operative report to determine the number of coronary venous grafts that were performed. Figure 4.13 illustrates the coronary arteries and stenosis.

> **Example:** CABG of two coronary arteries using saphenous vein grafts.
> The code reported is 33511.

The second series of codes (33517–33530) describes a CABG that uses both arterial and venous grafts. As already mentioned, the saphenous vein usually provides the venous grafts and the arterial graft is usually created from the internal mammary artery. To fully code arterial-venous bypass grafting, two codes must be assigned: one from the 33517 through 33523 series to identify the number of venous grafts performed, and one from the 33533 through 33536 series to identify the number of arterial grafts. Careful review of the operative report is required to determine the type and number of grafts performed.

Interventional Radiology Procedures for Cardiovascular Conditions

Coding interventional radiology procedures for cardiovascular conditions requires a thorough understanding of coding guidelines and anatomy. Coding professionals often refer to anatomic diagrams of the vascular families to assist with accurate coding assignment. Appendix L of the CPT book provides a reference list for the vascular families. The Society of Interventional Radiology publishes a book titled *The Interventional Radiology Coding Users' Guide,* and

Figure 4.13. Coronary arteries with stenosis

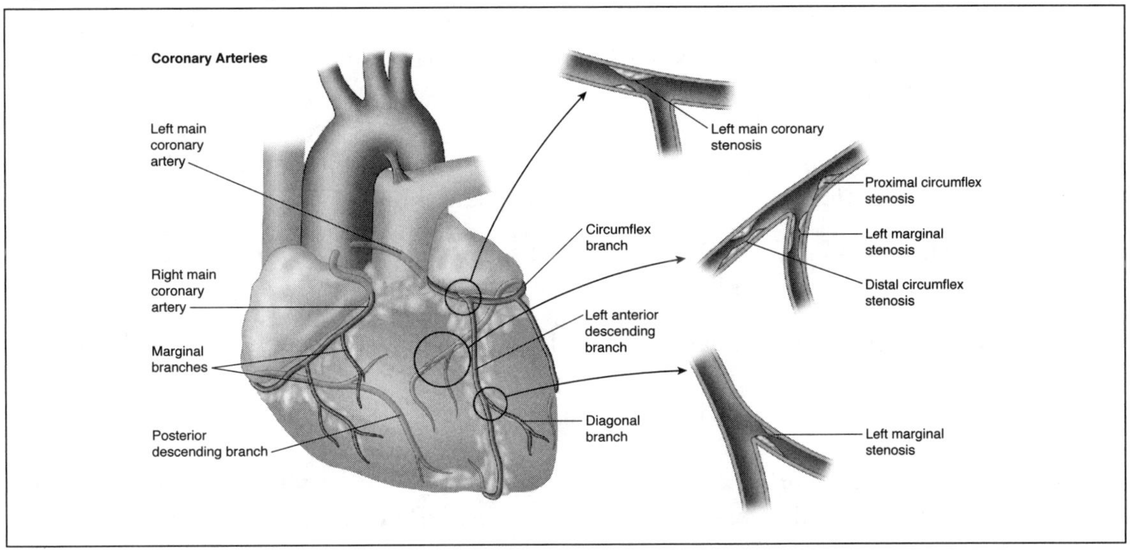

AHIMA has offered several audio seminars that concentrate on CPT coding in this area. The purpose of this lesson is to provide an overview of coding guidelines. In order to be proficient at interventional radiology coding, more advanced study and practice are necessary.

Angiography

Most interventional angiography procedures have two components: a surgical component (involving, for example, injection of contrast solutions, implantation of devices, and removal of strictures with angioplasty balloons), and an imaging (radiology) component, which includes supervision and interpretation (S&I) of images.

Codes for diagnostic radiology are in the 70000 series of the CPT codebook. Most interventional radiology procedures require at least two codes. Hospitals generally bill for both of the above-mentioned components, and radiologists bill for both components (provided they performed both components).

Coding guidelines state that codes must be assigned for both the catheter placement (surgical component) and the imaging procedure (S&I component). There is not always a one-to-one correlation between the number of surgical codes and the number of S&I codes. Several anatomic areas may be imaged from the same catheter placement; therefore, the number of S&I codes may exceed the number of surgical component codes.

CPT coding decisions for angiography are based on whether the physician performed a selective or nonselective catheter placement. Nonselective catheter placement is one in which the vascular catheter is left in the vessel it punctured and not advanced any further; or it is advanced into the aorta and not beyond. Examples of nonselective catheter placement CPT codes are as follows:

- 36120, Introduction of needle or intracatheter; retrograde brachial artery
- 36140, Introduction of needle or intracatheter, extremity artery
- 36147, Introduction of needle or intracatheter, arteriovenous shunt

Selective catheter placement is moved beyond the vessel punctured or beyond the aorta.

Review of the coding descriptions for selective catheter placement (36215–36248) reveals a reference to "order," such as first order, second order, and so on. It is important to emphasize the need to review anatomic diagrams/definitions and reference materials before attempting to code interventional radiology cases.

- CPT codes 36215 through 36218 are assigned for catheter placement in first-, second-, or third-order arteries (thoracic or brachiocephalic).
- CPT codes 36245 through 36248 are used for first-, second-, or third-order placement in abdominal, pelvic, and lower extremity arteries.
- Only two codes represent catheter placement on the venous side: 36011 and 36012.

The vascular family is divided into two parts:

- *Arterial vascular family:* A group of arteries fed by a primary branch of the aorta or a primary branch of the vessel punctured (that is, left common iliac artery, innominate artery, right renal artery)
- *Venous vascular family:* A group of veins that flows into a primary branch of the vena cava or a primary branch of the vessel punctured (that is, left iliac vein, right renal vein, left brachiocephalic vein)

Coding guidelines instruct coding professionals to assign a code to the highest-order catheter placement within a vascular family. Each vascular family that is catheterized is coded separately. A code for nonselective catheter placement should not be assigned in addition to a selective catheter placement code unless there are multiple accesses (punctures).

Example: A catheter is inserted in the femoral artery and passed into the aorta, into the brachiocephalic artery, and then further into the right common carotid artery.

The brachiocephalic is a first-order vessel and the right common carotid artery is a second-order vessel within the same vascular family. A code (36216) would be assigned for the second order only.

S&I codes are used to describe the imaging component of the procedure. S&I codes are assigned based on the vessels that are imaged, not the vessels that are catheterized.

Example: A catheter is inserted into the femoral artery and advanced into the right common carotid (second-order) and contrast injected, with imaging of the cervical and cerebral portions of the carotid circulation.

The correct coding assignment for this case would be 36216 for catheter placement; and 75665 (cerebral) and 75676 (cervical) imaging.

Arteriovenous Fistulas and Grafts

Creating an arteriovenous (AV) fistula is the most desirable method for hemodialysis access because AV fistulas are less likely to clot or become infected than other methods, and they last longer. See illustration in Figure 4.14. This procedure requires the surgeon to connect the artery to the vein. This abnormal connection between these two vessels causes more blood to flow from the artery directly to the vein under high arterial pressure. Eventually, the vein grows stronger and becomes thick-walled. This thick-walled vein becomes an ideal target to place the dialysis needles.

The CPT coding decision is based on whether the fistula was created by vein transposition or direct anastomosis. Codes for vein transposition are assigned according to the vein used:

- 36818 Upper arm (cephalic or brachiocephalic)
- 36819 Upper arm basilic vein
- 36820 Forearm vein (radio-cephalic)

The direct anastomosis method (36821) involves attaching an artery and a vein directly.

Figure 4.14. AV fistula

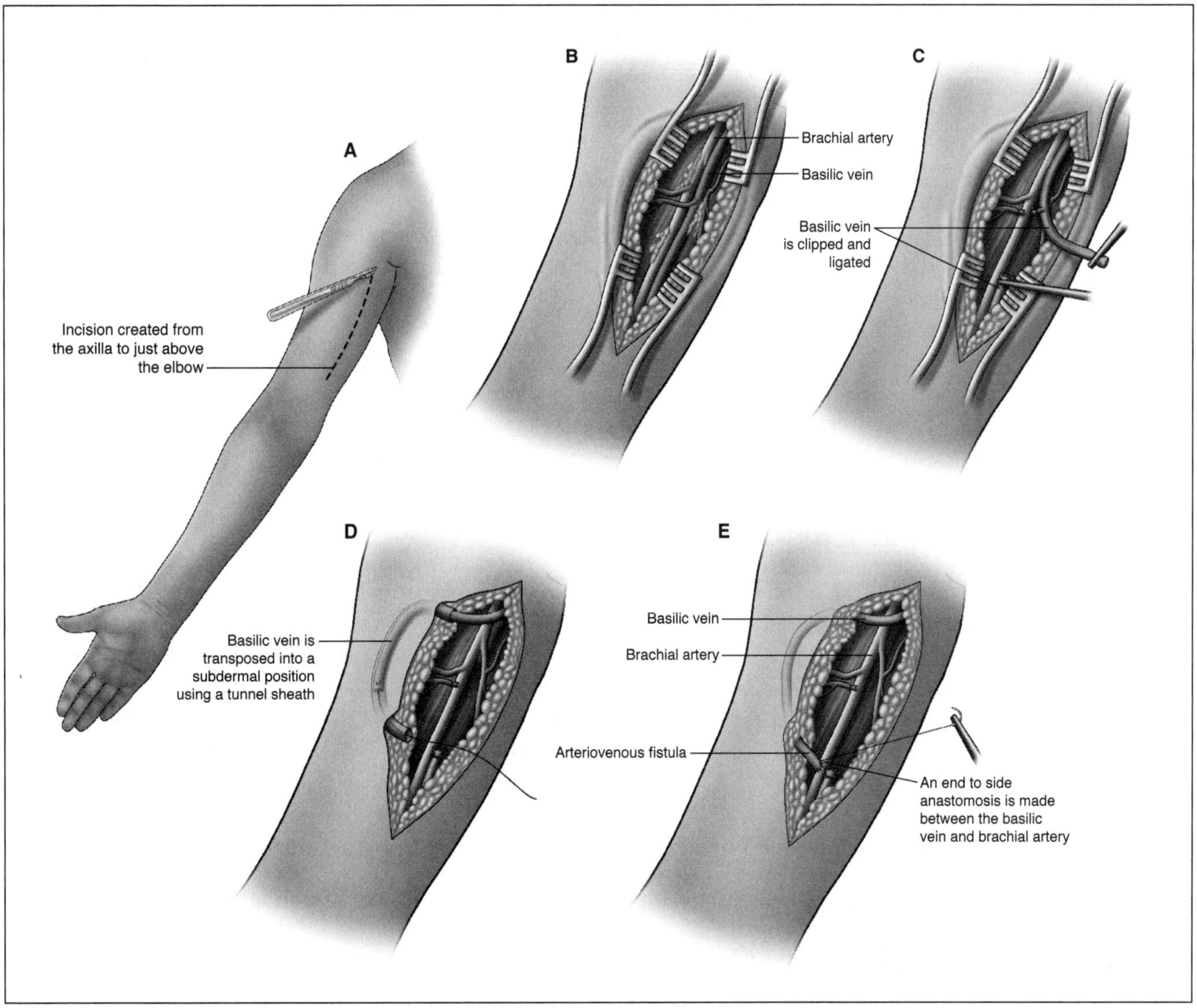

If an AV fistula is not possible because the patient's veins are too small or too far apart or there is not enough time to perform the procedure, the surgeon may elect to perform an AV graft (36825–36830) that connects the artery to the vein. AV fistulas require weeks or months to mature, but AV grafts require less time. A major disadvantage of AV grafts is that they often produce blood clots or become infected.

Complications of AV Fistulas and Grafts

Common complications of AV fistulas and grafts include clotting, obstruction, and narrowing of the access. Several CPT codes are provided for the procedures necessary to correct these complications.

There are several methods of treatment for stenosis, including angioplasty, stent placement, and thrombectomy. Thrombectomies can be performed with or without a revision of the graft, and CPT provides several codes to describe the various procedures:

- Thrombectomy, open, without revision (36831)
- Revision, open, without thrombectomy (36832)
- Revision, open, with thrombectomy (36833)

Percutaneous thrombectomy of a graft is coded with 36870, which includes all the work required to restore flow to the access. For this procedure, the thrombus may be removed pharmaceutically (that is, urokinase) or mechanically (AngioJet, small Fogarty-type balloons).

In addition to code 36870, additional procedures may be reported to identify the punctures of the graft. Two punctures are usually performed (both arterial and venous); each would be reported with CPT codes 36147 and 36148.

Because venous anastomotic stenosis is a common complication among hemodialysis patients, balloon angioplasties are often performed to restore patency and flow. CPT code 35476 (Transluminal balloon angioplasty, percutaneous; venous) is provided for this procedure.

Central Venous Access Procedures

Many therapies can be administered via various types of catheters and ports. CPT coding for catheterization procedures depends on the type and use of the catheter. In general, CPT codes are assigned only to catheters inserted by physicians and not to catheters inserted by nursing personnel.

Central venous access devices (CVADs) are small, flexible tubes placed in large veins for patients who require frequent access to their bloodstream. CVADs are commonly used for the following purposes:

- Administration of medications (for example, antibiotics, chemotherapy)
- Administration of fluids and nutritional compounds (for example, hyperalimentation)
- Transfusion of blood products
- Multiple blood draws for diagnostic testing

Before assigning codes in this section, coding professionals should read the note that precedes code 36555. First, CPT classifies venous access procedures into five distinct categories:

- Insertion
- Repair
- Partial replacement
- Complete replacement
- Removal

The definitions for each of these categories are provided in CPT. Additional information must be abstracted from the health record to determine the correct code. As an example, refer to the decision tree in Figure 4.15 for insertion of a central venous access device. From this decision tree, documentation is needed to determine the following:

- Catheter inserted centrally or peripherally
- Tunneled or nontunneled
- Pump or port
- Age of patient

A centrally inserted catheter is placed in the jugular, subclavian, or femoral vein, or inferior vena cava. The peripherally inserted catheters are typically placed in the arm and advanced forward into the larger subclavian vein. The documentation may state that the catheter was inserted into the basilic or cephalic vein. For the centrally inserted catheter, the coding professional must check the documentation to determine whether the catheter was tunneled. Tunneled catheters have an entrance site at a distance from where they enter the vascular system. These are "tunneled" through the skin and subcutaneous tissue to a great vein. Typically, these catheters are for long-term use. The code descriptions also differentiate between the use of subcutaneous ports or pumps. Implanted ports are placed below the skin, and blood is drawn or medication is delivered by placing a tiny needle through the overlying skin into the port or reservoir. See illustration in Figure 4.16. Pumps use a computerized mechanism for infusion.

Unlike centrally inserted central catheters, peripherally inserted central catheter (PICC) lines are not inserted into the central vein.

CPT provides codes for the removal of CVADs (36589–36590) but instructs the coding professional not to assign the codes for nontunneled central venous catheters. Removal of some catheters does not warrant a separate code when no surgical procedure is required and the catheter is simply pulled out.

Endovascular Revascularization (Open or Percutaneous, Transcatheter)

Peripheral artery disease (PAD) occurs when plaque builds up in the arteries and reduces the blood flow to the patient's limbs. With the advent of catheter-based interventional therapies, endovascular physicians have become able to improve arterial perfusion in lower extremities through the use of balloon angioplasty and stenting. A series of CPT codes (37220–37235) identify these procedures and are differentiated by site (for example, iliac, femoral/popliteal, or tibial/peroneal vascular territory) and by additional procedures performed during the revascularization procedure (stent placement, atherectomy).

Figure 4.15. Central venous access procedures coding decision tree

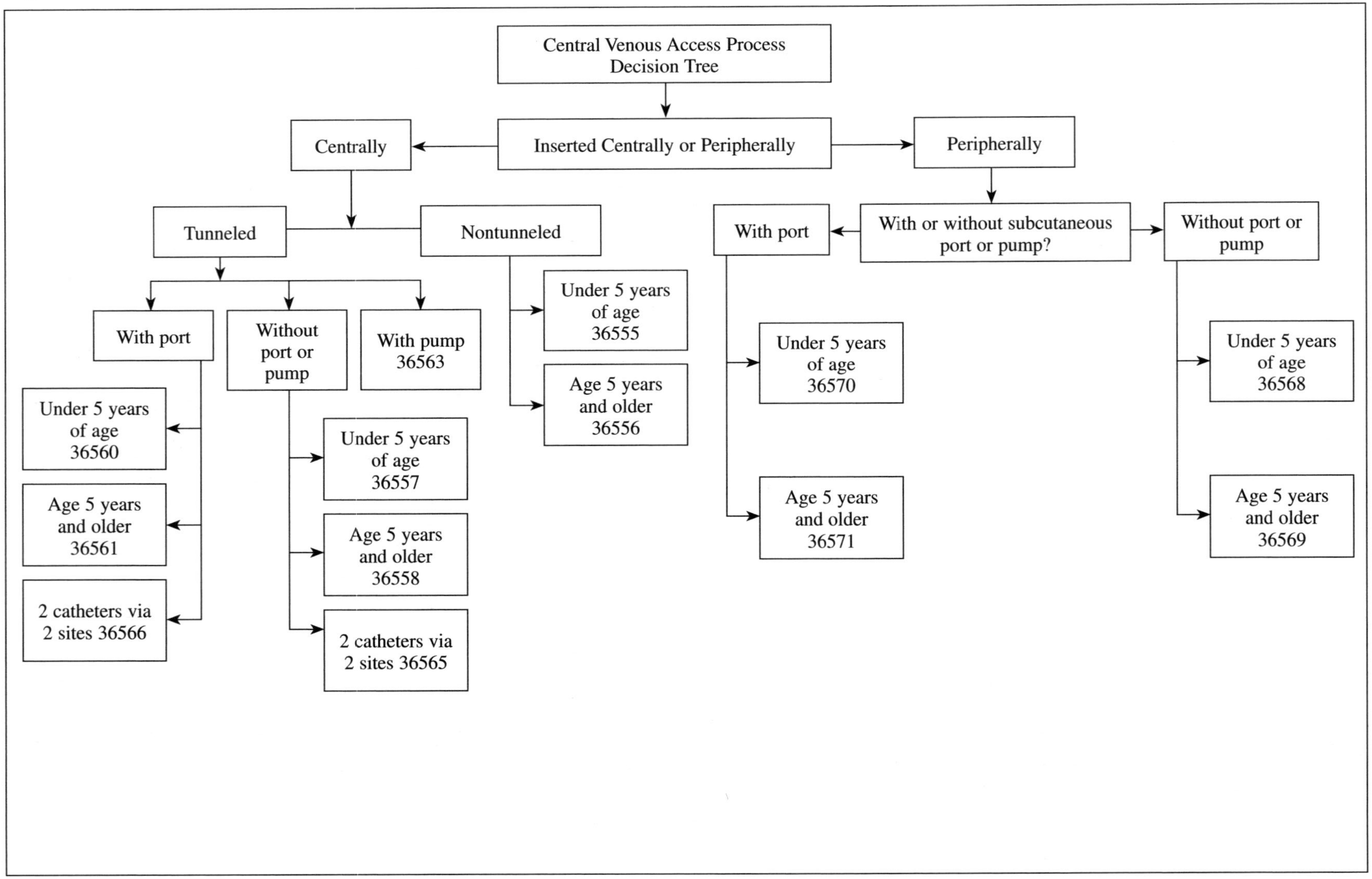

Figure 4.16. Port-a-cath

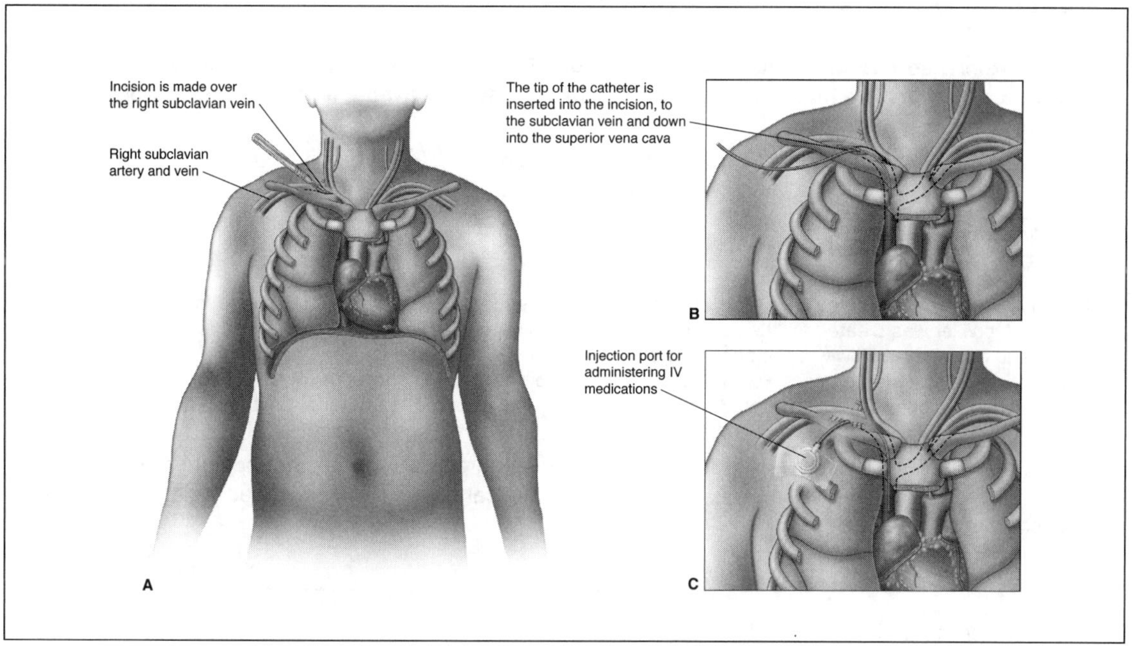

Coding professionals should carefully read the Notes section preceding code 37220 that provides guidance for selection of the appropriate code. General guidelines include:

- Only one code from the family should be reported for each lower extremity vessel.
- When coding for treatment of multiple territories in the same leg, one primary lower extremity code is used for each territory treated.
- Use add-on codes for additional vessels treated within the territory.
- If a lesion extends across the margins of one vessel vascular territory to another but can be opened with a single therapy, the single code should be reported.

Ligation, Division, and Stripping of Saphenous Veins

Varicose veins are gnarled, enlarged veins. Any vein may become varicose, but the veins most commonly affected are those in the saphenous veins of the leg. Surgical treatment includes ligation, division, and stripping of the affected veins (37718–37735). In ligation and division, the surgeon ties off all tributaries and then ties off the saphenous vein below the tributaries and divides it between the ligatures. Stripping involves completely removing the vein from the leg. Removing the veins does not affect the circulation of blood in the leg. Veins deeper in the leg take care of the larger volumes of blood.

Code 37700 is used for ligation and division of the long saphenous vein without stripping.

Exercise 4.30 Cardiovascular System

Unless otherwise noted, all answers can be found in appendix D of this book. Answers to selected exercises are located in the Instructor's Guide and available only to faculty of educational programs.

Operative Report

Preoperative Diagnosis:	Heart block
Postoperative Diagnosis:	Same
Procedure:	Insertion of permanent pacemaker

The patient was premedicated before arriving at the OR. The patient was prepared and draped in the usual manner. A pocket was created for the pacemaker. The bipolar electrode was introduced, taken to the pulmonary artery, and brought out slowly to the apex of the right ventricle. Measurements were taken, and the position was excellent. The electrode was anchored to the fascia over the sleeve and connected to the pacemaker battery. The wound was closed. Patient tolerated the procedure well and returned to the outpatient recovery area.

Assign appropriate CPT code(s) for the preceding procedure and indicate the index entries that were used to identify the code(s). Assign only CPT surgical codes (no E/M codes) and append any applicable modifiers.

1. Code(s): ____________________

   Index entries: ____________________

   ____

Exercise 4.31 Cardiovascular System

Unless otherwise noted, all answers can be found in appendix D of this book. Answers to selected exercises are located in the Instructor's Guide and available only to faculty of educational programs.

Operative Report

Preoperative Diagnosis:	Breast carcinoma
Postoperative Diagnosis:	Same
Operation:	Removal of venous access port

The patient is a 44-year-old woman who had a left, modified radical mastectomy in 2010. In August she had a Port-a-cath placed in the right side. However, it has caused an extreme amount of discomfort, so she has requested that it be removed.

The patient was taken to the OR and placed in a supine position on the table. She was then prepared and draped in the usual sterile fashion. The area was anesthetized with 1% Carbocaine. An incision was made over the venous access device and carried down to the place of the device. After freeing it up and cutting the retention sutures, the venous access device was removed. Hemostasis was obtained with cautery and pressure. The wound was then closed in layers and a dressing applied. The patient tolerated the procedure well and was returned to the surgicenter in stable condition.

Assign appropriate CPT code(s) for the preceding procedure and indicate the index entries that were used to identify the code(s). Assign only CPT surgical codes (no E/M codes) and append any applicable modifiers.

1. Code(s): ____________________

   Index entries: ____________________

   ____

Exercise 4.32 Cardiovascular System

Unless otherwise noted, all answers can be found in appendix D of this book. Answers to selected exercises are located in the Instructor's Guide and available only to faculty of educational programs.

Operative Report

Preoperative Diagnosis:	Renal failure
Postoperative Diagnosis:	Same
Operation:	Insertion of subclavian venous catheter

With this elderly patient in the head-down position, the entire left upper chest was prepared with Betadine scrub and draped in the usual sterile fashion. Then, 1% lidocaine was used for local anesthetic. A percutaneously subclavian venous catheter was inserted without difficulty and secured at the skin level with 3-0 nylon, and a sterile dressing was applied. The catheter also was irrigated with heparin solution. Patient tolerated the procedure well. Will follow with a chest x-ray.

Assign appropriate CPT code(s) for the preceding procedure and indicate the index entries that were used to identify the code(s). Assign only CPT surgical codes (no E/M codes) and append any applicable modifiers.

1. Code(s): ______________________

   Index entries: ______________________

   ____

Exercise 4.33 Cardiovascular System Review

Unless otherwise noted, all answers can be found in appendix D of this book. Answers to selected exercises are located in the Instructor's Guide and available only to faculty of educational programs.

Assign appropriate CPT code(s) for the following procedures and indicate the index entries that were used to identify the codes. Assign only CPT surgical codes (no E/M codes) and append any applicable modifiers.

1. Relocation of pacemaker pocket

   Code(s): ______________________

   Index entries: ______________________

   ____

2. Open revision of AV fistula with thrombectomy, patient receiving hemodialysis

   Code(s): ______________________

   Index entries: ______________________

   ____

3. Repair of patent ductus arteriosus by division (18-year-old patient)

   Code(s): ______________________

   Index entries: ______________________

   ____

(Continued on next page)

Exercise 4.33 (Continued)

4. Catheter placement into the brachiocephalic artery (first-order)

   Code(s): ______________________________

   Index entries: ______________________________

   ____

5. Complete replacement of tunneled centrally inserted central venous catheter with subcutaneous port; replacement performed through original access site (45-year-old patient)

   Code(s): ______________________________

   Index entries: ______________________________

   ____

Note: Answers to exercises 6 through 10 do not appear in appendix D of this text. They are located in the Instructor's Guide and available to faculty of educational programs.

6. Percutaneous thrombectomy of AV graft

   Code(s): ______________________________

   Index entries: ______________________________

   ____

7. Percutaneous transluminal femoropopliteal artery balloon angioplasty

   Code(s): ______________________________

   Index entries: ______________________________

   ____

8. Valvuloplasty of tricuspid valve with ring insertion

   Code(s): ______________________________

   Index entries: ______________________________

   ____

9. Insertion of dual chamber pacing cardioverter-defibrillator (transvenous electrode)

   Code(s): ______________________________

   Index entries: ______________________________

   ____

10. Long saphenous vein stripping from saphenofemoral junction to below knee of left and right legs

    Code(s): ______________________________

    Index entries: ______________________________

    ____

Digestive System

The digestive subsection includes surgical procedures involving the lips, mouth and tongue, palate and uvula, salivary glands and ducts, pharynx, adenoids and tonsils, esophagus, stomach, intestines, appendix, rectum, biliary tract, abdomen, peritoneum, and omentum. The codes are categorized first by body part involved and then by procedure, such as herniorrhaphy, esophagotomy, ileostomy, cholecystectomy, and hemorrhoidectomy. Figure 4.17 shows the digestive system.

Endoscopies

In general, gastrointestinal endoscopies are categorized by body part involved, type or purpose of endoscopy (diagnostic or surgical), and specific procedure performed, such as biopsy, ablation of tumor or polyp, and removal of foreign body. The endoscopy should always be coded as far as the scope was passed.

An esophagoscopy allows the physician to visualize the esophagus. Codes in the range 43200 through 43232 are used to report esophagoscopies.

Esophagogastroduodenoscopy

An upper gastrointestinal endoscopy, also known as an esophagogastroduodenoscopy (EGD), or upper endoscopy, involves the visual examination of the esophagus, stomach and upper duodenum, and/or jejunum. Indications for these procedures include gastrointestinal (GI) bleeding, ulceration, or inflammation; abdominal pain; narrowing of the esophagus; and suspected tumors or polyps. EGDs are reported with codes in the range 43234 through 43259. In the CPT format for upper GI endoscopic procedures, the diagnostic procedure is listed first, followed by a list of descriptions for surgical treatment. According to CPT endoscopy guidelines, it is appropriate to list multiple codes if the documentation supports the coding selection.

Example: During the EGD, the surgeon performs a snare removal of a polyp and removal of a foreign body.

Correct coding assignment: 43251 Snare removal
43247 Removal of foreign body

Note: For physician services, Modifier 51 (multiple procedures) would be appended to the second code to indicate that multiple procedures were performed by the same physician at the same session.

The code ranges can be located in the alphabetic index under Endoscopy, Gastrointestinal, Upper. There is no alphabetic entry for the abbreviation EGD. See figure 4.18 for illustration of upper GI endoscopy.

Esophageal Dilation

CPT provides for two methods for esophageal dilation:

- *Endoscopic:* Through the endoscopy the physician selects a dilating balloon (43220) or plastic dilators over the guiding wire to stretch the esophagus (43226).
- *Manipulation* (not with scope): Surgeon sprays the throat with local anesthesia to pass a tapered dilating instrument through the mouth and guide it into the esophagus (43450–43460). Hurst and Maloney are common types of bougies used for esophageal dilation (43450).

Figure 4.17. The digestive system

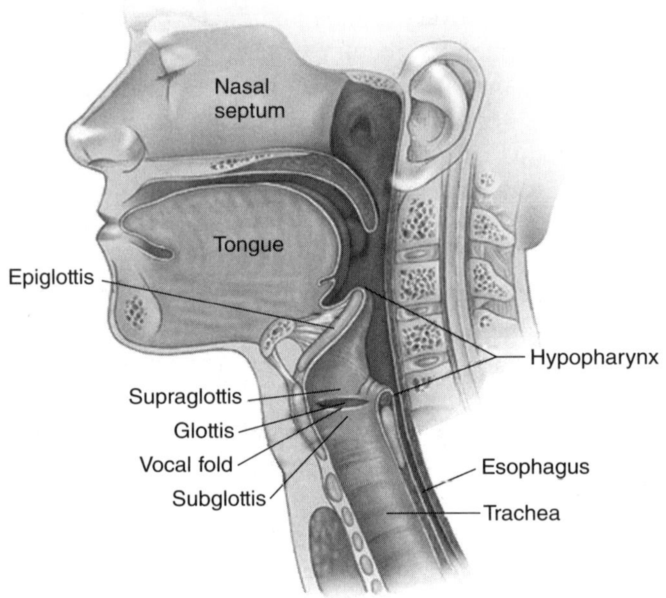

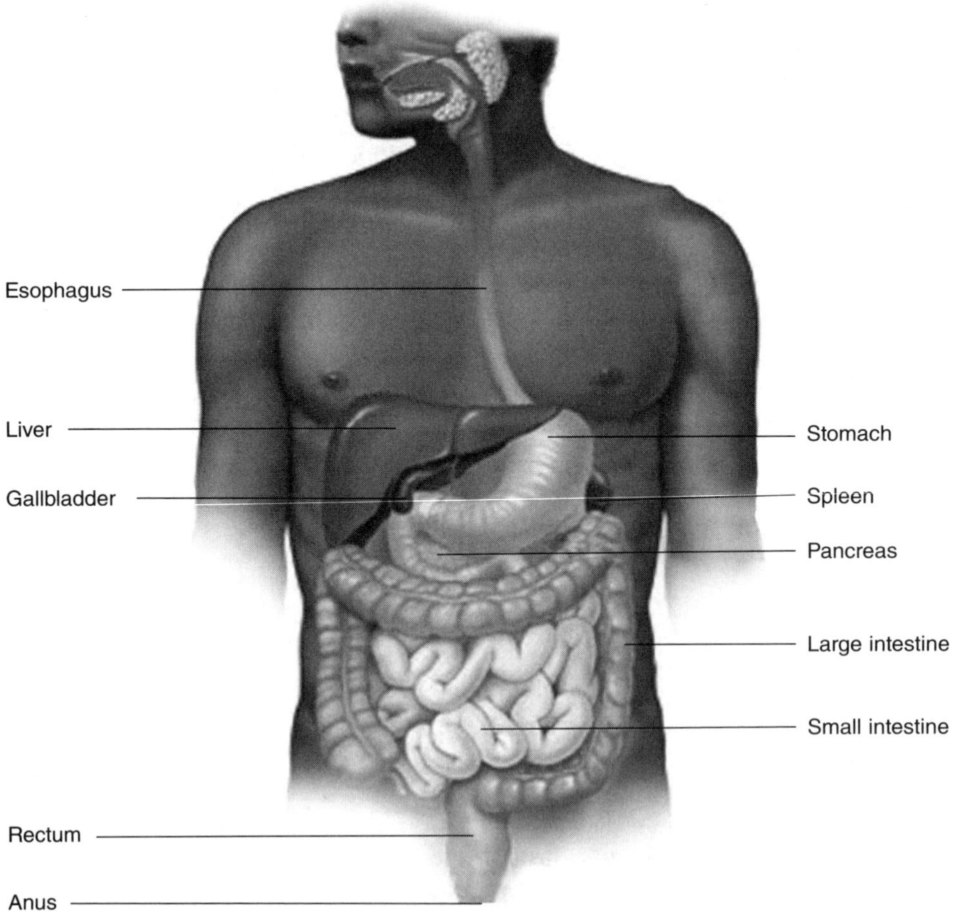

Figure 4.18. Upper GI endoscopy

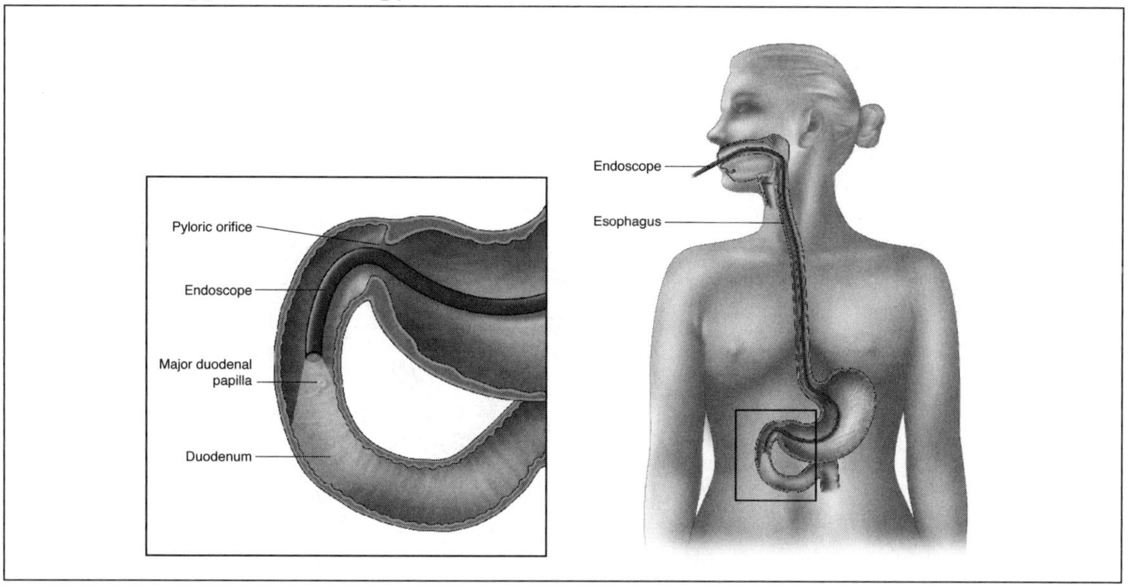

Endoscopic Retrograde Cholangiopancreatography

Endoscopic retrograde cholangiopancreatography (ERCP) is a procedure that is used to diagnose conditions in the liver, gallbladder, bile ducts, and pancreas. The liver is a large organ that, among other things, makes a liquid called bile that helps with digestion. The gallbladder is a small, pear-shaped organ that stores bile until it is needed for digestion. The bile ducts are tubes that carry bile from the liver to the gallbladder and small intestine. These ducts are sometimes called the biliary tree. The pancreas is a large gland that produces chemicals that help with digestion, and hormones such as insulin.

ERCP combines the use of x-rays and an endoscope. Through the endoscope, the physician can see the inside of the stomach and duodenum and inject dyes into the ducts in the biliary tree and pancreas so they can be seen on x-rays. The CPT code range for these procedures is 43260–43272. Note the reference to alert the coding professional to the radiological supervision and interpretation codes.

Lower Gastrointestinal System Endoscopies

Lower GI endoscopies can be classified by the area of the intestine examined, as follows:

- *Proctosigmoidoscopy:* An examination limited to the rectum and sigmoid colon (45300–45327)
- *Sigmoidoscopy:* An examination of the entire rectum and sigmoid colon that may also include a portion of the descending colon (45330–45345) (The depth visualization is typically 35 or 60 cm, depending on the instrument used.)
- *Colonoscopy:* An examination of the entire colon, from the rectum to the cecum, that may include the terminal ileum (45355–45392). In general, a colonoscopy examines the colon to a level of 60 cm or higher. Figure 4.19 illustrates the anatomy of the colon with colonoscopy procedure.

Indications for performing lower GI procedures include an abnormal barium enema, lower GI bleeding, iron deficiency anemia of unknown etiology, and diarrhea. They may also be performed for follow-up examination after removal of a neoplastic growth.

Figure 4.19. Anatomy of colon with colonoscopy procedure

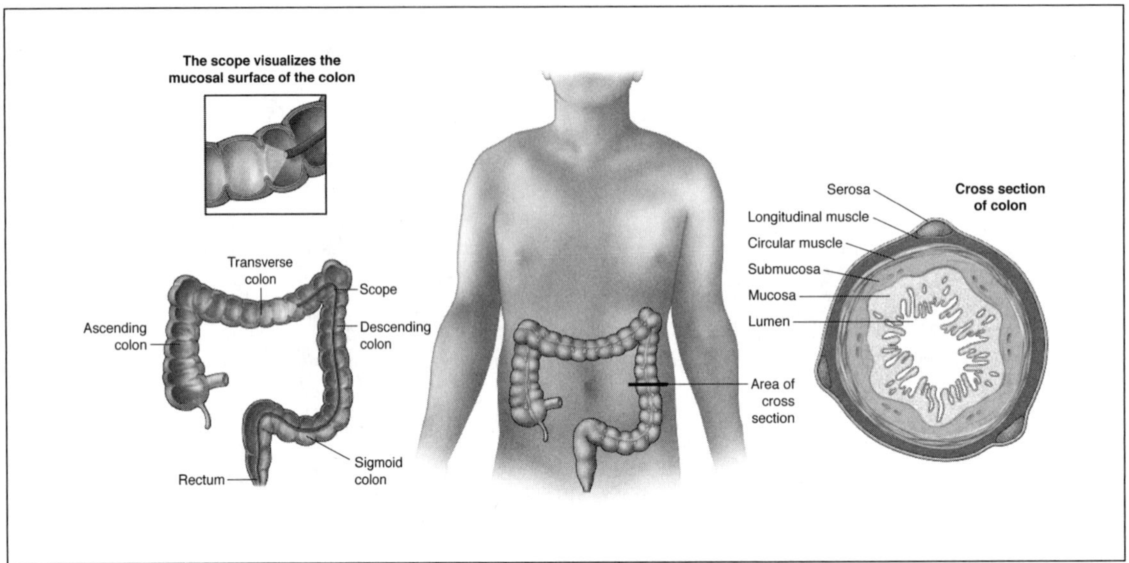

When coding a colonoscopy, the coding professional must review the operative report to determine the approach: through an existing colostomy (44388–44397), a colotomy (45355), or the rectum (45378–45392).

The following questions should be answered before a code is assigned for an endoscopy:

- *Was the diagnostic endoscopy performed as part of a surgical endoscopy?* If so, only the surgical endoscopy should be coded.
- *What was the purpose of the endoscopy?*
- *What approach was used to insert the endoscope?*

Removal of Tumors or Polyps

Because the endoscopic removal of a tumor or polyp can be accomplished with several techniques, the coding professional should review the documentation carefully before selecting a code. It is also possible for a physician to use different techniques to remove polyps during the same operative episode. In this case, an appropriate CPT code would be assigned to identify each technique.

One technique uses hot biopsy forceps or bipolar cautery. Hot biopsy forceps resemble tweezers connected to an electrosurgical unit. Grasping the polyp, the physician pulls the growth away from the wall of the structure. A portion of the neoplasm may be removed for pathological analysis. The remaining portion is destroyed with the electrocoagulation current. Bipolar cautery also uses electrical current to remove the polyp.

The snare technique uses a wire loop that is slipped over the polyp or tumor. The stalk is then cauterized and the growth removed.

Finally, the physician may elect to use a neodymium yttrium aluminum garnet (Nd:YAG) laser to remove the lesion. When a laser is used during the endoscopy, the coding professional should assign the code for the endoscopy that states "with ablation of tumor(s), polyp(s), or other lesion(s) not amenable to removal by hot biopsy forceps, bipolar cautery, or snare technique."

Incomplete Colonoscopies

Causes of incomplete colonoscopies include poor bowel preparation, obstructing disease, or patient's inability to tolerate the procedure. There are several guidelines for coding discontinued procedures for physicians and hospitals. (See chapter 3 of this book and appendix A of the CPT codebook for descriptions of modifiers 52, 53, 73, and 74.)

Coding Incomplete Colonoscopies for Physician Services

In the case of a colonoscopy, the procedure may be attempted, but circumstances may prevent the entire colon from being visualized (for instance, poor preparation). In this case, ***CPT guidelines*** instruct the coding professional to assign the colonoscopy code with modifier 53 for discontinued procedure (for physician services). See the note following the definition of Endoscopies (before code 45300).

Screening Colonoscopy (Medicare Guidelines)

Medicare covers colorectal cancer screening test/procedures for the early detection of colorectal cancer when coverage conditions are met. Among the screening procedures covered are screening colonoscopies:

- G0105 Colorectal cancer screening; colonoscopy on individual at high risk
- G0121 Colorectal screening; colonoscopy on individual not meeting criteria for high risk

These codes are to be assigned instead of 45378 (Diagnostic Colonoscopy) when there is no need for a therapeutic procedure (for example, polypectomy). Claims processing and payment of incomplete screening colonoscopies can be found in CMS Transmittal AB-03-114 (August 2003).

Modifier for Reporting of Colorectal Screening Tests (Coding Clinic for HCPCS 2011)

CMS created modifier PT, *Colorectal cancer screening test; converted to diagnostic test or other procedure,* for providers and practitioners to report the conversion of a screening colonoscopy or screening sigmoidoscopy to a diagnostic test or procedure provided on the same date and in the same encounter. In this instance modifier PT would be appended to the diagnostic procedure code that is reported instead of the HCPCS code for the screening colonoscopy or screening sigmoidoscopy. Additional details can be found in the transmittal R8640TN. Transmittals can be found on the CMS website.

Coding Incomplete Colonoscopies for Facility Services

For facility services coding of incomplete colonoscopies, CMS Transmittal 442 (January 2005) instructs the coding professional to append modifiers 73 (Discontinued Prior to Anesthesia) or 74 (Discontinued After Anesthesia) as appropriate.

Further clarification of use of modifiers 52, 73, and 74 can be found in the CMS Manual.

Biopsies and Lesion Removal

When performing a GI endoscopy, the physician may encounter one or many lesions. Biopsies of some or all lesions may be taken. Lesion removal may be performed after a biopsy or without a biopsy. Therefore, the following guidelines should be applied:

- When a biopsy of a lesion is taken and the remaining portion of the *same* lesion is excised during the same operative episode, assign a code for the excision only (*CPT Assistant,* February 1999).

- When one lesion is biopsied and a *different* lesion is excised, assign a code for the biopsy and a code for the excision. This rule is applicable unless the excision code narrative includes the phrase "with or without biopsy." In this case, only the excision code is assigned. It would be appropriate to append the biopsy code with modifier 59, Distinct Procedural Service.
- Biopsy codes use the terminology "with biopsy, single or multiple." These codes are to be used only once, regardless of the number of biopsies taken.

Exercise 4.34 Digestive System—Endoscopy

Unless otherwise noted, all answers can be found in appendix D of this book. Answers to selected exercises are located in the Instructor's Guide and available only to faculty of educational programs.

Assign appropriate CPT code(s) for the following procedures and indicate the index entries that were used to identify the codes. Assign only CPT surgical codes (no E/M codes) and append any applicable modifiers.

1. Esophagoscopy with biopsy of a small lesion in the esophagus and a snare removal of a polyp from another area of the esophagus

   Code(s): ______________________________

   Index entries: ______________________________

   ____

2. Proctosigmoidoscopy with biopsy of four separate lesions

   Code(s): ______________________________

   Index entries: ______________________________

   ____

3. EGD with laser removal of duodenal polyp

   Code(s): ______________________________

   Index entries: ______________________________

   ____

4. Endoscopic biopsy of a lesion of the transverse colon

   Code(s): ______________________________

   Index entries: ______________________________

   ____

5. ERCP with removal of bile duct stones

   Code(s): ______________________________

   Index entries: ______________________________

   ____

Exercise 4.35 Digestive System

Unless otherwise noted, all answers can be found in appendix D of this book. Answers to selected exercises are located in the Instructor's Guide and available only to faculty of educational programs.

Operative Note

Procedure: EGD with foreign body removal

Clinical Note: This patient is a 47-year-old man who experienced acute odynophagia after eating a meal consisting of fish. The patient felt a foreign body-like sensation in his proximal esophagus. He was evaluated with lateral cervical spine films and soft-tissue films without any evidence of perforation.

Findings: After obtaining informed consent, the patient underwent endoscopy. He was premedicated without any complication. Under direct visualization, an Olympus Q20 was introduced orally and the esophagus was intubated without any difficulty. The hypopharynx was carefully reviewed, and no abnormalities were noted. There were no foreign bodies and no lacerations to the hypopharynx. The proximal esophagus was normal. No active bleeding was noted. The endoscope was advanced farther into the esophagus, where careful review of the mucosa revealed no foreign bodies and no obstructions. However, the gastroesophageal junction did show a very small fish bone, which was removed without any complications. The endoscope was advanced into the stomach, where partially digested food was noted. The duodenum was normal. The endoscope was then removed. The patient tolerated the procedure well, and his postprocedural vital signs are stable.

Assign appropriate CPT code(s) for the preceding procedure and indicate the index entries that were used to identify the code(s). Assign only CPT surgical codes (no E/M codes) and append any applicable modifiers.

1. Code(s): ______________________________

   Index entries: ______________________________

   ____

Exercise 4.36 Digestive System

Unless otherwise noted, all answers can be found in appendix D of this book. Answers to selected exercises are located in the Instructor's Guide and available only to faculty of educational programs.

Operative Report

Procedure: Colonoscopy

Instrument Used: Olympus CF100L

Indications: The patient has a family history of carcinoma of the colon and colonic polyps.

The digital and anal examinations were normal. The colonoscope was inserted to the cecum. Preparation was good. Eight to 10 very sessile and diminutive polyps were identified, all but one located in the rectum. The other polyp was located in the proximal transverse colon. All were coagulated and removed with the hot biopsy forceps. No other mucosal lesions were identified.

Pathology Report

Results of Gross Examination:

1. The specimen labeled biopsy of polyp, transverse colon, consists of a pale tan, slightly firm tissue measuring 0.2 cm in greatest diameter; completely submitted.
2. The specimen labeled biopsy of polyp, rectum, consists of six pieces of slightly firm pinkish-tan tissue ranging from 0.2 to 0.3 cm in greatest diameter; completely submitted.

Results of Microscopic Examination:
No high-grade dysplasia or malignant change is seen in the colorectal polyps.

Pathological Diagnosis:

1. Biopsy of polyp, transverse colon: Hyperplastic polyp
2. Biopsy of polyp, rectum: Hyperplastic polyp

Assign appropriate CPT code(s) for the preceding procedure and indicate the index entries that were used to identify the code(s). Assign only CPT surgical codes (no E/M codes) and append any applicable modifiers.

1. Code(s): ______________________________

   Index entries: ______________________________

   ____

Exercise 4.37 Digestive System

Unless otherwise noted, all answers can be found in appendix D of this book. Answers to selected exercises are located in the Instructor's Guide and available only to faculty of educational programs.

Operative Report

Preoperative Diagnosis: Residual inflammatory changes

Postoperative Diagnosis: See below

Operation: Flexible fiberoptic sigmoidoscopy

The sigmoidoscope was inserted into the rectum and eventually advanced up to a level 60 cm from the anus. The mucosa throughout the colon and rectum were examined and appeared completely normal with no inflammation, ulceration, or exudate. There was no bleeding. I did not see any narrowed areas, polyps, or masses. I did see a few sigmoid diverticula.

With the exception of a few sigmoid diverticula, the examination up to a level of 60 cm from the anus was noted to be normal. The previous inflammatory changes have completely subsided.

Assign appropriate CPT code(s) for the preceding procedure and indicate the index entries that were used to identify the code(s). Assign only CPT surgical codes (no E/M codes) and append any applicable modifiers.

1. Code(s): ______________________________

   Index entries: ______________________________

   ____

Treatment of Hemorrhoids

There are a variety of CPT codes dedicated to the treatment of hemorrhoids. Hemorrhoids are swollen and inflamed veins in the anus and rectum. They may result from straining during bowel movements or the increased pressure on these veins during pregnancy. It is important to note that several codes in this section are not in numerical order. The symbol (#) identifies codes that are resequenced. Treatments are discussed in the following sections.

Incision of External Thrombosed Hemorrhoid (46083)

An incision is made over the thrombus, and the clot and diseased hemorrhoid plexus are removed in one piece.

Rubber Band Ligation (46221)

Hemorrhoidectomy, by simple ligature (without incision or excision), is a treatment for internal hemorrhoids that is sometimes referred to as "banding." The physician attaches tiny rubber bands to the base of hemorrhoids. With their circulation cut off, the hemorrhoids painlessly fall away after 7 to 10 days and are expelled with stool. The code is only assigned once per operative session regardless of how many hemorrhoids the physician bands at a time.

Destruction of Internal Hemorrhoid(s) by Thermal Energy (46930)

Methods for this procedure include cautery, radiofrequency, and infrared coagulation. Infrared coagulation involves a small probe with a light source that coagulates the veins above the hemorrhoid, causing it to shrink and recede.

Suture Ligation (46945–46946)

Suture ligation differs from hemorrhoidectomy by simple ligature in that the physician isolates the hemorrhoid and ties suture material to its base. For accurate code selection, documentation must support the number of columns/groups ligated.

Hemorrhoidectomy (46250–46262)

The surgical excision codes are differentiated by whether the hemorrhoids were internal, external, or both. In addition, codes are distinguished by the number of columns/groups (single vs. multiple).

Destruction by Cryosurgery (46999)

Coders are instructed to report an unlisted code of 46999 for destruction of hemorrhoids by cryosurgery.

Hernia Repairs

An abdominal hernia occurs when internal organs, such as the intestines, break through a hole or tear in the musculature of the abdominal wall. This protrusion produces a bulge that can be seen or felt. Symptoms include burning and pain with activity.

Codes 49491 through 49659 describe procedures related to hernia repair. To assign these codes accurately, the coding professional must be able to specify the type and/or site of the hernia, the history of the hernia, the age of the patient, and the clinical presentation of the hernia.

The following terms are used to describe the type and/or location of different hernias:

- *Inguinal hernia:* A common herniation of the inguinal canal in the groin area
- *Lumbar hernia:* A rare herniation in the lumbar region of the torso
- *Incisional hernia:* A herniation at the site of a previous surgical incision
- *Femoral hernia:* A common herniation in the femoral canal in the groin area

- *Epigastric hernia:* A herniation above the navel
- *Umbilical hernia:* A herniation at the navel
- *Spigelian hernia:* A herniation usually above the inferior epigastric vessel along the outer border of the rectus muscle

Some codes provide historical information specifying whether the hernia is an *initial* repair (first surgical repair of the hernia) or a *recurrent* repair (hernia has been surgically repaired previously). Other codes differentiate patients by age: any age, younger than 6 months, 6 months to younger than 5 years, or 5 years or older. Finally, a number of terms are used to describe the clinical presentation of hernias. These include:

- *Reducible:* The protruding organs can be returned to normal position by surgical (not medical) manipulation.
- *Sliding:* The colon or cecum is part of the hernia sac. (In some cases, the urinary bladder also may be involved.)
- *Incarcerated:* The hernia cannot be reduced without surgical intervention.
- *Strangulated:* The hernia is an incarcerated hernia in which the blood supply to the contained organ is reduced. A strangulated hernia presents a medical emergency.

The following example illustrates how the different variables describing hernias can be represented in a specific code assignment:

Example: 49550 Repair initial femoral hernia, any age; reducible
49553 incarcerated or strangulated

Traditional Hernia Repair (49491–49611)

A physician may perform one of three common types of repairs. The first type is the traditional or conventional repair. Under general anesthesia, the physician pushes the bulging tissue back into the abdominal cavity. The defect is closed by pulling together and stitching the surrounding muscles and ligaments. A recovery period of four to six weeks is usually needed.

Use of Mesh (49568)

The second type of herniorrhaphy uses mesh rather than stitches to repair the abdominal defect. Because stitches are not used, the patient experiences less postoperative pain. Commonly used meshes are Marlex and Prolene. When coding a mesh repair of an **incisional** or **ventral** hernia, code 49568, Implantation of mesh or other prosthesis for an open incisional or ventral hernia repair (or for closure of debridement for necrotizing soft tissue infection), must be assigned in addition to the repair code. The use of mesh with other hernia repairs is not coded.

Laparoscopic Hernia Repair (49650–49659)

The third type of hernia repair is performed by a laparoscope. A laparoscopic repair is commonly performed to repair bilateral and recurrent hernias. Less discomfort and faster recovery are the main advantages of this approach. As with other endoscopies, a surgical laparoscopy includes a diagnostic laparoscopy. See Figure 4.20 for a laparoscopic ventral hernia repair.

Paraesophageal Hiatal Hernia Repair (43332–43337)

A paraesophageal hernia occurs when part of the stomach pushes through the opening in the diaphragm. The repair codes in this section are differentiated by the surgical technique used (laparotomy, thoracotomy, and thoracoabdominal incision) and by whether the procedure involved implantation of mesh.

Figure 4.20. Laparoscopic ventral hernia repair

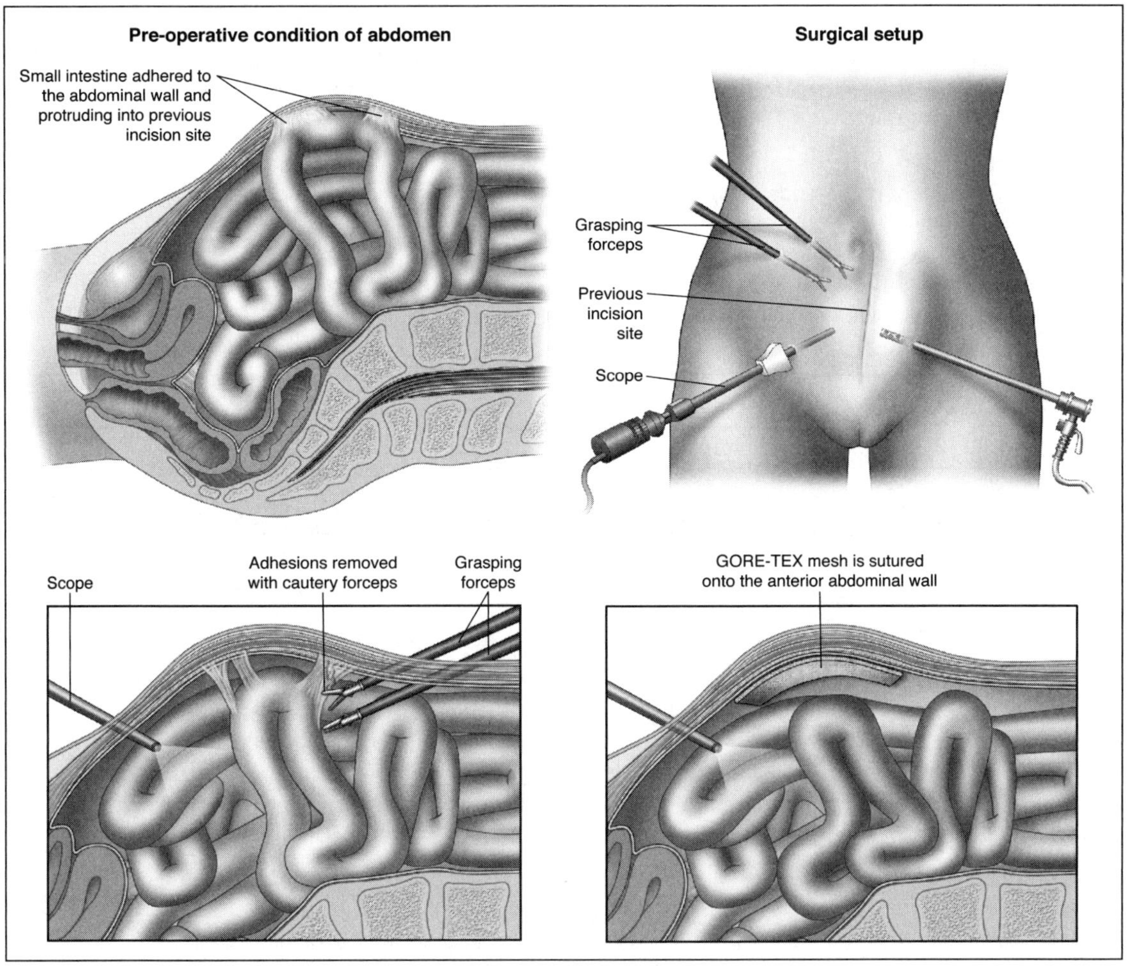

Other Laparoscopic Procedures of the Digestive System

Laparoscopic procedures are minimally invasive, requiring less recovery time than traditional open procedures.

Laparoscopy was long used by gynecologists for the diagnosis of diseases of the ovary and uterus. Technological improvements, such as use of video cameras, have permitted procedures on the smallest of structures, and the use of laparoscopy has been extended to surgical procedures involving the appendix, colon, and other areas of the body.

In earlier editions of CPT, laparoscopic procedures were consolidated into one section. Laparoscopic procedures currently have their own headings in the various surgical sections.

For example, note the following sampling of laparoscopic procedures in the digestive system:

- 43280 Laparoscopic fundoplasty
- 44970 Laparoscopic appendectomy
- 45400 Laparoscopic proctopexy

NOTE: The format of CPT provides for an "unlisted procedure" code in each of the Laparoscopic code ranges. Because of the advancements of surgical practice and technology, it is common for unlisted procedures to be assigned for new procedures.

Exercise 4.38 Digestive System—Hernia Repairs

Unless otherwise noted, all answers can be found in appendix D of this book. Answers to selected exercises are located in the Instructor's Guide and available only to faculty of educational programs.

Assign appropriate CPT code(s) for the following procedures and indicate the index entries that were used to identify the codes. Assign only CPT surgical codes (no E/M codes) and append any applicable modifiers.

1. Initial herniorrhaphy for repair of an inguinal hernia and a unilateral hydrocelectomy of the spermatic cord (4-year-old patient)

   Code(s): ______________________________

   Index entries: ______________________________

   ____

2. Right incarcerated initial incisional hernia repair with mesh (49-year-old patient)

   Code(s): ______________________________

   Index entries: ______________________________

   ____

3. Diagnosis: recurrent inguinal hernia; procedure: laparoscopic hernia repair

   Code(s): ______________________________

   Index entries: ______________________________

   ____

Note: Answers to exercises 4 through 6 do not appear in appendix D of this text. They are located in the Instructor's Guide and available to faculty of educational programs.

4. Recurrent incarcerated inguinal hernia repair with implantation of mesh (56-year-old patient)

   Code(s): ______________________________

   Index entries: ______________________________

   ____

5. Umbilical herniorrhaphy (35-year-old patient)

   Code(s): ______________________________

   Index entries: ______________________________

   ____

6. Laparoscopic repair of recurrent incisional hernia

   Code(s): ______________________________

   Index entries: ______________________________

   ____

Exercise 4.39 Digestive System

Unless otherwise noted, all answers can be found in appendix D of this book. Answers to selected exercises are located in the Instructor's Guide and available only to faculty of educational programs.

Operative Report

Preoperative Diagnosis:	Left inguinal hernia
Postoperative Diagnosis:	Same
Procedure:	Left initial inguinal hernia repair with mesh
Anesthesia:	General

The patient is a 23-year-old man who presented with several weeks' history of pain in his left groin associated with a bulge. Examination revealed that his left groin did indeed have a bulge and his right groin was normal. We discussed the procedure as well as the choice of anesthesia.

After preoperative evaluation and clearance, the patient was brought into the operating suite and placed in a comfortable supine position on the OR table. Monitoring equipment was attached, and general anesthesia was induced. His left groin was sterilely prepped and draped, and an inguinal incision made. This was carried down through the subcutaneous tissues until the external oblique fascia was reached. This was split in a direction parallel with its fibers, and the medial aspect of the opening included the external ring. The ileo-inguinal nerve was identified, and care was taken to retract this inferiorly out of the way. The cord structures were encircled and the cremasteric muscle fibers divided. At this point, we examined the floor of the inguinal canal, and the patient did appear to have a weakness here. We then explored the cord. There was no evidence of an indirect hernia. A piece of 3 × 5 mesh was obtained and trimmed to fit. It was placed down in the inguinal canal and tacked to the pubic tubercle. It was then run inferiorly along the pelvic shelving edge until lateral to the internal ring and tacked down superiorly using interrupted sutures of 0-Prolene. A single stitch was placed lateral to the cord to recreate the internal ring. Details of the mesh were tucked underneath the external oblique fascia. The cord and the nerve were allowed to drop back into the wound, and the wound was infiltrated with 30 cc of half percent Marcaine. The external oblique fascia was then closed with a running suture of 0-Vicryl. Subcutaneous tissues were approximated with interrupted sutures of 3-0 Vicryl. The skin was closed with a running subcuticular suture of 4-0 Vicryl. Benzoin and Steri-Strips and a dry sterile dressing were applied. All sponge, needle, and instrument counts were correct at the end of the procedure. The patient tolerated the procedure well and was taken to the recovery room in stable condition.

Assign appropriate CPT code(s) for the preceding procedure and indicate the index entries that were used to identify the code(s). Assign only CPT surgical codes (no E/M codes) and append any applicable modifiers.

1. Code(s): ______________________________

   Index entries: ______________________________

   ____

Exercise 4.40 Digestive System Review

Unless otherwise noted, all answers can be found in appendix D of this book. Answers to selected exercises are located in the Instructor's Guide and available only to faculty of educational programs.

Assign appropriate CPT code(s) for the following procedures and indicate the index entries that were used to identify the codes. Assign only CPT surgical codes (no E/M codes) and append any applicable modifiers.

1. Infrared coagulation of internal hemorrhoids

   Code(s): ____________________

   Index entries: ____________________

   ____

2. Laparoscopic gastric bypass and Roux-en-Y gastroenterostomy performed for obesity

   Code(s): ____________________

   Index entries: ____________________

   ____

3. EGD with balloon dilation of gastric outlet obstruction

   Code(s): ____________________

   Index entries: ____________________

   ____

4. Palatoplasty for cleft palate, soft

   Code(s): ____________________

   Index entries: ____________________

   ____

5. Colonoscopy with laser removal of lesions

   Code(s): ____________________

   Index entries: ____________________

   ____

Note: Answers to exercises 6 through 10 do not appear in appendix D of this text. They are located in the Instructor's Guide and available to faculty of educational programs.

6. Laparoscopic cholecystectomy with exploration of common duct

   Code(s): ____________________

   Index entries: ____________________

   ____

Exercise 4.40 (Continued)

7. Repair of recurrent, incarcerated inguinal hernia (34-year-old patient)

   Code(s): ______________________________

   Index entries: ______________________________

   ____

8. Laparoscopic aspiration of ovarian cyst

   Code(s): ______________________________

   Index entries: ______________________________

   ____

9. Anoscopy with removal of polyp via hot biopsy forceps

   Code(s): ______________________________

   Index entries: ______________________________

   ____

10. Removal of a chicken bone from pharynx

    Code(s): ______________________________

    Index entries: ______________________________

    ____

Urinary System

The urinary subsection includes surgical procedures involving the kidney, ureter, bladder, and urethra. These codes are categorized first by body part involved and then by procedure performed, such as cystourethroscopy, percutaneous renal biopsy, transurethral resection of the prostate, and urethroplasty. Figure 4.21 provides an illustration of the urinary system.

Urodynamics

Urodynamics is the investigation of the function of the lower urinary tract (the bladder and urethra) using physical measurements, such as urine pressure and flow rate, as well as clinical assessments. Codes 51725 through 51798 describe urodynamic procedures that may be reported separately or in combination when more than one procedure is performed. Modifier 51 should be reported when multiple procedures are performed (modifier 51 is for physician use only). These procedures are performed either by the physician or under his or her direction. The following services/supplies are considered part of the procedure and should not be reported separately: instruments, equipment, fluids, gases, probes, catheters, technicians' fees, medications, gloves, trays, tubing, and other sterile supplies.

Figure 4.21. The urinary system

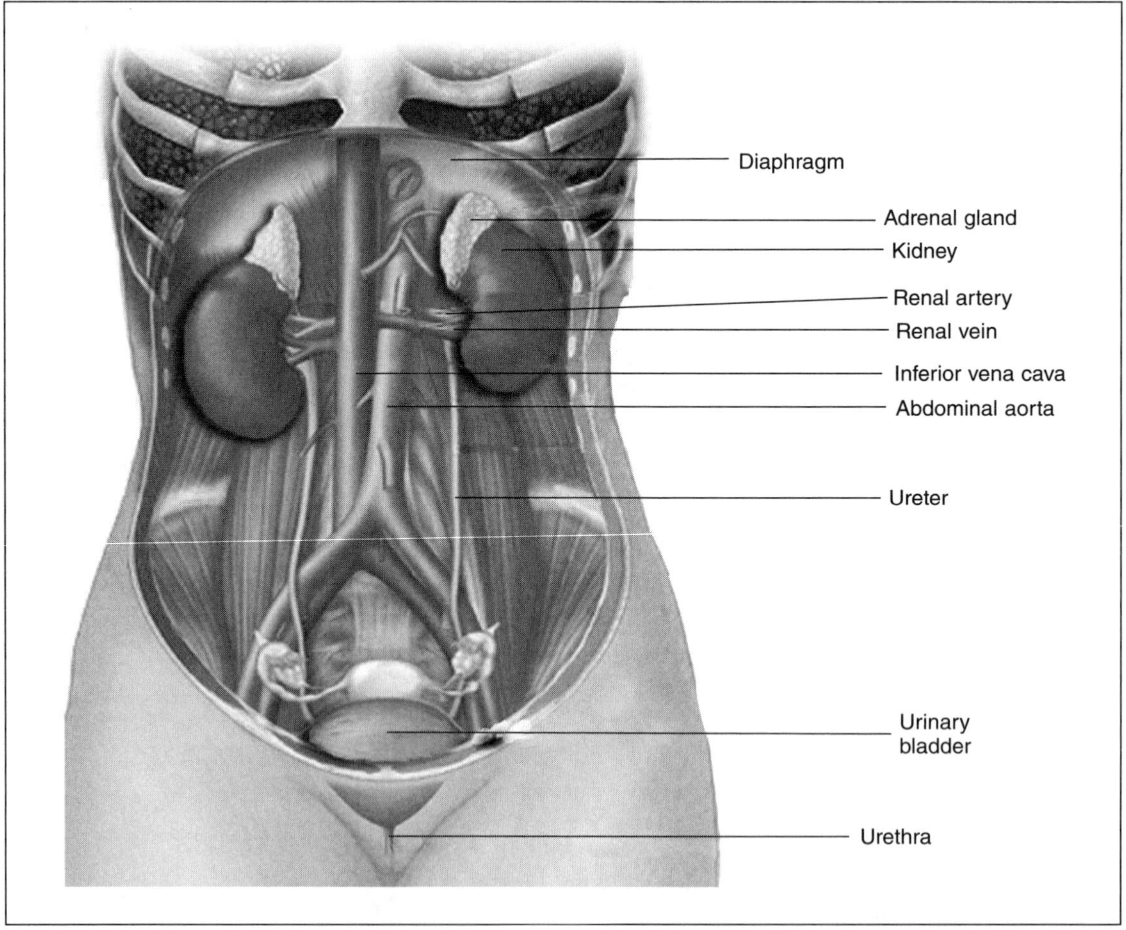

If the physician is providing only the professional component (that is, the supervision and interpretation), modifier 26 also should be reported for physician services.

The following definitions (Rogers 2004) describing the various urodynamic procedures will help the coding professional assign the appropriate CPT code:

- *Cystometrogram:* An examination performed to determine the capacity of the urinary bladder. A simple cystometrogram is the measurement of the bladder's capacity, sensation of filling, and intravesical pressure. A complex cystometrogram involves the measurement of the bladder's capacity, sensation of filling, and intravesical pressure using a rectal probe to distinguish between intra-abdominal pressure and bladder pressure.
- *Uroflowmetry:* An examination performed to determine the functional capacity of the urinary bladder. *Simple* uroflowmetry is the measurement of voiding time and peak flow. *Complex* uroflowmetry involves the measurement and recording of mean and peak flow and the time taken to reach peak flow during continuous urination.
- *Urethral pressure profile (UPP):* An examination that involves the recording of pressures along the urethra as a special catheter is slowly withdrawn.
- *Electromyography:* Studies performed to record muscle activity during voiding and to simultaneously record urine flow rate.

Genitourinary Endoscopies

In general, genitourinary endoscopies are categorized by body part involved—urethra, prostate, or ureter—and specific procedure performed, such as cystourethroscopy with biopsy of the bladder or urethra, transurethral incision of prostate, cystourethroscopy with ureteral meatotomy, and cystourethroscopy with insertion of indwelling ureteral stent. Cystourethroscopy, also known as cystoscopy, is an examination with a narrow, flexible tube-like instrument passed through the urethra to examine the bladder and urinary tract for structural abnormalities or obstructions, such as tumors or stones.

Many procedures are listed so that the main procedure can be identified without having to list all the minor related functions performed at the same time.

Example: Code 52647 describes laser coagulation of the prostate, including control of postoperative bleeding. The description indicates a complete procedure that includes vasectomy, meatotomy, cystourethroscopy, urethral calibration and dilatation, and internal urethrotomy. Minor procedures such as meatotomy, calibration, and so on are part of code 52647 and should not be reported separately.

Figure 4.22 illustrates a ureteral calculus with attempted ureteroscopy.

Figure 4.22. Ureteral calculus with attempted ureteroscopy

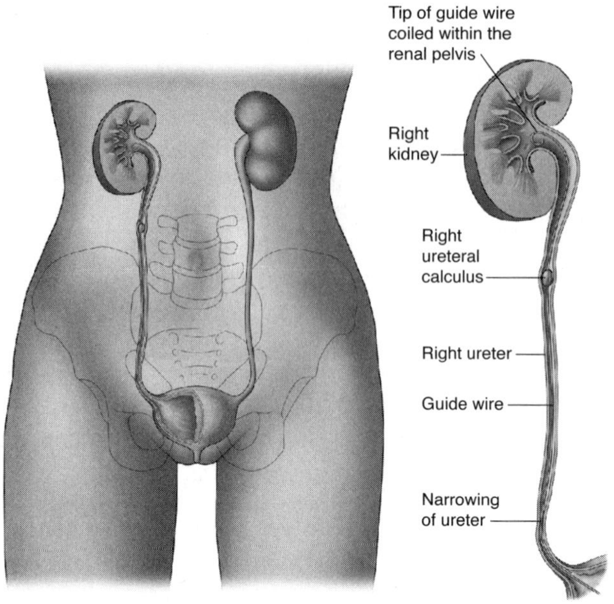

Exercise 4.41 Urinary System—Cystoscopy

Unless otherwise noted, all answers can be found in appendix D of this book. Answers to selected exercises are located in the Instructor's Guide and available only to faculty of educational programs.

Assign appropriate CPT code(s) for the following procedures and indicate the index entries that were used to identify the codes. Assign only CPT surgical codes (no E/M codes) and append any applicable modifiers.

1. Cystoscopy for insertion of double-J ureteral stent

   Code(s): ______________________________

   Index entries: ______________________________

   ____

2. Cystoscopy with fulguration of 1.0-cm lesion of bladder

   Code(s): ______________________________

   Index entries: ______________________________

   ____

3. Cystoscopy, left ureteroscopy with laser lithotripsy

   Code(s): ______________________________

   Index entries: ______________________________

   ____

4. Cystoscopy with insertion of permanent urethral stent

   Code(s): ______________________________

   Index entries: ______________________________

   ____

Exercise 4.42 Urinary System

Unless otherwise noted, all answers can be found in appendix D of this book. Answers to selected exercises are located in the Instructor's Guide and available only to faculty of educational programs.

Operative Report

Preoperative Diagnosis:	Right ureteral stone
Postoperative Diagnosis:	Same
Procedure:	Right ureteroscopy, stone extraction, stent

The patient was taken to the operating suite and placed in the dorsal lithotomy position, and then sterilely prepared and draped in the usual fashion. Cystoscope was then inserted into the urethra; it was normal. The prostate was nonobstructed, and the bladder was free of neoplasm, infection, or calculus. There was some edema of the right intramural ureter. A guide wire was introduced into the right ureteral orifice, and advanced to the right renal-collecting system without difficulty. A balloon was used to dilate the ureter, and a scope was introduced. The gravel was noted from the stone being fragmented from the balloon. This was washing out. The remainder of the ureter was examined and found to be free of neoplasm, perforation, or calculus. The stent was inserted. A string was kept attached. The patient was transferred to the recovery room in satisfactory condition.

Assign appropriate CPT code(s) for the preceding procedure and indicate the index entries that were used to identify the codes. Assign only CPT surgical codes (no E/M codes) and append any applicable modifiers.

1. Code(s) (physician services only): ______________________________

   Index entries: ______________________________

   ____

Exercise 4.43 Urinary System

Unless otherwise noted, all answers can be found in appendix D of this book. Answers to selected exercises are located in the Instructor's Guide and available only to faculty of educational programs.

Operative Report

Preoperative Diagnosis:	Recurrent bladder cancer
Postoperative Diagnosis:	Recurrent bladder cancer
Procedure:	Cystoscopy with bladder biopsies and fulguration
Anesthesia:	General

The patient has prior transitional cell carcinoma of the bladder and also carcinoma in situ. He has received MVAC therapy and BCG. Surveillance cystoscopy demonstrated erythema of the bladder wall. He is currently being admitted for cystoscopy, bladder biopsy, and fulguration. Procedure, reasons, risks, and complications were reviewed and consent was granted.

He was brought to the operating room under general anesthesia, placed in the dorsolithotomy position, and prepped and draped in a sterile manner. A #21 French cystoscope was inserted, urethra was normal, verumontanum intact. Prostate examination revealed evidence of prior transurethral resection and moderate outlet obstruction. There were erythematous areas throughout the bladder, and a 0.5-cm lesion was fulgurated. Both ureteric orifices were normal size, shape, and caliber with clear efflux. The erythematous areas were then biopsied with flexible biopsy forceps. After obtaining biopsies, the area was then fulgurated with a Bugbee electrode. Reinspection was carried out; no gross bleeding was noted. The bladder was drained, cystoscope was withdrawn, and the patient was transferred to the recovery room in satisfactory condition with all vital signs stable.

Pathology Report

Final Diagnosis: 1. Urothelial carcinoma in situ, focal
2. Chronic nonspecific cystitis

Assign appropriate CPT code(s) for the preceding procedure and indicate the index entries that were used to identify the codes. Assign only CPT surgical codes (no E/M codes) and append any applicable modifiers.

1. Code(s): ____________________

   Index entries: ____________________

   ____

Exercise 4.44 Urinary System Review

Unless otherwise noted, all answers can be found in appendix D of this book. Answers to selected exercises are located in the Instructor's Guide and available only to faculty of educational programs.

Assign appropriate CPT code(s) for the following procedures and indicate the index entries that were used to identify the codes. Assign only CPT surgical codes (no E/M codes) and append any applicable modifiers.

1. Laparoscopic sling procedure for stress incontinence

   Code(s): ____________________

   Index entries: ____________________

   ____

2. Excision of urethral polyp

   Code(s): ____________________

   Index entries: ____________________

   ____

Exercise 4.44 (Continued)

3. Cystoscopy with fulguration of 2.0-cm benign tumor

   Code(s): ____________________

   Index entries: ____________________

   ____

4. Cystotomy with excision of bladder diverticulum

   Code(s): ____________________

   Index entries: ____________________

   ____

5. Needle renal biopsy

   Code(s): ____________________

   Index entries: ____________________

   ____

Note: Answers to exercises 6 through 10 do not appear in appendix D of this text. They are located in the Instructor's Guide and available to faculty of educational programs.

6. Cystoscopy with ureteroscopy

   Code(s): ____________________

   Index entries: ____________________

   ____

7. Cystourethroscopy with bilateral ureteral meatotomy

   Code(s): ____________________

   Index entries: ____________________

   ____

8. Needle EMG studies of urethral sphincter

   Code(s): ____________________

   Index entries: ____________________

   ____

9. Insertion of straight catheter

   Code(s): ____________________

   Index entries: ____________________

   ____

10. Closure of ureterocutaneous fistula

    Code(s): ____________________

    Index entries: ____________________

    ____

Male Genital System

The codes in the male genital system subsection are used to report procedures on the penis, testis, epididymis, tunica vaginalis, scrotum, vas deferens, spermatic cord, seminal vesicle, and prostate gland. Figure 4.23 illustrates these structures.

Removal of Lesions

Removal of lesions (for example, condyloma, papilloma, molluscum contagiosum, herpetic vesicle) of the penis is not located in the integumentary system subsection but, rather, in the male genital system (54050–54065) subsection. The code selection is determined by the method of removal. For destruction or excision of other lesions, reference the integumentary system subsection of the surgery section.

Prostatectomy

The prostate gland lies under the bladder and surrounds the first part of the urethra, which carries urine to the penis. When the prostate becomes enlarged, it tends to obstruct the urethra and makes urination difficult. There are three common methods of prostatectomy, each involving a different approach: transurethral (most common), retropubic, and perineal. Transurethral resection of the prostate (52601–52640 and 53850–53853) uses a scope inserted through the urethra to remove the prostate tissue piece by piece. A perineal prostatectomy (55801–55815) requires an incision between the back of the scrotum and the anus. A retropubic prostatectomy (55821–55845) requires the surgeon to make an incision in the front wall of the abdomen, just above the pubic bone, to directly reach the prostate. CPT also provides a code for laparoscopic retropubic prostatectomy (55866).

Figure 4.23. The male genital system

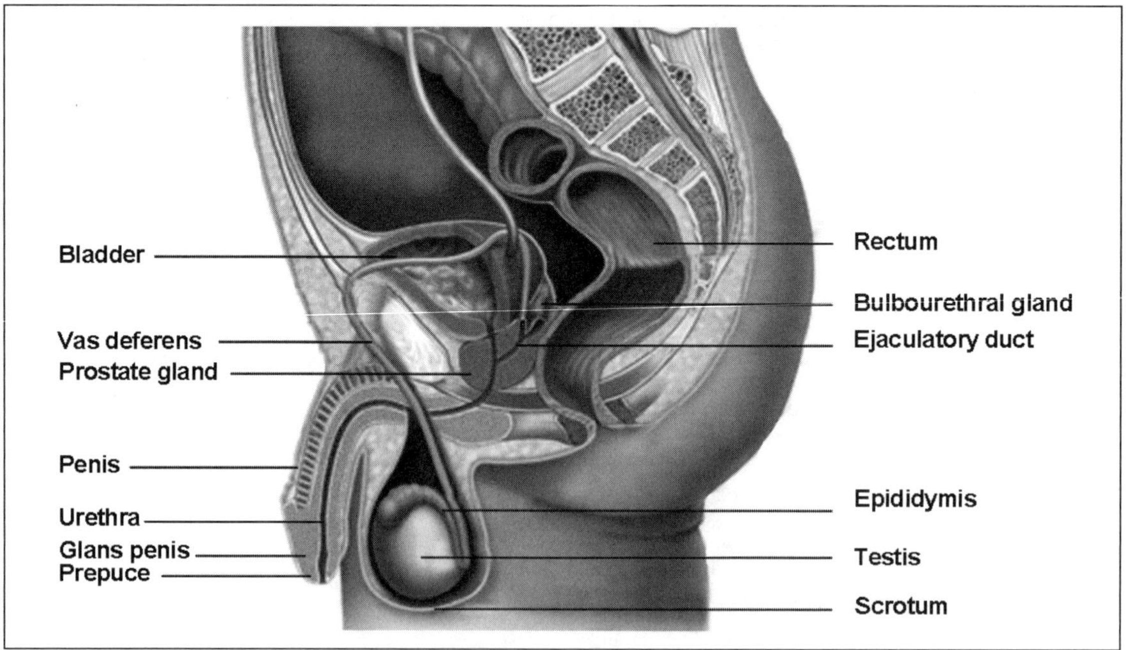

Exercise 4.45 Male Genital System

Unless otherwise noted, all answers can be found in appendix D of this book. Answers to selected exercises are located in the Instructor's Guide and available only to faculty of educational programs.

Assign appropriate CPT code(s) for the following procedures and indicate the index entries that were used to identify the codes. Assign only CPT surgical codes (no E/M codes) and append any applicable modifiers.

1. Laser destruction of four condylomas of the penis

   Code(s): ____________________

   Index entries: ____________________

   ____

2. Incision and drainage of subcutaneous abscess of the penis

   Code(s): ____________________

   Index entries: ____________________

   ____

3. Radical retropubic prostatectomy with excision of lymph nodes

   Code(s): ____________________

   Index entries: ____________________

   ____

4. Bilateral epididymectomy

   Code(s): ____________________

   Index entries: ____________________

   ____

5. Clamp circumcision, newborn

   Code(s): ____________________

   Index entries: ____________________

   ____

Exercise 4.46 Male Genital System

Unless otherwise noted, all answers can be found in appendix D of this book. Answers to selected exercises are located in the Instructor's Guide and available only to faculty of educational programs.

Operative Report

Preoperative Diagnosis:	Adenocarcinoma of the prostate
Postoperative Diagnosis:	Same
Procedure:	Transrectal ultrasound
	Transperineal implant of I–125 seeds into the prostate
Anesthesia:	General

The patient was brought to the cysto suite and placed in the lithotomy position at a 90-degree angle. General anesthesia was induced, and a Foley catheter was placed. The ultrasound probe was positioned in the rectum, and the appropriate reference points were identified and compared to his previous volumetric studies.

Under fluoroscopic and ultrasound guidance, 19 needles were inserted into the prostate based on a premeasured template. Approximately 70 seeds were placed.

A cystoscopic examination was performed at the end of the case, and no seeds were identified within the urinary bladder.

A Foley catheter was replaced into the bladder and will be removed later today. The appropriate postimplantation radiation and postoperative instructions were given. He tolerated the procedure well and was taken to the recovery room in satisfactory condition.

Assign appropriate CPT code(s) for the preceding procedure and indicate the index entries that were used to identify the codes. Assign only CPT surgical codes (no E/M codes) and append any applicable modifiers.

1. Code(s) for the physician's services:______________________________

   Index entries:____

   ____

Exercise 4.47 Male Genital System

Unless otherwise noted, all answers can be found in appendix D of this book. Answers to selected exercises are located in the Instructor's Guide and available only to faculty of educational programs.

Operative Report

Preoperative Diagnosis:	Chronic left orchialgia Chronic epididymitis
Procedure:	Left inguinal orchiectomy
Anesthesia:	Local standby; 0.25% Marcaine, 1% Xylocaine, 1/1 dilution. Total 25 cc used as inguinal block
Estimated Blood Loss:	Minimal

This is an 82-year-old man with chronic left gonadal pain due to chronic granulomatous epididymitis. This has failed to respond to conservative measures and has caused him marked discomfort in the left groin. As a result, we recommended that he consider outpatient orchiectomy. The risks and potential complications were discussed and informed consent obtained.

The patient was given Ancef IV as well as IV sedation and placed on the operating table in the supine position. The lower groin and abdomen were shaved, prepared, and draped in the standard fashion. The external inguinal ring was identified, and an area just distal to the external inguinal ring was anesthetized with the local anesthetic, and a small transverse incision was made down to the spermatic cord. The testis was then brought out through the inguinal incision after the spermatic cord blockade with local anesthetic. The testis was separated from the scrotum by incision in the gubernaculum with needle tip Bovie. The spermatic cord was identified, dissected back to the external inguinal ring, and bisected with a curved Kelly clamp and then clamped and transected with Metzenbaum scissors. The spermatic cord was closed with suture ligature of 0 Vicryl and a free tie of 0 Vicryl proximal to this on each side of the spermatic cord. The incision was inspected for hemostasis. No further bleeding was noted, and the testis was delivered for pathologic evaluation. The Scarpa's fascia was closed with interrupted 2-0 Vicryl, and the skin was closed with a running 4-0 Vicryl subcuticular closure. Steri-Strips and four by fours were applied as a dressing. He was returned to the recovery room in stable condition. Estimated blood loss was minimal.

Assign appropriate CPT code(s) for the preceding procedure and indicate the index entries that were used to identify the codes. Assign only CPT surgical codes (no E/M codes) and append any applicable modifiers.

1. Code(s) for the physician's services:______________________________

   Index entries:____

   ____

Exercise 4.48 Male Genital System Review

Unless otherwise noted, all answers can be found in appendix D of this book. Answers to selected exercises are located in the Instructor's Guide and available only to faculty of educational programs.

Assign appropriate CPT code(s) for the following procedures and indicate the index entries that were used to identify the codes. Assign only CPT surgical codes (no E/M codes) and append any applicable modifiers.

1. Excision of spermatocele with epididymectomy

   Code(s): ____

   Index entries: ____

   ____

(Continued on next page)

Exercise 4.48 (Continued)

2. Removal of inflatable penile prosthesis (no replacement)
   Code(s): ______________________
   Index entries: ______________________
   ____

3. Laparoscopic orchiectomy
   Code(s): ______________________
   Index entries: ______________________
   ____

4. One-stage distal hypospadias repair with simple meatal advancement
   Code(s): ______________________
   Index entries: ______________________
   ____

5. Biopsy and exploration of epididymis
   Code(s): ______________________
   Index entries: ______________________
   ____

Note: Answers to exercises 6 through 10 do not appear in appendix D of this text. They are located in the Instructor's Guide and available to faculty of educational programs.

6. Incision into abscess of scrotal wall to drain pus
   Code(s): ______________________
   Index entries: ______________________
   ____

7. Plethysmography of penis
   Code(s): ______________________
   Index entries: ______________________
   ____

8. Excision of condylomas of the penis
   Code(s): ______________________
   Index entries: ______________________
   ____

9. Bilateral orchiopexy, inguinal approach with hernia repair
   Code(s): ______________________
   Index entries: ______________________
   ____

10. Laparoscopic retropubic radical prostatectomy
    Code(s): ______________________
    Index entries: ______________________
    ____

Female Genital System

The female genital system subsection of the CPT surgery chapter includes codes for various surgical repairs, dilation and curettage (D&C), and hysterectomies and hysteroscopies. This section also contains codes for maternity care and delivery. Figure 4.24 provides an illustration of the female genital system.

Colposcopy

Colposcopy is a visual examination of the women's genital area, including the cervix, vagina, and vulva. CPT code ranges 57420–57421 and 57452–57461 are differentiated by the area visualized and additional procedures, such as biopsy, performed during the endoscopy.

Loop Electrode Biopsy (57460) vs. Loop Electrode Conization of Cervix (57461)

CPT code 57460, Colposcopy with loop electrode biopsy(s) of cervix, describes a procedure whereas the physician removes tissue (specimen) for examination by the pathologist. Code 57461 identifies the removal of a portion of the endocervix or transformation zone.

Laparoscopy

In a laparoscopic procedure, the surgeon first inserts a needle through the navel and the abdomen is filled with carbon dioxide gas. The gas pushes the internal organs away from the abdominal wall to decrease the risk of injury to surrounding organs. Next, the surgeon makes a small incision in the abdominal area (naval is common) and inserts a tube with a tiny video camera (laparoscope) to visualize the inside of the pelvis and abdomen. Additional small cuts

Figure 4.24. The female genital system

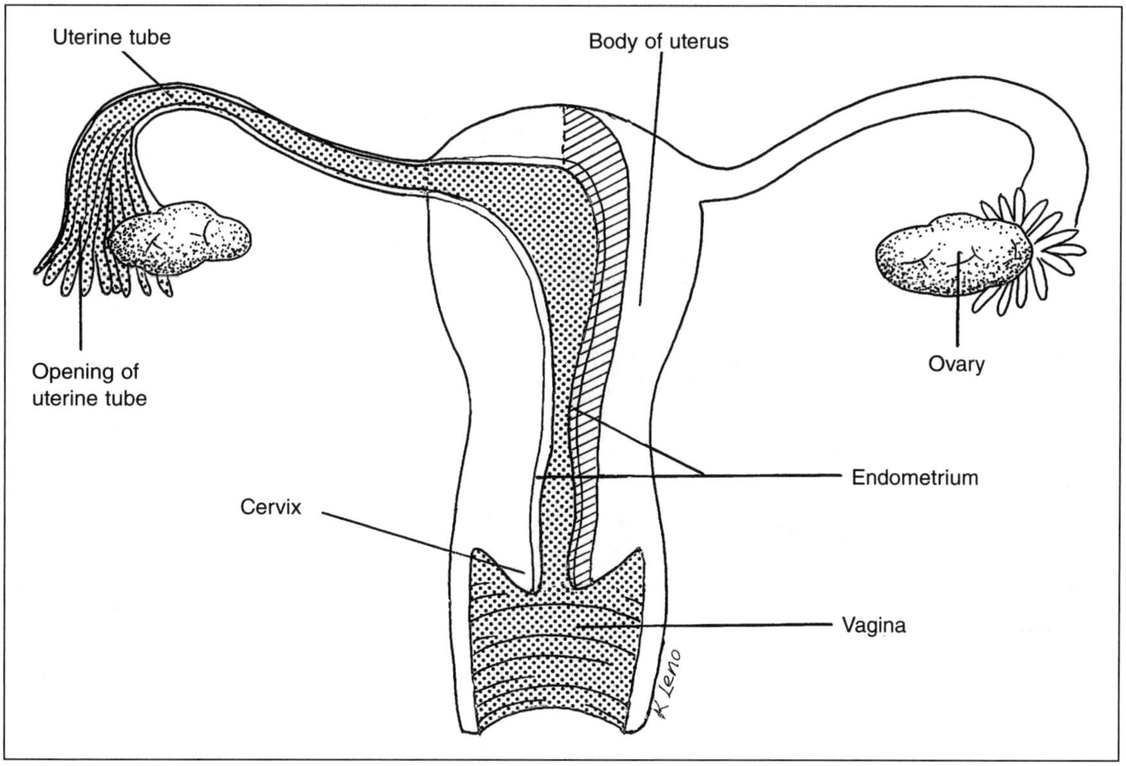

may be made if other instruments are needed such as a small probe for a clearer view. If defects or abnormalities are discovered, a diagnostic laparoscopy can become an operative laparoscopy. Figure 4.25 illustrates a laparoscopic procedure on a female patient.

Hysteroscopy

A hysteroscope is a thin, telescope-like instrument that allows the physician to look inside the uterus. After insufflation of the uterine cavity with CO_2, the hysteroscope is inserted through the cervical canal and into the uterus. This direct visualization improves the accuracy of diagnosis and treatment. Accessory instruments that may be used with a hysteroscope procedure include scissors, forceps, lasers, and various electrodes. A D&C is commonly performed with a hysteroscopic biopsy or polypectomy. Therefore, no additional code is assigned to identify the D&C. Codes for hysteroscopies are included in the range 58555 through 58579.

Hysterectomy

CPT bases the coding selection for hysterectomies on the surgical approach.

Laparoscopic Supracervical Hysterectomy (58541–58544)

This laparoscopic procedure removes the uterus but preserves the cervix. CPT codes differentiate between the weight of the uterus and whether or not the tubes and ovaries were removed.

Figure 4.25. Laparoscopy

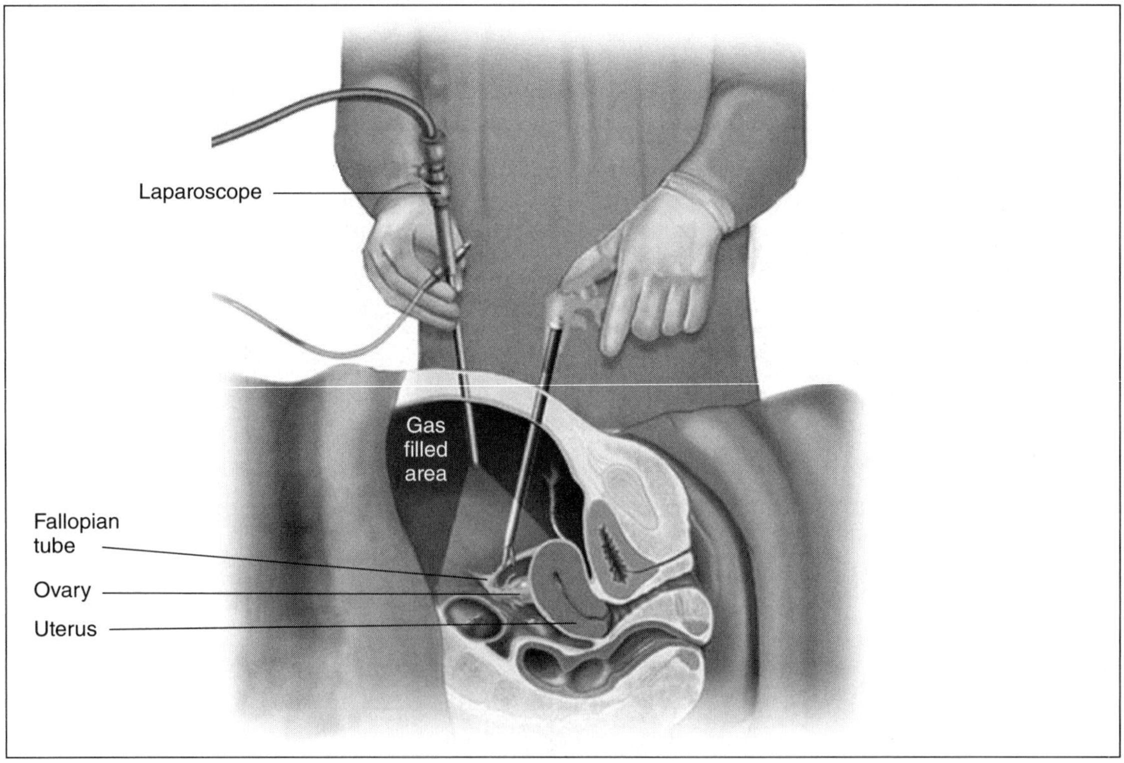

Laparoscopic Vaginal Hysterectomy (58550–58554)

Laparoscopically assisted vaginal hysterectomy (LAVH) is a surgical procedure using a laparoscope to remove the uterus and/or fallopian tubes and ovaries through the vagina.

Laparoscopic Total Hysterectomy (58570–58573)

For this procedure, the uterus and the cervix both are removed entirely through the scope. The code selection provides for the weight of the uterus and whether or not the tubes and ovaries were removed.

Excisional Approach (58150–58294)

The excisional operation can be performed through the vagina (58260–58294) or through a conventional incision in the front wall of the abdomen (58150–58240).

Maternity Care and Delivery Subsection (Guidelines for Physician Services)

Along with codes for surgery and other procedures involving the female reproductive organs, the female genital system subsection includes CPT codes for maternity care and delivery services. Antepartum care includes initial and subsequent history, physical examination, recording of clinical information, and monthly visits up to 28-week gestation, biweekly visits to 36-week gestation, and weekly visits until the time of delivery. According to the CPT codebook, any additional visits are to be coded separately using E/M codes. Health plans may have specific rules about the reporting of services beyond those included in the global service package that often accompanies maternity coverage. This may affect the reporting of services, particularly if more than one physician is required to care for the patient, as may occur with unexpected cesarean delivery.

Postpartum care codes include both hospital and office visit codes following either vaginal or cesarean delivery.

Some CPT codes address global care, and some are used to report only a portion of care.

> **Example:** CPT code 59425 is for antepartum care only, 4 to 6 visits. It may be used by a family practice physician who refers a patient in the second trimester of pregnancy to an obstetrician due to a high risk of complications.

Code 59510 would be reported by a physician providing global care for a cesarean delivery from start to finish.

Patients who attempt vaginal delivery after previous cesarean delivery or who successfully deliver vaginally after previous cesarean delivery have specific CPT codes assigned from the 59610 through 59622 range. These codes should always be used when they apply.

Exercise 4.49 Female Genital System

Unless otherwise noted, all answers can be found in appendix D of this book. Answers to selected exercises are located in the Instructor's Guide and available only to faculty of educational programs.

Assign appropriate CPT code(s) for the following procedures and indicate the index entries that were used to identify the codes. Assign only CPT surgical codes (no E/M codes) and append any applicable modifiers.

1. Laparoscopic fulguration of fallopian tubes

   Code(s): ______________________________

   Index entries: ______________________________

   ____

2. D&C performed for a patient with dysfunctional bleeding

   Code(s): ______________________________

   Index entries: ______________________________

   ____

3. D&C performed for a patient with diagnosis of incomplete abortion (8 weeks pregnant)

   Code(s): ______________________________

   Index entries: ______________________________

   ____

4. Laparoscopy with aspiration of ovarian cyst

   Code(s): ______________________________

   Index entries: ______________________________

   ____

5. Laparoscopic removal of two fibroids (total weight 150 g)

   Code(s): ______________________________

   Index entries: ______________________________

   ____

6. Vaginal hysterectomy with salpingo-oophorectomy (uterus weight 250 g)

   Code(s): ______________________________

   Index entries: ______________________________

   ____

Exercise 4.50 Female Genital System

Unless otherwise noted, all answers can be found in appendix D of this book. Answers to selected exercises are located in the Instructor's Guide and available only to faculty of educational programs.

Operative Report

Preoperative Diagnosis:	Moderate dysplasia of the cervix
Postoperative Diagnosis:	Same
Procedure:	Loop electrosurgical excision procedure (LEEP)
Anesthesia:	General inhalation anesthesia per mask

The patient was brought to the OR with IV fluids infusing and placed on the table in the supine position. General inhalation anesthesia per mask was administered after acquisition of an adequate anesthetic level, and the patient was placed in the lithotomy position. The perineum was draped. A laser speculum was placed in the vaginal vault. The cervix was rinsed with a solution of acetic acid, and colposcopic examination of the cervix showed areas of wide epithelium across the anterior lip of the cervix, consistent with the previous biopsy showing moderate dysplasia. Using the 2-cm electrosurgical loop excision, the endocervical canal was cauterized with bipolar cautery to remove all diseased tissue. Then the procedure was completed. The speculum was removed. The patient was taken out of the lithotomy position. Her anesthesia was reversed. She was awakened and taken to the recovery room in stable condition. Sponge, instrument, and needle counts were correct times three. Estimated blood loss was less than 25 cc.

Assign appropriate CPT code(s) for the preceding procedure and indicate the index entries that were used to identify the codes. Assign only CPT surgical codes (no E/M codes) and append any applicable modifiers.

1. Code(s) for the physician's services:________________________________

   Index entries:____

   ____

Exercise 4.51 Female Genital System

Unless otherwise noted, all answers can be found in appendix D of this book. Answers to selected exercises are located in the Instructor's Guide and available only to faculty of educational programs.

Operative Report

Preoperative Diagnosis:	Dysfunctional uterine bleeding, failed hormonal therapy
Postoperative Diagnosis:	Same
Procedure Performed:	Diagnostic hysteroscopy Fractional dilation and curettage

The patient is a 35-year-old Gravida V Para IV AB I female from the Towne Health Center. She has been bleeding the majority of each month over the past 4 months. She has been tried on Ortho-Novum 7/7 to control the bleeding, but this has been of no help. The patient is here for the above procedure.

Description of Procedure: With the patient under satisfactory general anesthesia in the dorsal lithotomy position, a pelvic examination revealed a cervix that came down to the introitus, constituting a second-degree uterine prolapse. The patient had many hymenal tags on both the right and left side. A large speculum was placed inside the vagina. The anterior lip of the cervix was grasped with a single-toothed tenaculum. The cervix was sounded to 8.5 cm. The endocervical canal was now serially dilated. Using the hysteroscope and lactated Ringer's solution as a distending solution, the hysteroscope was passed through the internal os into the uterine cavity. Inspection of the uterine contents revealed both right and left ostia identified. Some lining was on the floor of the uterus and some on the roof. The fundus was devoid of any lining. There were no submucosal fibroids and no submucosal septa. The hysteroscope was removed, and the next procedure was fractional dilation and curettage. Using a Kevorkian-Younge curette, the endocervical canal was curetted and the cervical canal was further dilated using a medium-sized curette. The endometrial cavity was curetted with moderate curettings obtained. These were sent for pathological diagnosis. The patient tolerated the procedure fairly well and was escorted to the recovery room in satisfactory condition.

Assign appropriate CPT code(s) for the preceding procedure and indicate the index entries that were used to identify the codes. Assign only CPT surgical codes (no E/M codes) and append any applicable modifiers.

1. Code(s) for the physician's services:____________________

   Index entries:____________________

   ____

Exercise 4.52 Female Genital System Review

Unless otherwise noted, all answers can be found in appendix D of this book. Answers to selected exercises are located in the Instructor's Guide and available only to faculty of educational programs.

Assign appropriate CPT code(s) for the following procedures and indicate the index entries that were used to identify the codes. Assign only CPT surgical codes (no E/M codes) and append any applicable modifiers.

1. Colposcopy with biopsy of cervix

   Code(s): ____________________

   Index entries: ____________________

   ____

Exercise 4.52 (Continued)

2. Vulvectomy, partial removal of skin and superficial subcutaneous tissues
   Code(s): ______________________________
   Index entries: ______________________________
   ____

3. Laparoscopy with fulguration of peritoneal lesions
   Code(s): ______________________________
   Index entries: ______________________________
   ____

4. Total abdominal hysterectomy with bilateral salpingo-oophorectomy
   Code(s): ______________________________
   Index entries: ______________________________
   ____

5. Incision and drainage of vaginal hematoma, posttrauma
   Code(s): ______________________________
   Index entries: ______________________________
   ____

Note: Answers to exercises 6 through 10 do not appear in appendix D of this text. They are located in the Instructor's Guide and available to faculty of educational programs.

6. Biopsy of two lesions, one from labia minora and another from the vaginal orifice, which required suture closure
   Code(s): ______________________________
   Index entries: ______________________________
   ____

7. Laparoscopic vaginal hysterectomy with bilateral salpingo-oophorectomy (uterus weighing 280 g)
   Code(s): ______________________________
   Index entries: ______________________________
   ____

8. Hysteroscopy with removal of fibroids
   Code(s): ______________________________
   Index entries: ______________________________
   ____

9. Vaginal hysterectomy (uterus weighing 260 g)
   Code(s): ______________________________
   Index entries: ______________________________
   ____

10. Endometrial cryoablation with ultrasonic guidance
   Code(s): ______________________________
   Index entries: ______________________________
   ____

Endocrine System

The endocrine system functions in the regulation of body activities. This ductless system acts through chemical messengers called hormones that influence growth, development, and metabolic activities. There are no specific coding guidelines applicable to this subsection, but knowledge of anatomy, physiology, and medical terminology is necessary for accurate code assignment.

Exercise 4.53 Endocrine System Review

Unless otherwise noted, all answers can be found in appendix D of this book. Answers to selected exercises are located in the Instructor's Guide and available only to faculty of educational programs.

Assign appropriate CPT code(s) for the following procedures and indicate the index entries that were used to identify the codes. Assign only CPT surgical codes (no E/M codes) and append any applicable modifiers.

1. Excision of thyroglossal duct cyst

   Code(s): ____________________

   Index entries: ____________________

   ____

2. Laparoscopic adrenalectomy, complete

   Code(s): ____________________

   Index entries: ____________________

   ____

3. Patient had a previous surgery for removal of part of thyroid; she now has a bilateral thyroidectomy for remaining tissue

   Code(s): ____________________

   Index entries: ____________________

   ____

4. Aspiration of thyroid cyst

   Code(s): ____________________

   Index entries: ____________________

   ____

5. Parathyroidectomy

   Code(s): ____________________

   Index entries: ____________________

   ____

Nervous System

The nervous system subsection of the CPT surgery chapter includes the procedures that involve the brain, spinal cord, and peripheral nerves. The CPT codes for procedures performed to manage pain, such as nerve blocks and epidural procedures, also are part of this subsection. Examples of procedures in this subsection include major brain operations such as craniectomies and craniotomies, as well as relatively minor spinal injections and catheter insertions into the nerves and the spinal cord.

Laminotomy and Laminectomy

Laminotomy and laminectomy procedures involve the nerves that occupy the space inside the vertebrae that make up the spinal column. (Figure 4.26 illustrates the sections of the spine.)

Figure 4.26. Sections of the spine

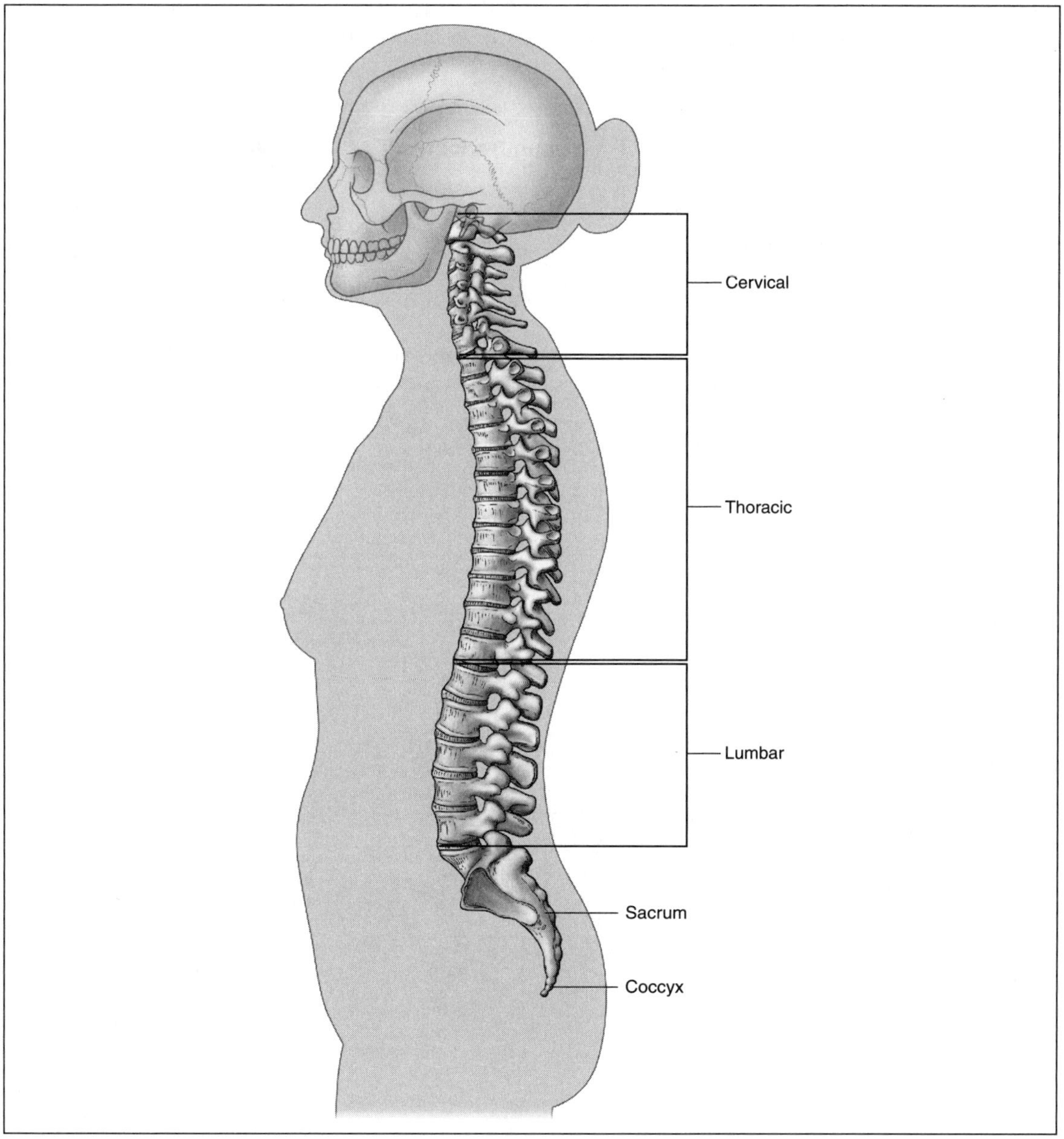

The CPT codes for surgical procedures involving the spine are based on the surgical approach, the anatomic location of the precipitating condition, and the specific procedures performed.

Laminotomy (hemilaminectomy) codes are based on the anatomic location of the specific interspace involved. When surgery is performed on more than one interspace, the coding professional should locate the appropriate code(s) in that section of CPT for each additional interspace. Figure 4.27 illustrates back surgery for a herniated disc.

Spinal Injections

Spinal injections, or infusions, are coded according to the site of the injection and the substance injected. Spinal injections deliver medications through a needle placed into a structure or space in the spine to allow the physician to identify the source of pain and/or to reduce it. Typical medications used include local anesthetics and corticosteroids. Local anesthetics numb the nerves and corticosteroids help reduce inflammation.

To accurately assign codes for these procedures, coding professionals must abstract documentation from the operative report to determine the injection site (cervical, lumbar) and the substance injected (neurolytic). For example, a single steroid injection into the lumbar spine would be assigned CPT code 62311.

Figure 4.27. Back surgery—L4-5 and L5-S1 laminectomy, discectomy, and spinal fusion

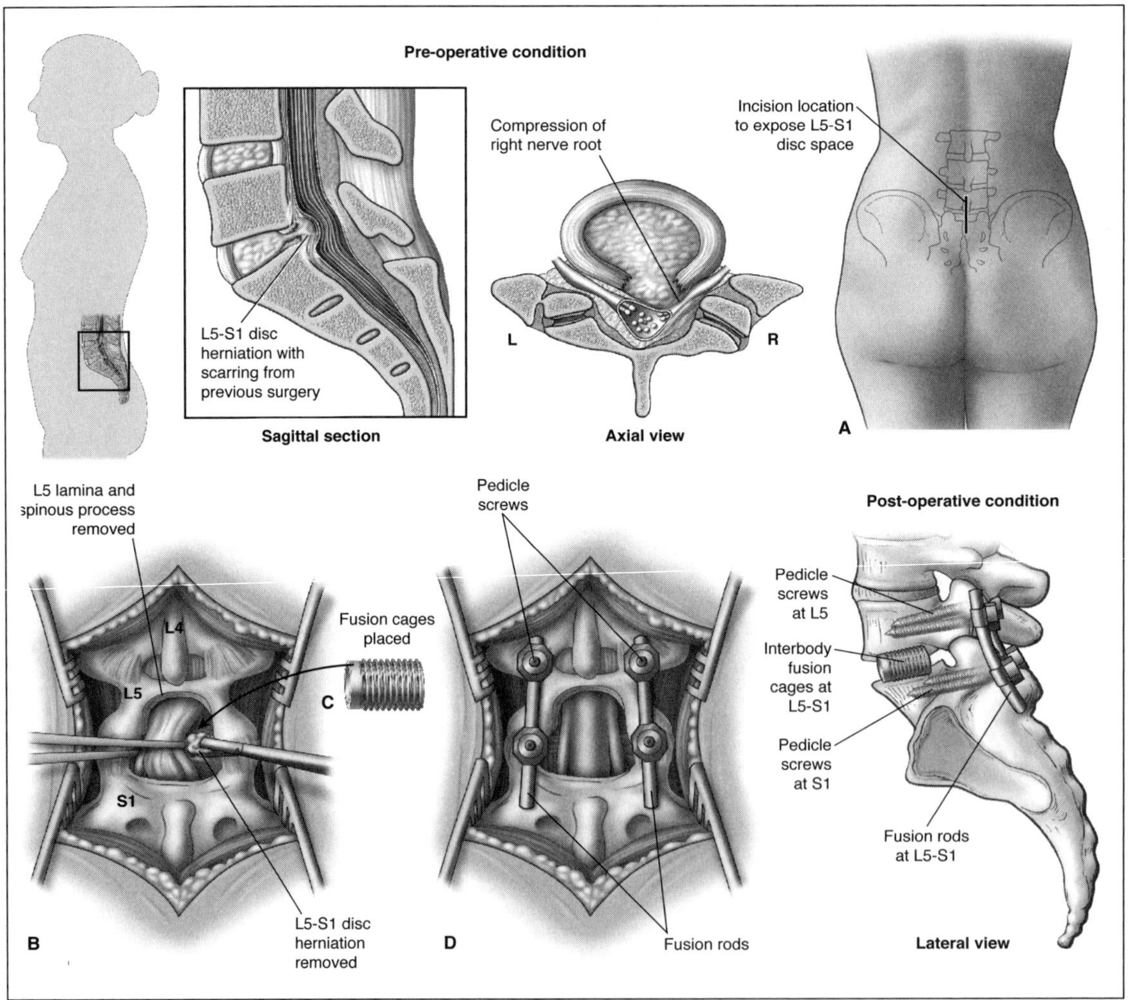

Exercise 4.54 Nervous System

Unless otherwise noted, all answers can be found in appendix D of this book. Answers to selected exercises are located in the Instructor's Guide and available only to faculty of educational programs.

Assign appropriate CPT code(s) for the following procedures and indicate the index entries that were used to identify the codes. Assign only CPT surgical codes (no E/M codes) and append any applicable modifiers.

1. Patient with chronic pain receives a nerve block; ropivacaine (anesthetic agent) injected into the branch of sciatic nerve

   Code(s): ______________________________

   Index entries: ______________________________

   ____

2. Using an operating microscope, the physician performs a neuroplasty of the right ring finger.

   Code(s): ______________________________

   Index entries: ______________________________

   ____

3. Cervical epidural spinal injection of phenol (neurolytic substance)

   Code(s): ______________________________

   Index entries: ______________________________

   ____

4. Neurorrhaphy of digital nerves of right thumb and ring finger

   Code(s): ______________________________

   Index entries: ______________________________

   ____

Exercise 4.55 Nervous System

Unless otherwise noted, all answers can be found in appendix D of this book. Answers to selected exercises are located in the Instructor's Guide and available only to faculty of educational programs.

Operative Report

Preoperative Diagnosis: C5–C6 disc herniation

Postoperative Diagnosis: Same

Procedure: Anterior cervical discectomy

This 45-year-old man presents with a 6-month history of neck pain, right shoulder pain, right intra-scapular pain, and pain radiating on the outer aspect of the right arm. He was found to have wasting of the supraspinatus and infraspinatus muscles, and EMG confirmed a C-6 radiculopathy.

MRI scan showed a lateral disc herniation at the level of C5–C6. The patient tried initial conservative measures, which did not help him; hence, recommendation of surgery was made. The risks and benefits included infection, hemorrhage, injury to the nerve roots, paralysis, injury to the spinal cord with paralysis, failure to improve, or even death. The patient fully understands and agrees to go ahead with the procedure.

The patient was anesthetized and positioned supine with a shoulder support, and the neck was prepared and draped in the usual manner. Midcervical crease incision was marked, both 4 cm. Incisions were placed transversely and the skin was sharply cut, and then the platysma was cut in the line of incision. The cervical fascia was dissected. Then we entered the plane between the trachea and the carotid sheath by blunt dissection reaching the prevertebral space. The prevertebral fascia was incised longitudinally. The disc bulge at C5–C6 was easily identified, and a spinal needle placed confirmed the position to be at C5–C6. The anterior osteophytes were prominent. They were removed and then we entered the disc space. The disc space itself had collapsed, and there was only desiccated disc material. We curetted out the disc and the cartilage plate, and the vertebral spreader was put in. More disc was removed from the lateral parts of the disc extending toward the uncus on both sides. As we moved posteriorly toward the ligament, there was subligamentous disc herniation to the right side. It was removed, and the ligament was reached. The ligament was lifted with a blunt hook and opened with micropunches. Using a Midas Rex drill, the posterior parts of the bone in this region were drilled doing a right foraminotomy on the right, and the nerve root was decompressed. A no-free fragment was identified inside the canal, and the entire ligamentum disc was removed over the nerve root. The bone was punched in those corners to give adequate space. The ligament was cut across the width of the space, and on the left side also foraminotomy was done removing the osteophytes in the corner and decompressing the nerve root. After we were satisfied with the decompression, the space was irrigated with antibiotic solution and hemostasis was achieved with some Gelfoam powder, and the wound was thoroughly irrigated. Hemostasis was achieved in the muscle plane, and closure was done with 3-0 Vicryl for the platysma and subcutaneous layer, and the skin was closed with 4-0 subcuticular Vicryl. Dressings were applied in the usual manner with Steri-Strips, Telfa gauze, and Tegaderm. The patient was reversed from anesthesia and had an uneventful recovery. He was moving all the limbs well and was transferred in stable condition to the recovery room.

Assign appropriate CPT code(s) for the preceding procedure and indicate the index entries that were used to identify the codes. Assign only CPT surgical codes (no E/M codes) and append any applicable modifiers.

1. Code(s): ______________________________

   Index entries: ______________________________

   ____

Exercise 4.56 Nervous System Review

Unless otherwise noted, all answers can be found in appendix D of this book. Answers to selected exercises are located in the Instructor's Guide and available only to faculty of educational programs.

Assign appropriate CPT code(s) for the following procedures and indicate the index entries that were used to identify the codes. Assign only CPT surgical codes (no E/M codes) and append any applicable modifiers.

1. Creation of ventriculo-atrial shunt for a patient with hydrocephalus

   Code(s): ______________________

   Index entries: ______________________

   ____

2. Sciatic neuroplasty, leg

   Code(s): ______________________

   Index entries: ______________________

   ____

3. Excision of neuroma of peripheral nerve of foot

   Code(s): ______________________

   Index entries: ______________________

   ____

4. Suture repair of posterior tibial nerve

   Code(s): ______________________

   Index entries: ______________________

   ____

5. Laminectomy and excision of intradural lumbar lesion

   Code(s): ______________________

   Index entries: ______________________

   ____

Note: Answers to exercises 6 through 10 do not appear in appendix D of this text. They are located in the Instructor's Guide and available to faculty of educational programs.

6. Lumbar epidural steroid injection, L5–S1 interspace

   Code(s): ______________________

   Index entries: ______________________

   ____

(Continued on next page)

Exercise 4.56 (Continued)

7. Removal of implanted spinal neurostimulator pulse generator

   Code(s): ____________________

   Index entries: ____________________

   ____

8. Repair of 6-cm myelomeningocele

   Code(s): ____________________

   Index entries: ____________________

   ____

9. Vagus nerve block injection—Naropin (anesthetic agent)

   Code(s): ____________________

   Index entries: ____________________

   ____

10. Craniotomy for evacuation of subdural hematoma

    Code(s): ____________________

    Index entries: ____________________

    ____

Eye and Ocular Adnexa

The eye and ocular adnexa subsection includes procedures involving the eyeball, anterior and posterior segment, ocular adnexa, and conjunctiva. (Figure 4.28 shows the structure of the eye.) The codes are categorized first by body part involved and then by type of procedure, such as retinal and choroid repair, conjunctivoplasty, cataract removal, and removal of foreign body. Many of the refractive procedures performed for vision correction (such as laser in-situ keratomileusis [LASIK] procedures) are categorized in the unlisted category for the anterior segment, CPT code 66999, rather than having specific CPT codes.

Cataract Extraction

The note at the beginning of the cataract extraction subsection (66830–66986) identifies the following procedures as part of the extraction: lateral canthotomy, iridectomy, iridotomy, anterior capsulotomy, posterior capsulotomy, use of viscoelastic agents, enzymatic zonulysis, use of other pharmacologic agents, and subconjunctival or sub-Tenon injections. When performed as part of the cataract extraction, these procedures should not be coded separately because they are incorporated into the bigger procedure of the cataract removal.

The two types of cataract extraction are extracapsular and intracapsular. Extracapsular extraction, which includes removal of the lens material without removing the posterior capsule, is reported with codes 66840 through 66852, 66940, 66982, and 66984. Intracapsular

Figure 4.28. Structure of the eye

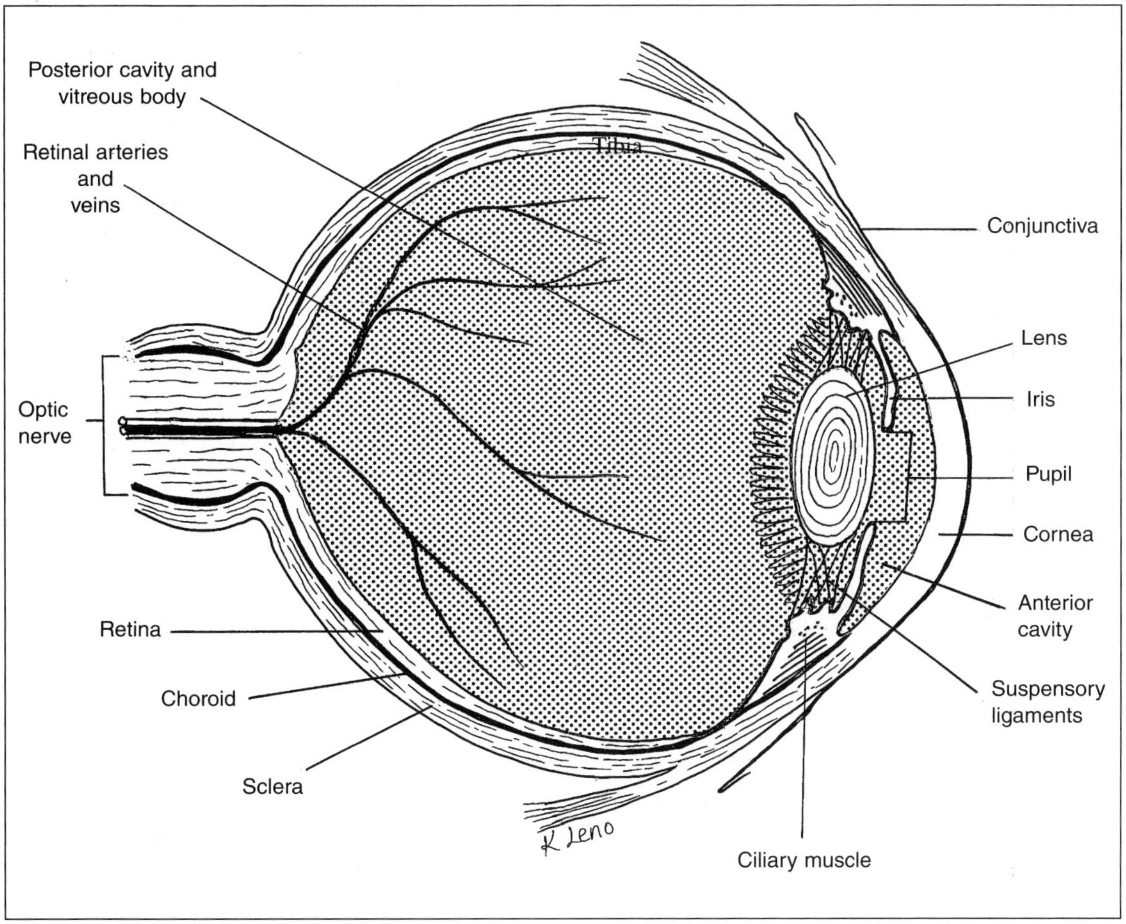

extraction, which involves removal of the entire lens including the capsule, is reported with codes 66920, 66930, and 66983.

Codes 66982, 66983, and 66984 describe cataract extraction with insertion of intraocular lens (IOL) prosthesis during the same operative episode. Insertion of IOL prosthesis performed during a subsequent encounter is reported with code 66985.

Exercise 4.57 Eye and Ocular Adnexa

Unless otherwise noted, all answers can be found in appendix D of this book. Answers to selected exercises are located in the Instructor's Guide and available only to faculty of educational programs.

Operative Report

Preoperative Diagnosis:	Cataract of the left eye
Postoperative Diagnosis:	Cataract of the left eye
Operative Procedure:	Phacoemulsification of cataract of the left eye with lens implantation
Complications:	None

The patient is a 77-year-old woman with a history of decreasing vision to a level of 20/100 in her left eye. Slit lamp examination showed a nuclear sclerotic cataract. Fundus examination view appeared to be normal. The patient requested removal of the cataract for improvement in her vision.

Procedure: The patient was brought to the OR and placed on the operating table in the supine position. A small amount of Brevital was given intravenously for relaxation, and then a local anesthetic using 0.75% Marcaine in a peribulbar manner and a modified Van Lint manner was administered. After obtaining proper anesthetic effect, the eye was prepared and draped in the usual manner. A blepharostat was placed between the lids of the eye, and a bridle suture using 4-0 silk was placed through the superior rectus tendon. A peritomy was performed from the 2 to 10 o'clock position superiorly with cautery used to obtain hemostasis. A 3.5-mm grooved incision was placed tangent to the limbus, approximately 2 mm posterior to the surgical limbus, and a scleral tunnel was formed anteriorly toward clear cornea. A stab incision was made at the 2 o'clock position in the limbus with a #75 Beaver blade, forming an irrigating peritomy site, and the anterior chamber was entered at the base of the scleral tunnel, using a #55 Keratome blade. Healon was instilled in the anterior chamber, and then an irrigating cystotome blade was used to perform a smooth capsulorrhexis opening of the anterior capsule. A balanced salt solution was used to perform hydrodissection, and the phacoemulsification tip was used to break up and remove the nucleus of the lens. The remaining cortical material was removed from the eye using the irrigation-aspiration tip. The posterior capsule of the lens was polished using a Kratz scratcher. The wound was extended very slightly, and then a 6-mm folding posterior chamber lens was placed in the eye with the lens within the capsular bag. Excess Healon was removed from the eye using the irrigation-aspiration tip.

The corneosclera was tested and found to be watertight and free of any iris incarceration. The conjunctiva was repositioned to its original site and tacked down using bipolar cautery. A collagen shield, which had been soaked in a suspension of Tobradex eyedrops, was then placed over the cornea, and one drop of Timoptic was instilled on the conjunctiva. The blepharostat and the bridle suture were removed from the eye, and a dry dressing and Fox shield were placed over the eye. The patient tolerated the procedure well and left the OR in good condition. She was instructed to leave the eye dressing intact for the remainder of the day and to return to the office the following day for follow-up care and instructions.

Assign appropriate CPT code(s) for the preceding procedure and indicate the index entries that were used to identify the codes. Assign only CPT surgical codes (no E/M codes) and append any applicable modifiers.

1. Code(s): ______________________________

   Index entries: ______________________________

   ____

Strabismus Surgery

Strabismus is a condition in which there is abnormal deviation of one eye in relation to the other. Surgical correction is performed on the muscles that regulate the movement of the eyeball. CPT codes from the series 67311 through 67318 require documentation of the number and types of muscles involved in the procedure. The procedure descriptions are considered to be unilateral. Note the following definitions:

- *Extraocular muscles:* Six extraocular muscles are attached to each eye, two horizontal and four vertical.
- *Horizontal muscles:* Two horizontal extraocular muscles—lateral rectus and medial rectus—move the eye from side to side.
- *Vertical muscles:* Four vertical extraocular muscles—inferior rectus, superior rectus, inferior oblique, and superior oblique—move the eye up and down. Figure 4.29 depicts the superior and inferior rectus muscles.

Figure 4.29. Movement of the eye

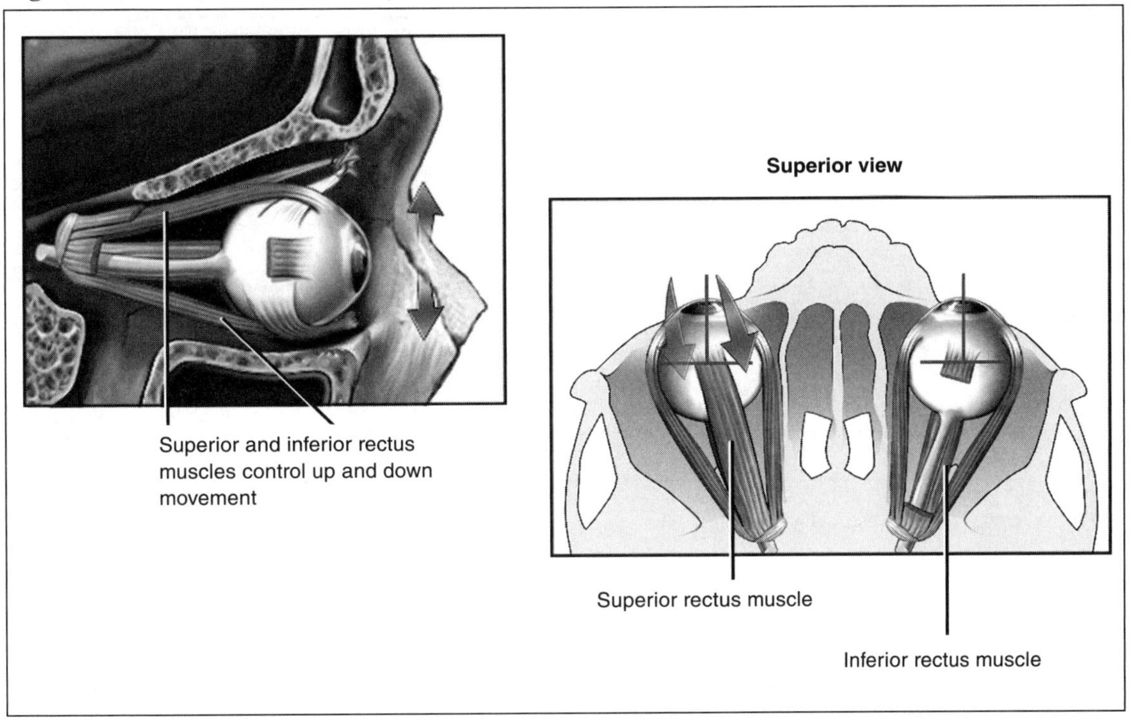

Exercise 4.58 Eye and Ocular Adnexa Review

Unless otherwise noted, all answers can be found in appendix D of this book. Answers to selected exercises are located in the Instructor's Guide and available only to faculty of educational programs.

Assign appropriate CPT code(s) for the following procedures and indicate the index entries that were used to identify the codes. Assign only CPT surgical codes (no E/M codes) and append any applicable modifiers.

1. With the use of a slit lamp, the physician removes a piece of metal from the patient's cornea.

   Code(s): ______________________________

   Index entries: ______________________________

   ____

2. Biopsy of left upper eyelid

   Code(s): ______________________________

   Index entries: ______________________________

   ____

3. Excision of 0.5-cm lesion of conjunctiva

   Code(s): ______________________________

   Index entries: ______________________________

   ____

4. Excision of a chalazion, right upper eyelid

   Code(s): ______________________________

   Index entries: ______________________________

   ____

5. Strabismus correction involving the lateral rectus muscle

   Code(s): ______________________________

   Index entries: ______________________________

   ____

Note: Answers to exercises 6 through 10 do not appear in appendix D of this text. They are located in the Instructor's Guide and available to faculty of educational programs.

6. Incision into upper right eyelid to drain abscess

   Code(s): ______________________________

   Index entries: ______________________________

   ____

Exercise 4.58 (Continued)

7. Repair of left blepharoptosis using superior rectus technique with fascial sling

   Code(s): ______________________________

   Index entries: ______________________________

   ____

8. Excisional transverse blepharotomy with one-quarter lid margin rotation graft

   Code(s): ______________________________

   Index entries: ______________________________

   ____

9. Ectropion repair using absorbable sutures

   Code(s): ______________________________

   Index entries: ______________________________

   ____

10. Orbitotomy of right eye to remove a piece of glass

   Code(s): ______________________________

   Index entries: ______________________________

   ____

Auditory System

The auditory system subsection includes codes for procedures performed on the inner, outer, and middle ear. (Figure 4.30 depicts the structure of the ear.) Diagnostic services such as audiometry and vestibular testing, however, are found in the medicine section of CPT. Surgical procedures are found in the code range from 69000 through 69979 and have no specific coding guidelines designated that impact code assignment.

One of the most commonly performed auditory surgical procedures is the tympanostomy for insertion of ventilating tubes for children with chronic ear infections. Under direct visualization with a microscope, the physician makes an incision in the eardrum (tympanum). The physician also may remove fluid from the middle ear. A ventilating tube is inserted through the opening in the tympanum. Coding professionals may be confused by the terminology when the physicians state that they performed a "myringotomy for insertion of ventilating tubes." For coding purposes, this describes a tympanostomy (code 69433 or 69436).

Figure 4.30. Structure of the ear

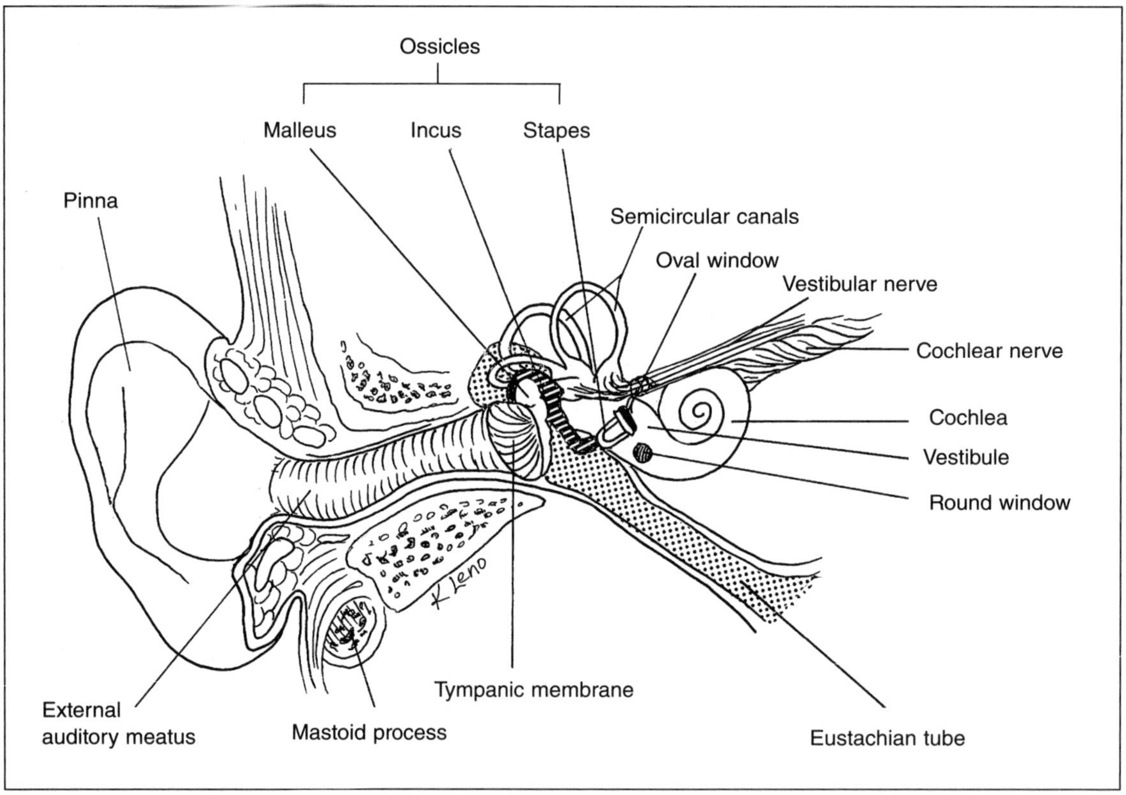

Exercise 4.59 Auditory System

Unless otherwise noted, all answers can be found in appendix D of this book. Answers to selected exercises are located in the Instructor's Guide and available only to faculty of educational programs.

Operative Report

Preoperative Diagnosis:	Bilateral otitis media
Postoperative Diagnosis:	Same
Procedure:	Bilateral myringotomy with tubes

The patient was brought to the operating room, placed in a supine position, and given a general anesthesia. Myringotomies were performed bilaterally in the anterior-superior quadrant of each tympanic membrane. The left middle ear cavity contained a mucopurulent material; the right middle ear cavity contained a thick mucoid material. Tympanostomy tubes were placed bilaterally without difficulty. The patient tolerated the procedure well and was discharged to the recovery area.

Assign appropriate CPT code(s) for the preceding procedure and indicate the index entries that were used to identify the codes. Assign only CPT surgical codes (no E/M codes) and append any applicable modifiers.

1. Code(s): ______________________________

   Index entries: ______________________________

   ____

Exercise 4.60 Auditory System Review

Unless otherwise noted, all answers can be found in appendix D of this book. Answers to selected exercises are located in the Instructor's Guide and available only to faculty of educational programs.

Assign appropriate CPT code(s) for the following procedures and indicate the index entries that were used to identify the codes. Assign only CPT surgical codes (no E/M codes) and append any applicable modifiers.

1. Labyrinthectomy with mastoidectomy

   Code(s): ______________________________

   Index entries: ______________________________

   ____

2. Under general anesthesia, a surgeon removes a pebble from the left external auditory canal of a 1-year-old child.

   Code(s): ______________________________

   Index entries: ______________________________

   ____

3. Tympanoplasty with mastoidotomy and ossicular chain reconstruction

   Code(s): ______________________________

   Index entries: ______________________________

   ____

4. Drainage of external left ear hematoma requiring an extensive amount of time

   Code(s): ______________________________

   Index entries: ______________________________

   ____

5. Physician inflates blocked eustachian tube by increasing air pressure in nasopharynx.

   Code(s): ______________________________

   Index entries: ______________________________

   ____

Exercise 4.61 Chapter 4 Review: Coding for Facility

Unless otherwise noted, all answers can be found in appendix D of this book. Answers to selected exercises are located in the Instructor's Guide and available only to faculty of educational programs.

Assume that the following procedures were performed in either the outpatient department or the emergency department of Central Hospital. Assign the appropriate CPT code(s) and modifiers that the hospital would submit to payers for reimbursement. Also indicate the index entries you used to find the codes.

1. Incision and drainage of complicated parotid gland abscess

   Code(s): ______________________________

   Index entries: ______________________________

   ____

2. Bilateral tympanostomy with insertion of ventilating tube, performed under general anesthesia

   Code(s): ______________________________

   Index entries: ______________________________

   ____

3. Colposcopy of cervix with biopsy

   Code(s): ______________________________

   Index entries: ______________________________

   ____

4. Cystourethroscopy with fulguration of bladder tumor (1.0 cm)

   Code(s): ______________________________

   Index entries: ______________________________

   ____

5. Open incisional biopsy of left breast (Medicare patient)

   Code(s): ______________________________

   Index entries: ______________________________

   ____

6. Intermediate wound repair of a 2-cm laceration of the face

   Code(s): ______________________________

   Index entries: ______________________________

   ____

(Continued on next page)

Exercise 4.61 (Continued)

7. Closed treatment of distal phalangeal fracture of right thumb without manipulation

   Code(s): ____________________

   Index entries: ____________________

   ____

8. Direct laryngoscopy with biopsy and use of operating microscope

   Code(s): ____________________

   Index entries: ____________________

   ____

9. Placement of central venous catheter via basilic vein in 50-year-old patient for hemodialysis

   Code(s): ____________________

   Index entries: ____________________

   ____

10. Flexible sigmoidoscopy with removal of polyp by hot biopsy forceps

   Code(s): ____________________

   Index entries: ____________________

   ____

Note: Answers to exercises 11 through 20 do not appear in appendix D of this text. They are located in the Instructor's Guide and available to faculty of educational programs.

11. Repair of bilateral, strangulated, initial inguinal hernia in a 10-year-old patient

   Code(s): ____________________

   Index entries: ____________________

   ____

12. Arthroscopy of the left elbow with removal of loose body

   Code(s): ____________________

   Index entries: ____________________

   ____

13. Drainage of abscess of left thumb and second finger

   Code(s): ____________________

   Index entries: ____________________

   ____

Exercise 4.61 (Continued)

14. Laminectomy for excision of thoracic extradural cyst

    Code(s): ____________________

    Index entries: ____________________

    ____

15. Repair of oval window fistula

    Code(s): ____________________

    Index entries: ____________________

    ____

16. Capsulotomy of midfoot with tendon lengthening

    Code(s): ____________________

    Index entries: ____________________

    ____

17. Excision of 2-mm papilloma of the penis

    Code(s): ____________________

    Index entries: ____________________

    ____

18. Shaving of 0.5-cm epidermal lesion of the left foot

    Code(s): ____________________

    Index entries: ____________________

    ____

19. Physician removes a small amount of amniotic fluid from the OB patient.

    Code(s): ____________________

    Index entries: ____________________

    ____

20. Hysteroscopy with removal of polyp

    Code(s): ____________________

    Index entries: ____________________

    ____

Exercise 4.62 Chapter 4 Review: Coding for Physician Services

Unless otherwise noted, all answers can be found in appendix D of this book. Answers to selected exercises are located in the Instructor's Guide and available only to faculty of educational programs.

Assume that the following procedures were performed by physicians in the surgery department of a hospital. Assign the appropriate CPT codes and modifiers for the physician services only. Also indicate which index entries you used to find the codes.

1. Craniectomy for excision of cerebellopontine angle tumor, a complex procedure that required the services of two neurosurgeons

   Code(s) for physician #1: ______________________

   Code(s) for physician #2: ______________________

   Index entries: ______________________

   ____

2. Induced abortion by dilation and curettage

   Code(s): ______________________

   Index entries: ______________________

   ____

3. Diagnostic and surgical arthroscopy of the right shoulder with complete synovectomy

   Code(s): ______________________

   Index entries: ______________________

   ____

4. Insertion of permanent cardiac pacemaker and atrial and ventricular transvenous electrodes; physician #1 provided the postoperative management for this patient; physician #2 provided the preoperative management and performed the procedure at a university hospital

   Code(s) for physician #1: ______________________

   Code(s) for physician #2: ______________________

   Index entries: ______________________

   ____

5. Endoscopic retrograde cholangiopancreatography (ERCP) with endoscopic retrograde insertion of tube into pancreatic duct

   Code(s): ______________________

   Index entries: ______________________

   ____

Exercise 4.62 (Continued)

Note: Answers to exercises 6–11 are located in the Instructor's Guide and available to faculty of educational programs.

6. Laparoscopy with removal of tubes and ovaries; the operative report indicates that the procedure was extremely difficult to perform and took two hours longer to complete than usual

   Code(s): ______________________________

   Index entries: ______________________________

   ____

7. Bilateral probing of lower nasolacrimal ducts with irrigation under general anesthesia

   Code(s): ______________________________

   Index entries: ______________________________

   ____

8. Bilateral sinus endoscopy with maxillary antrostomy and removal of maxillary sinus tissue

   Code(s): ______________________________

   Index entries: ______________________________

   ____

9. Total abdominal colectomy with continent ileostomy

   Code(s): ______________________________

   Index entries: ______________________________

   ____

10. Closed treatment of distal fibular fracture without manipulation; the patient was in the postoperative period for an arthroscopy of the shoulder performed 2 weeks ago; the same physician performed both surgeries

    Code(s): ______________________________

    Index entries: ______________________________

    ____

11. Microdermabrasion of the epidermis to remove tattoo of arm

    Code(s): ______________________________

    Index entries: ______________________________

    ____

Chapter 5
Radiology

The radiology section of CPT includes the following subsections:

Subsection	Code Range
Diagnostic Radiology (Diagnostic Imaging)	70010–76499
Diagnostic Ultrasound	76506–76999
Radiologic Guidance	77001–77032
Breast, Mammography	77051–77059
Bone/Joint Studies	77071–77084
Radiation Oncology	77261–77799
Nuclear Medicine	78000–79999

It is important to understand the differences between the subsections and not to assign codes based on the area of the body being treated or studied. Some of the subsections contain instructions that are unique to them, and notes are included throughout each subsection to explain important instructions, such as the definitions of A-mode, M-mode, or B-scan ultrasounds.

Many of the conventions and guidelines discussed in earlier chapters of *Basic Current Procedural Terminology and HCPCS Coding* also apply to this chapter. Specific conventions pertinent to the radiology section are included in this chapter.

Links to the Society of Interventional Radiology and MedLearn that are pertinent to the discussion in this chapter are located in the Web resources at the back of this book.

Hospital Billing and Radiology Code Reporting

When reporting radiological procedures, most hospitals use a computer program called a chargemaster. The chargemaster contain a computer-generated list of CPT/HCPCS codes, abbreviated definition descriptions, charges, and sometimes other information used by any given hospital, physician office, or clinic. (See table 5.1 for an example excerpt from a radiology chargemaster.) In addition, the file contains a revenue code (defined by CMS), which is assigned to each procedure, service, or supply to indicate the location or type of service provided to a patient. For example, in table 5.1, revenue code 320 describes Radiology-Diagnostic-General Classification. Revenue code 324 identifies Radiology-Diagnostic-Chest X-ray. Thus, whenever a radiologic procedure is ordered and performed, the computer automatically assigns the CPT code and applies the charge from the requisition form the physician used to order the service.

Table 5.1. Example excerpt from radiology chargemaster

Charge Seq Number	Revenue Center*		Description	CPT Code
	DEPT 721	RADIOLOGY—DIAGNOSTIC		
1700004 999	320	X RAY	NO CHARGE	
1701101 999	320	X RAY	MANDIBLE	70110
1701309 999	320	X RAY	MASTOIDS STENVERS LAWS	70130
1701341 999	320	X RAY	INT AUD CANAL	70134
1701341 999	320	X RAY	FACIAL BONES	70150
1701606 999	320	X RAY	NASAL BONES	70160
1701903 999	320	X RAY	OPTIC FORAMINA	70190
1702000 999	320	X RAY	ORBITS	70200
1702208 999	320	X RAY	SINUSES	70220
1702406 999	320	X RAY	SELLA TURCICA	70240
1702604 910	320	X RAY	SKULL	70260
1703305 999	320	X RAY	TEMPMAND JT BI	70330
1703552 999	320	X RAY	DENTAL PANOREX	70355
1703602 999	320	X RAY	NECK FOR SOFT TISSUE	70360
1703800 999	320	X RAY	SALIVARY GLAND	70380
1710102 910	324	X RAY	CHEST PA	71010

*73010320 = MDLAB, 910 = ER, 920 = OUTP, 921 = OUTP, 999 = INP

Assigning CPT codes for routine services (e.g. chest x-ray, EKG, CBC) is systematic and does not require decision making from the coding professional. The chargemaster is known by several other names, including charge description master (CDM), standard charge file, service item master, or charge compendium. In most cases, each ancillary department is responsible for maintaining its codes in the chargemaster. Requests for input, however, often are made to health information management (HIM) departments.

Periodic review of these systems is mandatory for correct reimbursement and data quality control. The wrong code attached to a procedure can result in significant revenue loss or overpayment for a hospital or large clinic. Inappropriate unbundling of codes can result in fraudulent charges to insurance companies, so the accuracy of any automated coding via a chargemaster program is an important data quality concern.

Physician Billing

When a radiology service is performed in a physician's office or a freestanding center owned by the radiologist, the Medicare Part B carrier will pay the radiologist for both the professional component (PC) and the technical component (TC). Payment for the technical component covers the cost for personnel, equipment, and supplies involved in the nonphysician portion of the services. Because many physicians do not have radiological equipment in their offices, they usually refer patients who need radiological procedures to the local hospital or a freestanding radiological center. In such cases, coding and billing professionals for referring physicians do not assign radiology codes unless the physicians or facilities provide supervision and interpretation. Usually, radiological procedures are reported by radiologists associated with a hospital, clinic, or freestanding radiology center. Individuals providing billing services for radiologists and radiation oncologists must have a thorough understanding of radiological procedures, ultrasound procedures, nuclear medicine procedures, and radiation therapy.

In some cases, hospitals employ radiologists and report both technical and professional components of procedures or, when available, CPT codes representing complete procedures or CPT codes without modifiers. Revisions have been made to CPT that have created fewer complete procedures and more procedures where the professional and technical components are reported using separate codes. The Medicare Physician Fee Schedule database contains a list of codes that have been approved for splitting.

Radiological Supervision and Interpretation

Many codes in the radiology section of CPT include the term *radiological supervision and interpretation* in their description. These codes are used to describe the radiological portion of a procedure that two physicians often perform. In situations where one physician performs the procedure and also provides the supervision and interpretation, two codes are reported: a radiological code and a code from another section of the CPT codebook, such as surgery. This is often referred to as a complete procedure.

Example: Unilateral lymphangiography of the extremity—complete procedure. The physician submits codes 75801 and 38790. Code 75801 identifies the radiological procedure, including interpretation of the results, and code 38790 identifies the injection provided for the lymphangiography.

It should be noted that the radiological supervision and interpretation codes do not apply to the radiation oncology subsection.

Modifiers in the Radiology Section

A complete listing of modifiers is in appendix A of the CPT codebook. Some of the common modifiers used with the radiology section follow:

22 **Increased Procedural Services:** This modifier is intended for physician use only when the service provided is greater than that usually required for the listed procedure. The CPT codebook states that modifier 22 may be reported with computerized tomography codes when additional slices are required or when a more detailed examination is necessary.

26 **Professional Component:** In circumstances where a radiological procedure includes both a physician (professional) component and a technical component, modifier 26 may be reported to identify the physician (professional) component. The professional component includes supervising the procedure, reading and interpreting the results, and documenting the interpretation in a report. This service can be provided by the physician who ordered the procedure or by the radiologist on staff at the hospital or freestanding radiology clinic. The technical component includes performance of the actual procedure and expenses for supplies and equipment. Usually, this service is provided by a radiologic technician at a hospital or a freestanding radiology clinic. The physician reports the professional component by attaching modifier 26 to the appropriate radiologic procedure. The freestanding radiology clinic reports the technical component by attaching modifier TC (technical component) to the same procedure. Modifier TC is a Level II HCPCS modifier that may not be recognized by all payers.

Example: Code 74220, Radiologic examination of the esophagus. The physician should report 74220–26, and the clinic should report 74220–TC.

When reporting a code that includes "radiologic supervision and interpretation" in the description, modifier 26 should not be appended to the procedure code. Because the radiologic supervision and interpretation code already describes the professional component, the modifier is unnecessary.

Example: Cervical myelography with the physician providing only the supervision and interpretation of this procedure. The physician should report as follows: 72240, Myelography, cervical, radiological supervision and interpretation.

In this example, modifier 26 is inappropriate because the descriptor for code 72240 already indicates that the physician provided only supervision and interpretation of the procedure.

51 **Multiple Procedures:** Modifier 51 (for physician use only) may be reported to identify that multiple radiological procedures were performed on the same day or during the same radiological episode by the same provider. The first procedure listed should identify the major procedure or the one that is most resource intensive.

52 **Reduced Services:** Modifier 52 may be reported by hospitals or physicians to indicate that a radiological procedure has been partially reduced or eliminated at the discretion of the physician.

The CPT codebook states that modifier 52 may be reported with computerized tomography codes for a limited study or a follow-up study.

53 **Discontinued Procedure:** Modifier 53 is appropriate in circumstances where the physician elected to terminate or discontinue a diagnostic procedure, usually because of risk to the patient's well-being. Modifier 73 or 74 would be used for hospital reporting.

Example: A patient planned to have urography with KUB, which would be reported with code 74400. Because the patient fainted during the procedure, it was discontinued before completion. The physician should report 74400–53.

59 **Distinct Procedural Services:** Modifier 59 may be used by both hospitals and physicians to identify that a procedure or service was distinct or independent from other services provided on the same day. Modifier 59 is appropriate for procedures that have been performed together because of specific circumstances, although they usually are not integral to one another or not performed together.

A patient is seen in radiology for a single cervical spine x-ray (72020) due to an injury. Later in the day, the patient returns complaining of severe pain. The physician orders a complete examination (72052). Codes 72020 and 72052–59 should be reported.

GH **Diagnostic Mammogram Converted from Screening Mammogram on the Same Day**

RT/LT Modifiers: Modifiers RT and LT are Level II HCPCS modifiers that should be reported when bilateral radiological procedures are performed. To report these modifiers to reflect a bilateral radiological procedure, the procedure code should be assigned twice and RT attached to one code and LT to the other.

Example: 73650–RT and 73650–LT, Radiologic examination of the calcaneus with a minimum of 2 views, bilateral

Both of these modifiers apply to Medicare claims, and their use varies according to the reporting requirements of Medicaid programs and other third-party payers. The CMS guidelines for hospitals state that RT and LT are not to be used to report bilateral surgical procedures. Instead, modifier 50 is to be used because of the effect on payment.

TC **Technical Component:** HCPCS Level II Modifier that indicates only the technical component was provided.

Diagnostic Radiology (Diagnostic Imaging)

Codes 70010 through 76499 describe diagnostic radiology services and are subdivided first by anatomic site and then by specific type of procedure performed:

- *X-ray:* An x-ray is a test that uses radiation to take pictures inside the body.
- *Computed tomography (CT) scan:* The CT scan can produce detailed pictures of slices of body structures and organs. For some types of CT scans, a dye substance (ingested or introduced via IV) is used to make the structures more easily seen. For example, the dye (contrast material) can be used to check blood flow or help to visualize tumors. Combination CPT codes are provided for CT scans of the abdomen and pelvis performed during the same session. Coding professionals are to reference the table (before code 74176) that outlines the stand-alone codes when the procedures are performed during the same session.

  Example: Patient has a CT scan of the abdomen and pelvis (without contrast); the correct code assignment is 74176.

- *Magnetic resonance imaging (MRI) scan:* In this test, images are obtained with the use of high-powered magnets and radio waves.
- *Magnetic resonance angiography (MRA) scan:* This test uses a magnetic field and radio waves to provide pictures of blood vessels. In many situations, MRAs can provide information that cannot be obtained from many of the other types of tests (for example, CT scans).

These radiology procedures may be found in the alphabetic index of the CPT codebook by referencing the following main entries: x-ray, CT scan, Magnetic Resonance Imaging, and Magnetic Resonance Angiography. They also may be referenced under the specific site with a subterm identifying the specific procedure.

Contrast Material

The CPT codebook differentiates between radiologic procedures with and without contrast material. Contrast material consists of radiopaque substances that obstruct the passage of x-rays and cause the areas containing the material to appear white on the x-ray film, thus outlining the contour of body structures and permitting the identification of abnormal growths. Contrast material may be administered orally or intravenously. Examples of contrast agents include barium or Gastrografin, iohexol, iopamidol, ioxaglate, Hypaque, and Renografin. Commonly performed radiologic examinations using contrast material include barium enema, angiography, cystogram, endoscopic retrograde cholangiopancreatogram, fistulogram, intravenous pyelogram, excretory urogram, lymphangiography, oral cholecystogram, retrograde pyelogram, and voiding cystourethrogram.

CT scans also may be performed with or without contrast material. Although this radiological procedure can scan any body part, it is most helpful in evaluating the brain, lung, mediastinum, retroperitoneum, and liver.

When coverage requirements are met, reimbursement for the supply of contrast media may be obtained by reporting the appropriate HCPCS code.

MRI scans are almost equal to CT scans, although they are considered superior for scanning the brain, spinal cord, soft tissues, and adrenal and renal masses. This radiological procedure is contraindicated for patients who have metallic objects in their bodies such as pacemakers, shrapnel, cochlear implants, metallic eye fragments, and vascular clips in the central nervous system. Contrast material also can be used when performing MRI scans. Gadolinium (gadopentetate dimeglumine) is the contrast agent most often used.

Exercise 5.1 Diagnostic Radiology

Unless otherwise noted, all answers can be found in appendix D of this book. Answers to selected exercises are located in the Instructor's Guide and available only to faculty of educational programs.

Assign the appropriate codes for the following procedure(s). Append modifiers if applicable.

1. MRI of abdomen with contrast

   ____

2. CT scan of lumbar spine without contrast

   ____

3. X-ray of pelvis, AP

   ____

4. Upper GI x-ray exam with KUB

   ____

5. Cystography, three views, supervision and interpretation only

   ____

6. CT scan of the colon without contrast

   ____

7. CT scan of the abdomen and pelvis (with contrast)

   ____

Interventional Radiology

Interventional radiology is the branch of medicine that diagnoses and treats diseases using percutaneous or minimally invasive techniques with the use of imaging guidance. Assigning codes for interventional radiology requires advanced study and thorough knowledge of anatomy and physiology. Suggested references are provided in this book.

Diagnostic Ultrasound

The subsection of diagnostic ultrasound includes codes 76506 through 76999, which are subdivided by anatomic site. The diagnostic ultrasound codes can be found in the alphabetic index of the CPT codebook by referencing the main entries of Ultrasound or Echography. Diagnostic ultrasound involves the use of ultrasonic waves, or high-frequency sound waves, to visualize internal structures of the body. Ultrasounds are commonly performed for evaluation of the abdomen, the pelvis (for both gynecologic and obstetric diagnoses), and the heart.

Four types of diagnostic ultrasounds are recognized:

- *An A-mode ultrasound* is a one-dimensional ultrasonic measurement procedure.
- *An M-mode ultrasound* is a one-dimensional ultrasonic measurement procedure with movement of the trace to record amplitude and velocity of moving echo-producing structures.
- *A B-scan ultrasound* is a two-dimensional ultrasonic scanning procedure with a two-dimensional display.
- *A real-time scan* is a two-dimensional ultrasonic scanning procedure with display of both two-dimensional structure and motion with time.

The medicine section of the CPT codebook includes ultrasounds involving the following areas:

- Cerebrovascular arterial studies (93875–93893)
- Arterial studies of the extremities (93922–93931)
- Venous studies of the extremities (93965–93971)
- Visceral and penile vascular studies (93975–93982)
- Arterial-venous studies of the extremities (93990)
- Ultrasounds of the heart (echocardiography) (93303–93352)

Complete vs. Limited Examination

Several CPT descriptions require the coding professional to differentiate between "complete" and "limited." For those anatomic regions that have "complete" or "limited" ultrasound codes, the elements that comprise the examination are contained in the notes preceding the codes. For example, the note referenced before CPT code 76700 describes a complete examination of the abdomen as real time scans of the liver, gallbladder, common bile duct, pancreas, spleen, kidneys, and the upper abdominal aorta and inferior vena cava including any demonstrated abdominal abnormality.

Exercise 5.2 Diagnostic Ultrasound

Unless otherwise noted, all answers can be found in appendix D of this book. Answers to selected exercises are located in the Instructor's Guide and available only to faculty of educational programs.

Assign the appropriate codes for the following procedure(s). Append modifiers if applicable.

1. Saline infusion hysterosonography with color flow Doppler

   ____

2. Limited ultrasound of pregnant uterus to determine fetal position

   ____

3. Bilateral ultrasound of breasts (real time)

   ____

Radiation Oncology

The radiation oncology codes (77261–77799) describe the therapeutic use of radiation to treat diseases, especially neoplastic tumors. Radiation therapy may be used as primary therapy to treat certain types of malignancies, such as early stages of Hodgkin's disease. It also may be used:

- As adjuvant treatment in small-cell lung cancer and head and neck cancers
- As palliative treatment to alleviate pain caused by metastasis to bone
- To control bleeding caused by gynecologic malignancies
- To relieve obstruction and compression from advanced lung cancer, brain lesions, and spinal cord lesions

The most common type of radiation used in the treatment is electromagnetic radiation with x-rays and gamma rays. X-rays are photons generated inside a machine; gamma rays are photons emitted from a radioactive source. Radiation is measured in units known as the radiation-absorbed dose (rad) or the gray (Gy). The Gy is equal to 100 rad.

The delivery of radiation therapy may be external or internal. *External* radiation therapy involves delivery of a beam of ionizing radiation from an external source through the patient's skin toward the tumor region. *Internal* radiation therapy, also known as brachytherapy, involves applying a radioactive material inside the patient or in close proximity. This material may be contained in various types of devices, including tubes, needles, wires, seeds, and other small containers. Common radioactive materials used in brachytherapy include radium-226, cobalt-60, cesium-137, and iodine-125. Three types of brachytherapy are recognized in the CPT codebook:

- *Interstitial brachytherapy* involves placing a radiation source directly into tissues.
- *Intracavitary (intraluminal) brachytherapy* utilizes radiation source(s) placed in special devices and then implanted in body cavities, such as vagina, uterus, bronchus, or esophagus. Code selection is based on the number of radioactive sources used to produce the localized dose of radiation.

- *Surface application brachytherapy* uses radioactive material that is contained on the surface of a plaque or mold and applied directly or close to the surface of the patient.

Radiation Consultation (Clinical Management), Clinical Treatment Planning, and Radiation Treatment Delivery

Radiation oncology involves a variety of specialized planning, management, and treatment delivery services that physicians provide to patients throughout the course of radiation therapy. Accurate coding in these areas requires careful attention to the type, level, and extent of services provided.

Consultation: Clinical Management

Radiation oncologists often provide consultative services before a treatment plan is developed for the patient. Such treatment planning consultations should be reported with the appropriate E/M, medicine, or surgery code.

Clinical Treatment Planning

The planning that occurs before treatment involves a complex decision-making process that includes interpretation of testing, choice of treatment modality, selection of treatment devices, and so forth. Codes for treatment planning (77261–77263), simulation-aided field setting (77280–77299), and medical radiation physics, dosimetry, treatment devices, and special services (77300–77370) often require the coding professional to distinguish between "simple," "intermediate," and "complex." The definitions for each are provided in the Notes section before the CPT codes. For example, *simple* therapeutic radiology treatment planning requires a single treatment area of interest encompassed in a single port or simple parallel opposed ports with simple or no blocking.

Stereotactic Radiation Treatment

Stereotactic radiotherapy (77371–77373) uses multiple small fractions of radiation as opposed to one large dose. Stereotactic radiotherapy is frequently used to treat tumors in the brain as well as other parts of the body.

Radiation Treatment Delivery

Codes 77401 through 77425 describe the technical component of delivering the radiation treatment, as well as the various energy levels administered. To assign the appropriate code, the following information is needed:

- Number of treatment areas involved
- Number of ports involved
- Number of shielding blocks used
- Total million electron volts (MeV) administered

New in CPT 2012 are two codes associated with delivery of intraoperative radiation treatment (77424–77425).

Neutron Beam Treatment Delivery

This code selection (77422–77423) identifies a specialized form of radiation therapy that is often used to treat inoperable tumors or tumors that are resistant to other types of conventional radiation therapy.

Radiation Treatment Management

The actual management of radiation treatment services is reported in units of five fractions or treatment sessions, regardless of the actual time period in which the services are furnished. The services need not be furnished on consecutive days. Multiple fractions representing two or more treatment sessions furnished on the same day may be counted as long as there has been a distinct break in therapy sessions and the fractions are of the character usually furnished on different days.

Hyperthermia Treatment

Hyperthermia involves the use of heat to raise the temperature of a specific area of the body to increase cell metabolism and destroy cancer cells. Usually, it is performed as an adjunct to radiation therapy or chemotherapy. The hyperthermia codes (77600–77615) in the CPT codebook include external, interstitial, and intracavitary treatment. If administered at the same time, radiation therapy should be reported separately.

Codes 77600 through 77615 include management during the hyperthermia treatment and follow-up care for three months after completion.

Clinical Brachytherapy

Clinical brachytherapy uses natural or manufactured radioactive elements that are applied in or around a particular treatment field. A therapeutic radiologist supervises the use of radioactive elements and interprets appropriate dosage. When the services of a surgeon are needed, modifiers 66 or 62 may be reported to ensure that both physicians are reimbursed.

Codes 77750 through 77799 include admission to the hospital and daily visits by the physician. The codes differentiate between interstitial and intracavitary brachytherapy, and are subdivided further to identify the number of sources/ribbons applied: simple, intermediate, or complex. The CPT codebook includes definitions for each of these levels. (In the context of clinical brachytherapy, the term *sources* refers to intracavitary or permanent interstitial placement of radioactive material, and the term *ribbons* refers to temporary interstitial placement of radioactive material.)

Nuclear Medicine

Nuclear medicine involves the administration of radioisotopes, which are radioactive elements that diagnose diseases. The radioactive isotope deteriorates spontaneously and emits gamma rays from inside the body that enable the physician to view internal abnormalities. Some radioisotopes are selectively absorbed by tumors or specific organs in the body, making them visible on the scan.

Nuclear medicine procedures are organized in codes 78000 through 79999 according to body systems, such as the cardiovascular system. The provision of radium or other radioelements is not included in the services listed in this section. These procedures may be found in the alphabetic index of the CPT codebook by referencing Nuclear Imaging or Nuclear Medicine.

Some of the more common diagnostic nuclear medicine scans include the following:

- *Bone scans* are performed as part of metastatic workups to identify infections such as osteomyelitis, to evaluate hip prostheses, to distinguish pathologic fractures from traumatic fractures, and to evaluate delayed union of fractures.

- *Cardiac scans* are performed for diagnosis of myocardial infarction, stress testing, ejection fraction, measurement of cardiac output, and diagnosis of ventricular aneurysms.

  —The thallium 201 scan examines myocardial perfusion, with normal myocardium appearing as "hot" and ischemic or infarcted areas appearing as "cold."

  —The technetium 99m pyrophosphate scan identifies recently damaged myocardial tissue and is most sensitive 24 to 72 hours after an acute myocardial infarction.

  —The technetium 99m ventriculogram scan identifies abnormal wall motion, cardiac shunts, size and function of heart chambers, cardiac output, and ejection fraction. The multigated acquisition (MUGA) scan is another form of this type of study.

- *Hepatobiliary scans,* or hydroxyiminodiacetic acid (HIDA) scans, are performed for diagnosis of biliary obstruction, acute cholecystitis, or biliary atresia.
- *Lung scans* (ventilation-perfusion [V/Q] scans) can reveal pulmonary disease, chronic obstructive pulmonary disease, and emphysema. When performed along with chest x-rays, these scans are important tools in evaluating pulmonary emboli.
- *Renal scans* are performed to evaluate the overall function of the kidneys.
- *Thyroid scans* are most commonly performed with technetium 99m pertechnetate and are useful in detecting nodules.

Exercise 5.3 Chapter 5 Review

Unless otherwise noted, all answers can be found in appendix D of this book. Answers to selected exercises are located in the Instructor's Guide and available only to faculty of educational programs.

Assign the appropriate codes for the following procedure(s). Include CPT modifiers and HCPCS Level II modifiers when applicable.

1. Radiological examination (x-ray) of the forearm, anteroposterior (AP), and lateral views. What code(s) should be submitted on the claim form if the physician provided only the supervision and interpretation (professional component) for this procedure?

   ____

2. MRI of the cervical spine with contrast material. The MRI is performed at an independent radiology facility, and the facility sends the images to an independent radiologist who will read and write a report of the findings. What code(s) should be submitted on the claim form for the radiologist to receive payment?

   ____

3. Physician performed the radiological supervision and interpretation for cystography (minimum of three views). What code(s) should be submitted?

   ____

4. Myocardial perfusion imaging tomographic (SPECT) (nuclear medicine) single study performed at rest. What code(s) should be submitted?

   ____

5. Bilateral screening mammogram. What code(s) should be submitted?

   ____

6. CT scan of the abdomen with contrast and the pelvis without contrast (same session). What code(s) should be submitted?

   ____

7. CT scan of the head with contrast material. The scan was performed at an independent radiology facility, and it was sent to an independent radiologist who reads and writes the report of the findings. What code(s) and modifier should the independent radiology facility report on the claim it submits?

   ____

8. Pelvic ultrasound, pregnant uterus. Real-time with image documentation, transvaginal. What code(s) should be submitted?

   ____

9. Radiologist provided radiological supervision and interpretation for ultrasonic guidance needle biopsy. What code(s) should be submitted?

   ____

10. Whole-body bone scan (nuclear medicine). What code(s) should be submitted?

    ____

Exercise 5.3 (Continued)

Note: Answers to exercises 11 through 25 do not appear in appendix D of this text. They are located in the Instructor's Guide and available to faculty of educational programs.

11. Barium enema with KUB (using contrast). What code(s) should be submitted?

    ____

12. SPECT liver imaging. What code(s) should be submitted?

    ____

13. Delivery of radiation therapy to single area with single port and simple blocks–13 MeV. What code(s) should be submitted?

    ____

14. Renal scan with vascular flow and function study (nuclear medicine) without pharmacologic intervention. What code(s) should be submitted?

    ____

15. Chest x-ray, two views. What code(s) should be submitted?

    ____

16. Intracavitary placement of four radioelement sources. What code(s) should be submitted?

    ____

17. Cervical myelogram (S&I). What code(s) should be submitted?

    ____

18. Retroperitoneal ultrasound, limited study. What code(s) should be submitted?

    ____

19. X-ray of the hips and pelvis in a 5-year-old, with two views. What code(s) should be submitted?

    ____

20. Gastroesophageal reflux study. What code(s) should be submitted?

    ____

Assign the appropriate CPT codes to the following reports. Assume that you are billing for the professional and technical component.

21. RENAL ULTRASOUND

    History: Pyelonephritis

    Findings: The right kidney measures 11.1 cm and left measures 11.5 Both kidneys are normal in echo texture and smooth in contour. There is no mass, calcification, or evidence of hydronephrosis. There is no perinephric fluid collection or abscess. There is no evidence of focal nephronia.

    There is a cyst in the upper pole of the right kidney. This measures just under 2 cm. It has typical ultrasound characteristics of a benign renal cyst.

    ____

(Continued on next page)

Exercise 5.3 (Continued)

22. AP PELVIS AND LEFT HIP X-RAYS

    There is generalized demineralization of the bone.

    There is an intertrochanteric fracture of the left hip with moderate angulation and displacement present. There is a free fracture fragment of the lesser trochanter.

    ____

23. PA AND LATERAL CHEST X-RAYS

    Coronary artery bypass graft changes are noted. The heart is mildly enlarged in size. The lung fields are clear, without infiltrate or effusion. Moderate spondylitic changes are noted in the thoracic spine.

    ____

24. KUB, UPPER GI X-RAY SERIES

    A preliminary KUB study reveals a large amount of fecal matter present in the colon. Staples are seen in the right upper quadrant.

    A barium swallow reveals a normal filling of the esophagus. The stomach is high and transverse in type. There is a small sliding hiatal hernia and there is small gastroesophageal reflux. The duodenal bulb fills without ulceration. The stomach empties well.

    Opinion: Small sliding hiatal hernia with intermittent gastroesophageal reflux

    ____

25. CT SCAN OF THE HEAD WITHOUT INTRAVENOUS CONTRAST

    Reveals a diffuse, moderately large area of localized atrophy involving the superiormost portion of the left parietal region. This is seen on images #14, 15, and 16. There is no extra-axial fluid collection, acute intracranial bleeding, midline shift, mass effect, or other significant abnormality.

    IMPRESSION: Localized atrophy involving the superiormost portion of the left parietal lobe as described above. This could be old or recent. Short-term interval follow-up CT scan is suggested for further evaluation.

    ____

Chapter 6

Pathology and Laboratory Services

The pathology and laboratory section of the CPT codebook includes services provided by physicians, including pathologists and technologists under the supervision of a pathologist or other physician. It includes codes for services and procedures such as organ or disease panel tests, automated multichannel tests, urinalysis, hematologic and immunologic studies, and surgical and anatomic pathologic examinations. This chapter discusses specific subsections of the pathology and laboratory section.

Subsection	**Code Range**
Organ or Disease Oriented Panels	80047–80076
Drug Testing	80100–80104
Therapeutic Drug Assays	80150–80299
Evocative/Suppression Testing	80400–80440
Consultations (Clinical Pathology)	80500–80502
Urinalysis	81000–81099
Molecular Pathology	81200-81099
Chemistry	82000–84999
Hematology and Coagulation	85002–85999
Immunology	86000–86849
Transfusion Medicine	86850–86999
Microbiology	87001–87999
Anatomic Pathology	88000–88099
Cytopathology	88104–88199
Cytogenetic Studies	88230–88299
Surgical Pathology	88300–88399
In Vivo Laboratory Procedures	88720–88749
Other Procedures	89049–89240
Reproductive Medicine Procedures	89250–89398

Alphabetic Index

Laboratory and pathology procedures/services are listed in the alphabetic index of the CPT codebook under the following main terms:

- Specific name of the test, such as urinalysis, evocative/suppression test, and fertility test

- Specific substance/specimen/sample, such as glucose, CPK, cyanide, enterovirus, bone marrow, and nasal smear
- Specific method used, such as culture, fine needle aspiration, and microbiology

Hospital Billing for Laboratory and Pathology Procedures

In the hospital setting, the chargemaster is used to automate the billing of laboratory and pathology services. (See table 6.1 for an example excerpt from a laboratory chargemaster.) As mentioned in chapter 5, the chargemaster is a computer program containing codes, abbreviated definition descriptions, charges, and possibly other information used by a given hospital. Therefore, when patients visit the outpatient department with a requisition from their physician for laboratory work, the computer automatically assigns the appropriate code and charge for that particular service. Although coding professionals are not really involved in the actual coding of these services, the health information management (HIM) department may be asked to help the laboratory and pathology department update its portion of the chargemaster.

Physician Billing

When reporting laboratory services provided by a physician, the coding professional must determine whether the physician performed the complete procedure or only a component of it. Some physician offices and physician-owned clinics have sophisticated laboratory equipment on the premises that enables the physicians to provide complete laboratory testing. A complete test would involve ordering the test, obtaining the sample (for example, blood or urine), handling the specimen, performing the actual test or procedure, and analyzing and interpreting the results. However, most physicians typically send the sample to a freestanding or hospital-based laboratory for testing and analysis. In this instance, the physician may report only the collection and handling of the blood sample or specimen.

Physicians also may send the patient for laboratory testing to a local hospital, where the sample or specimen is taken, the test or procedure is performed, and the results are analyzed and interpreted. The physician may seek reimbursement for these tests from some insurance

Table 6.1. Excerpt from a laboratory chargemaster in numeric order by department

Charge Seq Number	Revenue Center*	Description	CPT Code
		DEPT 703 CHEMISTRY	
2120053 320	301	HEPATITIS B CORE HBcAb	86704
2120053 910	301	HEPATITIS B CORE IgM antibody	86705
2120103 320	301	ELECTROLYTES PROFILE I	80051
2120111 999	301	BASIC METABOLIC PANEL	80048
2120129 320	301	GLUCOSE FASTING	82947
2120137 320	301	ACETONE SERUM	82009
2120145 320	301	GLUCOSE 1HR PP	82950
2120152 999	301	HDL CHOLESTEROL	83718
2120186 999	301	UREA NITROGEN	84540

*320 = MDLAB, 999 = INP

plans when the tests are purchased from a reference laboratory or a hospital acting as a reference laboratory. Medicare, however, does not allow any provider who does not perform the test to bill for it. The reporting of laboratory tests depends on the organizations involved and the health plan guidelines applicable to the patient.

Example: Dr. Reynolds performed a bone marrow needle biopsy in an oncology clinic and sent the specimen to a pathologist for review and interpretation. Dr. Reynolds reports 38221 for the actual biopsy of the bone marrow, and the pathologist reports 88305 for the review and interpretation of the specimen. If Dr. Reynolds pays the pathologist for the interpretation, he may report both codes, depending on the guidelines of the health plan involved.

Quantitative and Qualitative Studies

Throughout the laboratory and pathology section of the CPT codebook, code descriptions state whether the test performed is quantitative or qualitative in nature. *Qualitative* screening refers to tests that detect the presence of a particular analyte, constituent, or condition. Typically, qualitative studies are performed to determine whether a particular substance is present in the sample being evaluated. In contrast, *quantitative* studies provide results expressing specific numerical amounts of an analyte in a specimen. Usually, these tests are performed after a qualitative study to identify the specific amount of a particular substance in the sample.

Modifiers in the Laboratory Section

Because most of the commonly used modifiers in the pathology and laboratory section have been discussed in earlier chapters, only a brief summary of each is offered here.

22 **Increased Procedural Services:** This modifier is intended for use by physicians when the service provided is greater than the one usually required for the listed procedure.

26 **Professional Component:** In circumstances where a laboratory or pathology procedure includes both a physician (professional) component and a technical component, modifier 26 can be reported to identify the physician component.

32 **Mandated Services:** Modifier 32 may be reported when a group such as a third-party payer or a PRO mandates a service.

52 **Reduced Services:** Modifier 52 may be reported by both hospitals and physicians to indicate that a laboratory or pathology procedure was partially reduced or eliminated at the discretion of the physician.

53 **Discontinued Procedure:** Modifier 53 may be reported by physicians only to indicate that the physician elected to terminate a procedure due to circumstances that put the patient's well-being at risk.

59 **Distinct Procedural Service:** Modifier 59 may be used by both hospitals and physicians to identify that a procedure or service was distinct or independent from other services provided on the same day. This modifier may be used when procedures are performed together because of specific circumstances, even though they usually are not.

90 **Reference (Outside) Laboratory:** Modifier 90 may be reported by physicians to indicate performance of the test by a party other than the treating or reporting physician.

91 **Repeat Clinical Diagnostic Laboratory Test:** Modifier 91 shows the need to repeat the same laboratory test on the same day to obtain multiple test results. It may be used by both hospitals and physicians. It is not to be used to confirm initial results due to testing problems with specimens or equipment or for any reason when a normal one-time reportable result is all that is required. In addition, it is inappropriate for tests where codes describe a series of test results, such as with glucose tolerance or evocative suppression testing.

Example: Dr. Reynolds performed a venipuncture to obtain a blood sample for a lipid panel. He prepared the sample for transport and had it sent to an outside laboratory for testing, analysis, and interpretation. Dr. Reynolds should report 80061–90 to describe the laboratory test with the interpretation and analysis being performed at an off-site laboratory, along with code 36415 for the venipuncture. If this were a Medicare patient, HCPCS code G0001 would be used to report the venipuncture and the off-site laboratory would report code 80061 for the lipid panel.

92 **Alternative Laboratory Platform Testing:** This modifier describes when laboratory testing is being performed using a kit or transportable instrument that wholly or in part consists of a single use, disposable analytical chamber. The service may be appended with use of modifier 92 appended to the codes (HIV testing 86701–86703 and 87389).

Organ- or Disease-Oriented Panels

The organ- or disease-oriented panels describe the laboratory procedures performed most commonly for specific diseases, such as hepatitis and arthritis, or for specific organs, such as thyroid and hepatic function. All the tests listed in a panel must be performed for that code to be reported. When additional tests are performed that are not part of that particular panel, the codes describing those tests also must be reported. When some, but not all, of the tests in the panel are performed, the individual CPT codes should be reported, rather than the panel code. The introductory section of the Organ- or Disease-Oriented Panels subsection states that coders should not report multiple panel codes that include any of the same constituent tests performed from the same patient collection. In the index, reference the main term Organ for a list of the panels.

Example: Code 80051 describes an electrolyte panel and includes the following tests: carbon dioxide, chloride, potassium, and sodium. For code 80051 to be reported, all four tests must be performed. If the carbon dioxide test is omitted, separate codes must be assigned for the remaining tests: chloride (82435), potassium (84132), and sodium (84295). Code 80051 should not be reported.

If a glucose test is performed in addition to the electrolyte panel, a separate code is reported for the glucose test (82947), along with the electrolyte panel (80051).

Evocative/Suppression Testing

The codes used for evocative/suppression testing (80400–80440) allow the physician to determine a baseline and the effects on the body after evocative or suppressive agents are administered. In reviewing the codes in this series, it should be noted that the description for each panel identifies the type of test(s) included in that panel and the number of times a specific test must be performed.

Example: Code 80420, Dexamethasone suppression panel, 48-hour. This panel must include:
Free cortisol, urine (82530 × 2)
Cortisol (82533 × 2)
Volume measurement for timed collection (81050 × 2)

Physician attendance and monitoring during the test should be reported with the appropriate E/M services code, as well as the prolonged physician care codes, if they apply.

Overview of Urinalysis and Chemistry Subsections

A variety of tests can be found in the urinalysis and chemistry subsections. Urinalysis tests are performed from a urine sample. Chemistry tests can be performed on several types of specimens, such as urine, blood, sputum, and feces. For this subsection of CPT, accurate coding requires identification of the specific tests performed. In some cases, the codes differentiate between qualitative/quantitative and automated versus nonautomated.

Molecular Pathology (81200–81408)

New in CPT 2012 is a subsection related to procedures that aid in the discovery of disease-associated genes. Technological advances have permitted the identification of molecular mechanisms of numerous diseases.

Chemistry

This series of codes (82000–84999) is used to report individual chemistry tests that are not performed as part of the automated organ- or disease-oriented panels (80047–80076). Unless otherwise noted in the code description, these tests are quantitative in nature.

Example: Patient was seen in the laboratory department and the calcium level test was performed. Results: total calcium: 82310

Hematology and Coagulation

The codes in the hematology and coagulation subsection (85002–85999) are used to report hematological procedures, such as complete blood count (CBC), and coagulation procedures, such as clotting factor and prothrombin time.

To assign the appropriate code, careful attention must be paid to the specific type of procedure performed. Collaboration with the medical laboratory director or technician is helpful in ensuring that CPT codes are correct and consistent with the equipment available and the actual test performed.

Surgical Pathology

In surgical pathology coding (88300–88399), the unit of service is known as the specimen. The CPT codebook defines a specimen as tissue or tissues submitted for individual and separate attention, requiring individual examination and pathologic diagnosis. Codes are differentiated by six levels. Level I (88300) identifies the gross examination of tissue only. Levels II through VI (88302–88309) refer to the gross and microscopic examination of tissue. Selection of a level between II and VI is made based on the type of specimen submitted. When two or more specimens are obtained from one patient, separate codes identifying the appropriate level for each should be reported.

Example #1: Gross examination of a gallstone. The pathologist reports code 88300.

Example #2: Gross and microscopic examination of a pituitary adenoma. The pathologist reports code 88305.

Example #3: Gross and microscopic examination of two separate colon polyps. The pathologist reports codes 88305 and 88305 to identify examination of two separate specimens.

It should be noted that codes 88300 through 88309 include the accession or acquisition, examination, and reporting of a specimen.

Exercise 6.1 Chapter 6 Review

Unless otherwise noted, all answers can be found in appendix D of this book. Answers to selected exercises are located in the Instructor's Guide and available only to faculty of educational programs.

Assign the appropriate codes for the following pathology and laboratory procedures.

1. Gross and pathologic examination of transurethral resection of the prostate

   ____

2. Natriuretic peptide

   ____

3. ACTH stimulation panel for 21-hydroxylase deficiency

   ____

4. Automated urinalysis (dip stick), without microscopy

   ____

5. Reticulated platelet assay

   ____

6. Gross and microscopic examination of left mastectomy with regional lymph nodes

   ____

7. Candida skin test

   ____

8. Confirmatory test for HTLV antibody

   ____

Exercise 6.1 (Continued)

9. The following tests were performed as a group from one blood sample: (lipid panel) total serum cholesterol, high-density lipoprotein and triglycerides; (electrolyte panel) carbon dioxide, chloride, potassium, and sodium.

____

10. Quantitative testing (therapeutic drug assay) of theophylline level

____

Note: Answers to exercises 11 through 15 do not appear in appendix D of this text. They are located in the Instructor's Guide and available to faculty of educational programs.

11. Evaluation of blood gases—pH, pCO_2, pO_2, CO_2, and HCO_3

____

12. Hepatitis B surface antibody (HBsAb)

____

13. Partial thromboplastin time (PTT) of whole blood and prothrombin time (PT)

____

14. Gross and microscopic autopsy, including brain and spinal cord

____

15. Pathology consultation provided during surgery with frozen section of single specimen

____

Chapter 7

Evaluation and Management Services

The section dedicated to evaluation and management (E/M) services was added to the CPT codebook in 1992. The E/M codes are designed to classify the cognitive services provided by physicians during hospital and office visits, skilled nursing facility (SNF) visits, and consultations. The various levels of the E/M codes describe the wide variety of skills and the amount of effort, time, responsibility, and medical knowledge that physicians dedicate to the prevention, diagnosis, and treatment of illnesses and injuries as well as the promotion of optimal health. Healthcare facilities such as hospitals also report E/M codes to designate encounters or visits for outpatient services.

In claims processing for physicians, E/M codes are reported to document the professional services provided to patients. The level of medical decision making is a key factor in the selection of appropriate E/M codes, but the level of decision making is sometimes difficult to quantify in documentation. Generally, it is preferable that physicians select E/M codes. Coding professionals can then validate and verify the physicians' code selections according to the documentation guidelines developed jointly by the American Medical Association (AMA) and the Centers for Medicare and Medicaid Services (CMS).

Assignment of an E/M code for hospital services is required in most of the prospective payment systems developed by third-party payers, such as ambulatory payment group (APG) or ambulatory payment classification (APC) systems. E/M code assignment helps distinguish medical services from surgical services when assigning patients to a particular payment group. It also facilitates data collection by counting patients rather than services for outpatient reporting because one patient may have a number of outpatient services during a single visit. Under the prospective payment system, CMS instructed hospitals to develop their own method for assignment of the facility E/M codes.

CMS and the American Academy of Family Physicians Web sites provide additional information pertinent to E/M coding. (See appendix A of this workbook for a list of relevant Web sites.)

Classification of the Evaluation and Management Services

The E/M services section of CPT is divided into broad subsections that are further divided into subcategories. The E/M subsections are outlined below:

Office or Other Outpatient Services	99201–99215
Hospital Observation Services	99217–99226

Hospital Inpatient Services	99221–99239
Consultations	99241–99255
Emergency Department Services	99281–99288
Critical Care Services	99291–99292
Nursing Facility Services	99304–99318
Domiciliary, Rest Home or Custodial Care Services	99324–99337
Domiciliary, Rest Home or Home Care Plan Oversight Services	99339–99340
Home Services	99341–99350
Prolonged Services	99354–99360
Case Management Services	99363–99368
Care Plan Oversight Services	99374–99380
Preventive Medicine Services	99381–99429
Non Face–to–Face Physician Services	99441–99444
Special Evaluation and Management Services	99450–99456
Newborn Care Services	99460–99465
Inpatient Neonatal Intensive Care Services and Pediatric and Neonatal Critical Care Services	99466–99480
Other Evaluation and Management Services	99499

Format of Evaluation and Management Codes

The basic format of the E/M service codes followed in most of the categories in the section consists of five elements:

1. A unique code number beginning with 99
2. The place or type of service (for example, physician office or other outpatient service; initial or subsequent hospital care)
3. The extent or level of service (for example, detailed history and detailed examination)
4. The nature of the presenting problem (for example, moderate severity)
5. The amount of time typically required to provide a service

Documentation Guidelines for Evaluation and Management Services

Documentation is the basis for all coding, including E/M services. In the fall of 1994, the AMA and CMS developed documentation guidelines for E/M reporting in an effort to clarify code assignment for both physicians and claims reviewers. These guidelines were implemented in 1995.

In 1997, CMS and the AMA collaborated again on a revised edition of the guidelines that includes specific elements that should be performed and documented for general multisystem and selected single-specialty examinations. However, the 1997 revised version did not replace the 1995 documentation guidelines. Physicians may use either set of guidelines, whichever is more advantageous to the individual physician. (See appendix B of this workbook, which includes an excerpt from the 1997 documentation guidelines for E/M. A complete set of the 1995 and

1997 documentation guidelines is available on the CMS Web site: http://www.cms.hhs.gov/MLNEdWebGuide/25_EMDOC.asp.)

Code Assignment for Evaluation and Management Services

Before an E/M service code can be assigned, the coding professional should review the documentation and answer three groups of questions:

- *What type of service did the patient receive? Was the encounter an initial or a subsequent episode of care? Did the patient receive a critical care service?*
- *Where was the service provided? A physician's office or clinic? A hospital inpatient or outpatient department? Observation unit? An emergency department? A nursing facility or rehabilitation unit?*
- *Was the recipient of the service a new patient or one of the physician's established patients?*

The following subsections describe the factors that should be considered in determining code assignments for E/M services.

New or Established Patient

Some of the E/M categories provide separate code ranges to identify new and established patients:

Office or Other Outpatient Services New patient range is 99201–99205	99201–99215
Domiciliary, Rest Home, or Custodial Care Services New patient range is 99324–99328	99324–99337
Home Services New patient range is 99341–99345	99341–99350
Preventive Medicine Services New patient range is 99381–99387	99381–99397

In this context, a patient who has not received any professional services from the physician (or another physician of the exact same specialty and subspecialty who belongs to the same group practice) within the past three years is considered a *new patient.* Professional services are those face-to-face services rendered by a physician and reported by a specific CPT code or codes. An *established patient* is a patient who has received professional services from the physician (or another physician of the exact same specialty and subspecialty who belongs to the same group practice) within the past three years. In the E/M Services Guidelines, a decision tree is provided to aid in distinguishing between a new or established patient encounter.

Concurrent Care and Transfer of Care

The CPT codebook defines *concurrent care* as the circumstance in which more than one physician provides similar services (for example, hospital visits or consultations) to the same patient on the same day. Health plans often limit reimbursement to one physician per day unless the physicians have different specialties and the services of more than one physician are medically necessary. CMS assigns a specialty number that is used for this purpose.

Correct assignment of ICD-9-CM codes also plays an important role in billing and receiving payment for concurrent care services. The physicians involved in the concurrent care episode must identify the appropriate ICD-9-CM code for each service provided. Assigning the same ICD-9-CM code could result in one of the physicians being denied payment, usually the one who submitted the claim last.

Example: Patient is admitted to the hospital complaining of unstable angina and uncontrolled type 2 diabetes mellitus. Dr. Smith treats the patient's angina, and Dr. Reynolds follows the patient's diabetes. The following codes should be reported:

Dr. Smith: 411.1, Intermediate coronary syndrome, and the appropriate E/M level of service code from the hospital inpatient services category

Dr. Reynolds: 250.02, Diabetes mellitus, uncontrolled, and the appropriate E/M level of service code from the hospital inpatient services category

Transfer of care is the process whereby a physician who is providing management for some or all of a patient's problems relinquishes this responsibility to another physician who explicitly agrees to accept this responsibility and who, from the initial encounter, is not providing consultative services. An extended definition is found in the guidelines at the beginning of the E/M Section. In addition, all of the sections of CPT have "Coding Tip" elements disseminated throughout the book that provide guidance.

Seven Factors in Evaluation and Management Services

Three key factors and four contributing factors determine appropriate E/M code assignment. The key factors are *history, examination, and medical decision making.* The contributing factors include *counseling, coordination of care, presenting problem,* and *time.* Information about the three key factors should be documented in the patient's health record as should information pertaining to any or all of the other four factors when they apply to a case. All applicable factors must be considered in code assignment.

History, examination, and medical decision making are essential factors because they represent the amount of resources expended by a provider in rendering a service to a patient. For example, when counseling and coordination comprise more than 50 percent of a physician–patient or physician–family encounter, time is considered the controlling factor for determining the correct code.

Example: Established patient seen in the physician's office for disease management. The physician documents that 40 minutes of the 60-minute visit were devoted to counseling and coordination. With time as the controlling factor, the appropriate code assignment would be 99215.

Documentation in the health record must support code-level selection by describing the key components and the pertinent contributing factors. Physician selection of E/M codes is recommended to ensure clinical validity for service levels. Coding professionals may validate code selection with documentation and assist physicians in meeting the current guidelines for code selection. Facility use of E/M coding is usually assigned via a chargemaster, which is a computerized program that contains codes, abbreviated definition descriptions, and charges. (Chargemaster programs are discussed further in chapters 5 and 6.)

Appendix C of the CPT codebook includes a supplement of clinical examples illustrating the appropriate selection of E/M services codes for specific medical specialties. However, these examples are only guidelines, and the documentation in the health record remains the most authoritative and final source when assigning a code for a particular level of service.

The CPT codebook defines each level of E/M services by basing it on a unique combination of the three essential factors. The key elements that define E/M services, and the variation within these elements, are reflected in table 7.1.

History

The following types of histories are recognized. The level of complexity is based on the amount of information (number of elements) obtained by the physician:

- *Problem-focused:* Limited to a chief complaint and a brief history of the present illness or condition
- *Expanded problem-focused:* A chief complaint, brief history, and a problem-pertinent system review
- *Detailed:* A chief complaint, expanded history of the present illness, a system review, and one item from any of the following: past, family, or social history
- *Comprehensive:* A chief complaint, extended history of present illness, extended system review, and one item from at least two (or in some cases three, depending on the E/M category) of the following: past, family, and/or social history

Each type of history includes some or all of the following elements:

- Chief complaint
- History of present illness
- Review of systems
- Past, family, and/or social history

Chief Complaint

The chief complaint (CC) is a concise statement describing the symptom, problem, condition, diagnosis, a return visit recommended by the physician, or other factor as the reason for the visit.

Table 7.1. Key elements that define E/M services

History	Examination	Medical Decision Making
Problem-focused	Problem-focused	Straightforward
Expanded problem-focused	Expanded problem-focused	Low complexity
Detailed	Detailed	Moderate complexity
Comprehensive	Comprehensive	High complexity

History of Present Illness

The history of present illness (HPI) describes the patient's developing condition/problem from the first sign and/or symptom in chronological order, starting from the initial visit to the present. Table 7.2 reflects the elements included in the HPI.

There are two types of HPI: a brief HPI and an extended HPI. A *brief HPI* refers to the documentation of no more than one to three HPI elements. It may involve a single problem without any complicating factors or symptoms. An *extended HPI* refers to the documentation of four or more HPI elements. It may be appropriate when multiple, confusing, or complex symptoms are present; when the symptoms are prolonged in development; when the history is obtained from an individual other than the patient; and when other complicating factors are present.

Example: A patient is seen in the physician's office with influenza-like symptoms (chief complaint). For the past 2 days (duration), she has had chills, fever, and muscle aches (associated signs). She feels worse in the evening (timing).

In the above example, three HPI elements are documented (duration, associated signs, and timing). Therefore, this would be considered a brief HPI.

Review of Systems

A review of systems (ROS) is an inventory of body systems obtained by the physician through a series of questions seeking to identify signs and/or symptoms the patient may be experiencing or has experienced. An ROS includes the following 14 systems:

- Constitutional symptoms (fever, weight loss, and so on)
- Eyes
- Ears, nose, mouth, throat
- Cardiovascular

Table 7.2. Elements included in the HPI

HPI Element	Examples
Location	Abdomen, chest, leg, head
Severity	Bad, intolerable, minimal, slight
Timing	Two hours after eating, 1 hour after waking
Quality	Burning, dull, puffy, pus-filled, red
Duration	For two months, since prescription began
Associated signs/manifestations	Rash with blistering, nausea and vomiting, abdominal pain
Context	When walking in company of smokers
Modifying factors	Improves when lying down, worse after eating

- Respiratory
- Gastrointestinal
- Genitourinary
- Musculoskeletal
- Integumentary (skin and/or breast)
- Neurologic
- Psychiatric
- Endocrine
- Hematologic/lymphatic
- Allergic/immunologic

Three types of ROS are recognized:

- A *problem-pertinent ROS* is directly related to the problem(s) identified in the HPI. The patient's positive responses and pertinent negatives for the system related to the problem should be documented.
- An *extended ROS* is directly related to the problem(s) identified in the HPI and a limited number of additional systems. The patient's positive responses and pertinent negatives for two to nine systems should be documented.
- A *complete ROS* is directly related to the problem(s) identified in the HPI and all additional body systems. At least 10 organ systems must be reviewed. Those systems with positive or pertinent negative responses should be documented individually. For the remaining systems, a notation indicating that all other systems are negative is permissible. In the absence of such a notation, at least 10 systems must be documented individually.

  Example: A patient presents with nausea (chief complaint). She has lost seven pounds in the past month (constitutional). She denies abdominal pain, diarrhea, and vomiting (gastrointestinal).

According to documentation guidelines, the preceding example would demonstrate an extended ROS because two systems are documented.

Past, Family, and/or Social History

The past, family, and/or social history (PFSH) element is broken down as follows:

- A *past history* consists of the patient's past experiences with illnesses, operations, injuries, and treatments (including medications). For pediatric populations, the past history also should include prenatal and birth history, feedings, food intolerance, and immunization history.
- A *family history* consists of a review of medical events in the patient's family, including diseases that may be hereditary or may place the patient at risk, as well as the age and status (alive or dead) of blood relatives.

- A *social history* consists of an age-appropriate review of past and current social activities. It also may include the patient's marital status and number of children, present and past employment, exposure to environmental agents, religion, hobbies, living conditions, water supply, and daily habits such as alcohol, tobacco, drug, and caffeine use. For veterans, it includes military service history. For pediatric populations, it may include school grades and sleep/play habits.

There are two types of PFSH:

- A *pertinent PFSH* includes the documentation of at least one specific item from any of the three history areas.
- A *complete PFSH* refers to the documentation of at least one specific item from two of the three history areas for the following E/M categories: office or other outpatient services, established patient; emergency department; subsequent nursing facility care; domiciliary care, established patient; and home care, established patient.

At least one specific item from each of the three history areas must be documented for a complete PFSH for the following E/M categories: office or other outpatient services, new patient; hospital observation services; hospital inpatient services, initial care; consultations; comprehensive nursing facility assessments; domiciliary care, new patient; and home care, new patient.

Table 7.3 incorporates all the elements of a history. All three levels must be met to qualify for a specific level. A CC is required for all levels.

Table 7.3. Elements of a history

History Component (equal to lowest category documented)	Problem-Focused	Expanded Problem-Focused	Detailed	Comprehensive
Chief Complaint ________________ HPI—History of Present Illness __ Location __ Duration __ Severity __ Quality __ Context __ Timing __ Modifying factors __ Associated signs and symptoms	Brief: one to three HPI elements documented	Brief: one to three HPI elements documented	Extended: four or more HPI or status of three or more chronic conditions documented	Extended: four or more HPI or status of three or more chronic conditions documented
ROS—Review of System(s) __ Constitutional (wt loss, etc.) __ Integumentary __ Endocrine __ Eyes __ GI __ Hem/lymph __ ENT, mouth __ GU __ Allergy/Immun __ Respiratory __ MS __ Cardiovascular __ Neuro __ Psychiatric	None	Problem specific: one system	Extended: two to nine systems	Complete: more than 10 systems or some with all others negative
PFSH (past medical, family, and social histories) __Previous medical (past experience with illness, injury, surgery, medical treatments, and so on) __Family medical history (diseases, which may be hereditary or with increased risk of occurrence) __Social (relationships, diet, exercise, occupation, and so on)	None	None	Pertinent: at least one item from at least one history area	Complete: specifics of at least two history areas documented

Note: A chief complaint (CC) is required for all history types.

Following are some history documentation guidelines:

- The CC, ROS, and PFSH may be listed as separate elements of the history or included in the description of the HPI.
- An ROS and/or PFSH obtained during an earlier encounter do not need to be redocumented if there is evidence that the physician has reviewed and updated the previous information. The review and update may be documented by:

  —Describing any new ROS and/or PFSH information or noting that no change in the previous information has occurred

  —Noting the date and location of the earlier ROS and/or PFSH
- The ROS and/or PFSH may be recorded by ancillary staff or the patient on a completed form. To indicate that the physician has reviewed the information, a notation must supplement or confirm the documentation recorded by the other parties.
- If the physician is unable to obtain a history from the patient or other source, the documentation in the record should describe the patient's condition or other circumstance that precludes obtaining a history.

Exercise 7.1 Evaluation and Management (History)

Unless otherwise noted, all answers can be found in appendix D of this book. Answers to selected exercises are located in the Instructor's Guide and available only to faculty of educational programs.

Using table 7.3 and applying the documentation guidelines, assign the history level (problem-focused, expanded problem-focused, detailed, comprehensive) to the following scenarios.

1. Patient seen in the physician's office complaining of a right eye that is itchy, watery, and red. Symptoms began on Saturday. Patient denies any loss of vision.

   ____

2. Patient seen in the clinic complaining of irritated throat, runny nose, and pressure in the cheek area for the past three days. Pressure seems to be worse today. Patient reports some coughing but denies headaches, just pressure in cheeks. Temperature has been normal. No daily meds. Takes Claritin 10 mg as needed.

   ____

3. Patient seen in the urgent care center for back pain extending down in both legs and feeling numb at times. This has been going on for about five months but has become intolerable. She notices it more when she is driving the car. The patient denies any trauma. She recently started a new job. She denies any sense of weakness. No bowel or bladder habit changes. She is not allergic to any medications. Has a history of diabetes and takes glucose tablets. She smokes two packs of cigarettes a day and drinks alcohol occasionally.

   ____

Examination

The physical examination is the objective description of the patient's chief complaint, illness, or injury. Four types of examinations are recognized:

- *Problem-focused:* Examination limited to the affected body area or organ system
- *Expanded problem-focused:* Examination of affected body area or organ system, as well as symptomatic or related organ systems
- *Detailed:* Extended examination of affected body area(s) and other symptomatic or related organ system(s)
- *Comprehensive:* A general multisystem examination or complete examination of a single-organ system and other symptomatic or related body area(s) or organ system(s)

The types of examination have been defined by the revised guidelines for general multi-systems as well as the following single-organ systems:

- Cardiovascular
- Ears, nose, mouth, and throat
- Eyes
- Genitourinary (female)
- Genitourinary (male)
- Hematologic/lymphatic/immunologic
- Musculoskeletal
- Neurological
- Psychiatric
- Respiratory
- Skin

The following areas of the body are examined:

- Head, including the face
- Genitalia, groin, buttocks
- Neck
- Back, including spine
- Chest, including breasts and axillae
- Each extremity
- Abdomen

The following systems are examined:

- Constitutional (vital signs, general appearance)
- Genitourinary
- Eyes
- Musculoskeletal
- Ears, nose, mouth, and throat
- Skin
- Cardiovascular
- Neurologic
- Respiratory
- Psychiatric
- Hematologic/lymphatic/immunologic
- Gastrointestinal

Table 7.4 lists all the components of an examination.

Table 7.4. Components of an examination

Examination Component			Problem-Focused	Expanded Problem-Focused*	Detailed	Comprehensive
Body Areas	**Organ Systems**		One body area or system	Two to four body systems or two to seven basic systems, including affected area	Two to seven detailed systems, including affected area	Eight or more systems
__ Head, face	__ Const. (vitals, general appearance)					
__ Neck	__ Eyes	__ GU				
__ Chest, breasts	__ ENT, mouth	__ Skin				
__ Abdomen	__ Respiratory	__ Integumentary				
__ Genit, groin	__ Cardiovascular	__ MS				
__ Back, spine	__ Gastrointestinal	__ Neurological				
__ Each extremity	__ Lymph/hem/immun	__ Psychiatric				

*Some texts use two to four body systems for expanded problem-focused and five to seven body systems for detailed. Both methods have been published in CMS publications. This is a controversy in the industry, and CMS will not give an opinion on whether one method is more acceptable than the other. Physicians frequently find that the two–four and five–seven distinction is easier to understand and follow.

Exercise 7.2 Evaluation and Management (Physical Examination)

Unless otherwise noted, all answers can be found in appendix D of this book. Answers to selected exercises are located in the Instructor's Guide and available only to faculty of educational programs.

Using table 7.4 as a guide, assign the level of examination based on the documentation in the following scenarios.

1. Vital signs: temperature is 98.4° F, respirations 16, and blood pressure is 119/81. General: well-nourished, well-developed female in no apparent distress. HEENT: normocephalic, atraumatic. Mucous membranes appear moist. Lungs: clear. Heart: regular rate and rhythm. Abdomen: positive bowel sounds, soft, nontender, and nondistended. Back: no swelling, bruising, or erythema. Extremities: lower extremities show no muscle wasting. Patient has 2+ patellar and ankle jerks, 5/5 muscle strength bilaterally, and a negative straight leg raise bilaterally.

   ____

2. Alert 16-year-old boy. Temperature: 98.6° F; pulse: 86; respirations: 14; blood pressure: 126/80. Has 2-cm laceration of chin.

   ____

3. Temperature: 98; pulse 86; respirations 16; blood pressure 150/65. General: Patient is a well-nourished female who is wearing corrective lenses and looks to be somewhat uncomfortable. HEENT: head examination is normocephalic, atraumatic. Eyes: clear. Pupils equally round and reactive to light and accommodation. Discs sharp bilaterally. Ears, tympanic membranes pearly white bilaterally. Negative fluid. Neck: trachea midline, supple, no adenopathy. Cervical spine shows no swelling, bruising, or erythema. She had tenderness in the sternocleidomastoid muscle. C-spine itself was nontender to palpation.

   ____

Medical Decision Making

Medical decision making involves the complexity of establishing a diagnosis and/or selecting a management opinion or treatment plan as measured by the following:

- The number of possible diagnoses and/or management options or treatment plans to be considered
- The amount and/or complexity of the data (health records, diagnostic tests, and/or other information) to be obtained, reviewed, and analyzed
- The risk of significant complications, morbidity, and/or mortality associated with the patient's presenting condition, the diagnostic procedure(s), and/or the possible management options or treatment plans

Number of Possible Diagnoses and/or Management Options

The number of possible diagnoses and/or management options is based on the number and types of problems addressed during the encounter, the complexity of establishing a diagnosis, and the management decisions made by the physician.

The following documentation guidelines apply:

- For each encounter, an assessment, clinical impression, or diagnosis should be documented. It may be stated explicitly or implied in documented decisions regarding management plans and/or further evaluation.
- For a presenting problem with an established diagnosis, the record should reflect whether the problem is improving, well-controlled, resolving, or resolved; or inadequately controlled, worsening, or failing to change as expected.
- For a presenting problem without an established diagnosis, the assessment or clinical impression may be stated in the form of a differential diagnosis, or as a possible, probable, or rule-out diagnosis.
- The initiation of, or changes in, treatment should be documented clearly. Treatment involves a wide range of management options, including patient instructions, nursing instructions, therapies, and medications.
- The record should indicate whether referrals are made and where, whether consultations are requested and with whom, and whether advice is sought and from whom.

Amount and/or Complexity of Data for Review

The amount and/or complexity of data for review is based on the types of diagnostic testing ordered or reviewed. A decision to obtain and review old health records and/or to obtain history from sources other than the patient increases the amount and complexity of data to be reviewed.

The following documentation guidelines apply:

- When a diagnostic service (test or procedure) is ordered, planned, scheduled, or performed at the time of the E/M encounter, the type of diagnostic service should be documented.
- The review of laboratory, radiology, and/or other diagnostic tests should be documented. An entry in a progress note (for example, "WBC elevated" or "chest x-ray unremarkable") is acceptable. Alternatively, the review may be documented by initialing and dating the report containing the test results.
- Relevant findings from any review of old records and/or the receipt of additional history from the family, caretaker, or other sources should be documented. If nothing exists beyond the relevant information that already has been obtained, that fact should be documented. A notation of "old records reviewed" or "additional history obtained from family" without further specification is insufficient.
- Documentation of discussions with the physician(s) who performed or interpreted laboratory, radiology, or other diagnostic tests should be included.
- The direct visualization and independent interpretation of an image, tracing, or specimen previously or subsequently interpreted by another physician should be documented.

Risk of Significant Complications, Morbidity, and/or Mortality

The risk of significant complications, morbidity, and/or mortality is based on the risks associated with the presenting problem(s), the diagnostic procedure(s), and the possible management options. The determination of risk is complex and not readily quantifiable.

The risk assessment of the presenting problem(s) is based on the risk related to the disease process anticipated between the present and the next encounter. The risk assessment of selecting diagnostic procedures and management options is based on the risk during and immediately following any procedures or treatment. The highest level of risk in any one category (presenting problem, diagnostic procedure, or management option) determines the overall risk.

Figure 7.1 outlines the factors that determine medical decision making. Two of the three elements in table 7.5 must be met or exceeded before selecting a type of medical decision making.

Counseling and Coordination of Care

Both counseling and coordination of care are contributing factors in the selection of an E/M level of service. Counseling involves discussion of the patient's care with the patient and/or his or her family. Examples of counseling/coordination of care activities include discussions about results of diagnostic studies, treatment options, and instructions. An often overlooked coding guidcline states:

> When counseling and coordination of care constitute more than 50% of the physician/patient and/or family encounter (face-to-face time in the office or other outpatient setting or unit/floor time in the hospital or nursing facility), time may be considered the **key or controlling factor** to qualify for a particular level of E/M service.

Time can only be used as a key factor when the E/M codes include typical times, such as 99201–99215. There are no typical times for emergency department services (99281–99285), which eliminates the option of code selection based on time.

There are two important documentation guidelines to support use of counseling and coordination as a key factor for selection of E/M code:

- Physician must include a record of the total time of the visit
- Physician must include the specific time spent in counseling and coordination of care activities

For example, the physician could document, "The established office visit of Mrs. Lee was 25 minutes in duration, and 15 minutes of the visit was spent in discussing her treatment options for cancer treatment."

Analysis of this documentation:

- Did counseling and coordination dominate the visit? Answer: Yes (15 of the 25 minutes)
- Because counseling and coordination dominated the visits, refer to the times stated in the E/M codes for established patients for office visits (99211–99215). Code 99214 would be selected based on the total time of the encounter.

Note that elements of the visit that are not involved in face-to-face time (reviewing lab results, telephone calls) are not reflected in the time stated.

Figure 7.1. Decision-making process

Number of Diagnosis or Treatment Options

A × B = C

Problem Status	**Number**	**Point**	**Result**
Self-limited or minor	(max. two)	1	
Established problem; stable, improving		1	
Established problem; worsening		2	
New problem; no additional workup planned	(max. one)	3	
New problem; additional workup planned		4	
		Total _________	

Amount and/or Complexity of Data Reviewed

Reviewed Data	**Points**
Review and/or order clinical lab tests	1
Review and/or order tests in the radiology section of CPT	1
Review and/or order tests in the medicine section of CPT	1
Discussion of test results with performing provider	1
Decision to obtain old records/obtain history from other than patient/discuss case with other provider	2
Independent visualization of image, tracing, or specimen itself (not simply review of report)	2
	Total _________

Risk Factors

Level of Risk	**Presenting Problem**	**Dx Procedures Ordered**	**Management Options**
Minimal	One self-limited or minor problem	Lab tests, x-rays, EKG, EEG	Rest, superficial dressings, none required
Low	• Two or more self-limited or minor problems • One stable chronic illness • Acute uncomplicated illness or injury	• Physiologic tests w/o stress • Imaging studies w/contrast • Superficial needle biopsy • Skin biopsy • Arterial blood draw	• Over-the-counter remedy • Minor surgery w/o risk factor • Physical, occupational therapy • IV fluids w/o additive
Moderate	• One or more chronic illness with exacerbation, progression, or treatment side effects • Undiagnosed new problem with uncertain prognosis • Acute complicated injury • Acute illness with systemic symptoms	• Stress tests • Endoscopies w/o risk factor • Cardiovascular imaging study w/o identified risk factors • Deep needle or incisional biopsy • Centesis of body cavity fluid	• Minor surgery with identifiable risk factors • Elective major surgery without identifiable risk factors • Prescription drug management • Therapeutic radiology • IV fluids with additives • Closed treatment of skeletal injury
High	• One or more chronic illness with severe exacerbation, progression, or Tx side effects • Acute or chronic illness or injury that may pose a threat to life or bodily function • An abrupt change to mental status	• Cardiovascular imaging studies with identifiable risk factors • Cardiac electrophysiological tests • Endoscopy with identifiable risk factors	• Elective major surgery with identifiable risk factors • Emergency major surgery • Parenteral-controlled substances • Drug therapy requiring intensive monitoring • DNR status

Tabulation of Medical Decision-Making Elements: Highest Two of Three

Diagnosis/Management Options	Minimal (one or none)	Limited (two)	Multiple (three)	Extensive (four or more)
Amount/Complexity of Data	Minimal/Low (one or none)	Limited (two)	Moderate (three)	Extensive (four or more)
Highest Risk (from any category)	Minimal	Low	Moderate	High
Medical Decision Making	**Straightforward**	**Low Complexity**	**Moderate Complexity**	**High Complexity**

Table 7.5. Selection of level of E/M service

All three of the key components must meet or exceed the stated requirements to qualify for a particular level of E/M services code.	Two of the three components must meet or exceed the stated requirements to qualify for a particular level of E/M services code.	Time
Office or other outpatient services, new patient Initial observation care Initial hospital care Office or other outpatient consultations Initial inpatient consultations ED services Comprehensive nursing facility assessments Domiciliary, rest home, or custodial care, new patient Home services, new patient	Office or other outpatient services, established patient Subsequent hospital care Subsequent nursing facility care Domiciliary, rest home, or custodial care, established patient Home services, established patient	When counseling and/or coordination of care dominates, or is more than 50 percent of, the face-to-face physician–patient encounter, time is considered the key factor to qualify for a particular level of E/M services code.

Nature of Presenting Problem

CPT defines presenting problems as diseases, conditions, illnesses, injuries, symptoms, signs, findings, complaints, or other reasons for an encounter, regardless of whether a diagnosis is established at the time of the encounter.

Five types of presenting problems are identified:

- *Minimal:* A problem that does not require the presence of a physician, although care is provided under a physician's supervision (for example, a blood pressure check).
- *Self-limited or minor:* A temporary problem with a definite and prescribed course and good prognosis (for example, an upper respiratory infection). The conditions are typically transient in nature.
- *Low severity:* With no treatment, this problem carries a low risk of morbidity and little or no risk of mortality (for example, a teenager with acne that does not respond to over-the-counter medications). A patient with this type of problem can expect full recovery without impairments.
- *Moderate severity:* With no treatment, this problem carries a moderate risk of morbidity and mortality (for example, Dupuytren's contracture of the hand involving several fingers). The patient's prognosis may be uncertain, or the probability of prolonged functional impairment is increased.
- *High severity:* With no treatment, the risk of morbidity is high and a high probability exists for severe, prolonged functional impairment or moderate to high risk of mortality (for example, Type 1 diabetes mellitus, uncontrolled, with chronic renal failure requiring dialysis).

Exercise 7.3 Evaluation and Management (Medical Decision Making)

Unless otherwise noted, all answers can be found in appendix D of this book. Answers to selected exercises are located in the Instructor's Guide and available only to faculty of educational programs.

Using Figure 7.1 as a reference, assign the level of medical decision making for the following case studies.

1. Patient seen in the emergency department after an automobile accident. She is complaining of pain in her back and right leg. X-rays, UA, and CBC were normal. Discharge diagnosis: Thoracic/rib cage strain and contusion. Right leg contusion. Discharged on Voltaren 50 mg three times a day for pain and Robaxin 750 mg three times a day for muscle spasms. She is to return to work in a couple of days and follow up with her family doctor as necessary.

   ____

2. Physician office progress note: Follow-up appointment for bronchitis. Patient reports that she feels tired and weak, and the bronchitis is lingering. Impression: Questionable resolution of her bronchitis. Plan: Refill Tessalon Perles and continue with amoxicillin. Will call if not improved.

   ____

3. Mother brings 4-year-old child to urgent care after the child sustained a cut on the bottom of the foot. A 2-inch laceration was cleaned and sutured. Tylenol given for pain. Referred to family physician.

   ____

Exercise 7.4 Evaluation and Management Case Study

Unless otherwise noted, all answers can be found in appendix D of this book. Answers to selected exercises are located in the Instructor's Guide and available only to faculty of educational programs.

Case Study: Established Patient

This 56-year-old woman has been my patient for three years. She complains of cough, congestion, stuffy nose over the past 3 to 4 days; feels worse today. Denies any fever, chills, but has occasional yellow productive sputum. Denies any chest pain, nausea, vomiting, or diarrhea.

Past Medical History: Cholecystectomy

Medications: None

Allergies: None

Social History: Smoker

Physical Examination:
- General: Alert woman in no apparent distress
- Vital signs: Blood pressure 152/84, temperature 99.2, pulse 84, respirations 18
- HEENT: Pupils equal, round and reactive to light and accommodation. Extraocular movements intact
- Neck: Supple, nontender
- Lungs: Breath sounds are equal. No rales or wheezes.
- Heart: S1, S2, no murmur
- Abdomen: Soft, nontender. Bowel sounds present in all quadrants.
- Extremities: Pulses equal
- Skin: Warm and dry

Studies: Chest x-ray is negative.

Diagnosis: Acute bronchitis

Plan: Zithromax Z-Pak. Follow-up in one week. Call if symptoms worse.

1. Refer to previous tables and apply the documentation guidelines to assign the E/M code for the preceding case.

   ____

Time

The 1992 edition of *Current Procedural Terminology* introduced the notion of time as a separate contributing factor for selecting the appropriate E/M level of service codes. Prior editions had been based on the idea that time was an implicit factor in the definition of each level of service. In the current system, the specific times included in the level of service codes are averages and, as such, may vary according to the actual clinical circumstances. Details about use of time with counseling and coordination of care were discussed previously.

Face-to-Face Time

Face-to-face time is the amount of time the physician spends face-to-face with the patient and/or his or her family. This includes the period during which the physician obtains a history, performs an examination, and counsels the patient. Face-to-face time applies to the following subsections and subcategories: Office and Other Outpatient Visits and Office Consultations.

Unit/Floor Time

Unit/floor time is the amount of time the physician is present on the patient's hospital unit and rendering services for the patient at the bedside. This includes the period when the physician establishes and/or reviews the patient's health record, examines the patient, writes notes, and communicates with other professionals and the patient's family regarding the patient's care. Unit/floor time applies to the following four subsections and subcategories: Hospital Observation Services, Inpatient Hospital Care, Inpatient Consultations, and Nursing Facility Care.

Instructions for Selection and/or Validation of E/M Service Levels

The following steps should be followed in selecting and/or validating a level of E/M services:

1. Identify the category and subcategory of service. Is this an office visit with an established patient? Inpatient consultation? Comprehensive nursing facility assessment? New patient home service? Individual counseling for preventive medicine services? Visit to the emergency department? Hospital outpatient service?
2. Review specific notes and instructions for the selected category and subcategory.
3. Review the narrative descriptors within the category and subcategory of the E/M services. The seven components should be reviewed in selecting the appropriate level of service code.
4. Using the definitions provided under each level of service, determine the extent of history obtained.
5. Determine the extent of examination performed using the definitions provided under each level of service.
6. Determine the complexity of medical decision making.
7. Select or verify the appropriate level of E/M services.

Selection of Modifiers

Under certain circumstances, a listed service may be modified slightly without changing its basic definition. In these situations, several modifiers are available for use with E/M services codes. Modifiers are reported as two-digit numbers attached to the main code.

The following modifiers are available for use with E/M codes:

24 Unrelated Evaluation and Management Service by the Same Physician during a Postoperative Period: Modifier 24 can be reported by physicians with an E/M service provided during the postoperative period by the same physician who performed the original procedure. The E/M service must be unrelated to the condition for which the original procedure was performed.

Example: Office visit provided to a patient who is in the postoperative period for a cholecystectomy performed three weeks earlier. The patient's current complaint is a possible infection of a finger that was lacerated four days ago. The physician may report the appropriate office visit code and attach modifier 24 to identify this activity as an unrelated service provided during the postoperative period of the cholecystectomy.

25 Significant, Separately Identifiable Evaluation and Management Service by the Same Physician on the Same Day of the Procedure or Other Service: Modifier 25 may be reported by hospitals and physicians to indicate that the patient's condition required a separate E/M service on the day a procedure or other service was performed because the care provided went beyond the usual procedures associated with the activity. By definition, CPT guidelines state that this modifier is not to be reported with an E/M service that resulted in a decision to perform surgery.

Example: Office visit is provided to a patient for evaluation of diabetes and associated chronic renal failure, as well as a mole on the arm that has increased in size. Suspecting the mole is malignant, the physician excises it. The pathology report confirms a 1.1-cm malignant lesion. The physician can bill for the malignant lesion removal and use the office visit code accompanied by modifier 25 to identify that, during the visit, a separate condition was addressed (in this example, the diabetes and the renal failure). Generally, two diagnosis codes are required to explain the reporting of two separate services during the same encounter, although CPT guidelines do not require it.

It is important to note that CMS and other payers may have guidelines for use of this modifier.

Example: A patient is seen in the emergency department for chest pains. An EKG is performed. The hospital would report the emergency department E/M code of 99283–25 with 93005 (EKG).

27 Multiple Outpatient Hospital E/M Encounters on the Same Date: Modifier 27 was developed to allow hospitals to report multiple outpatient hospital E/M encounters on the same date. The modifier is appended to the second encounter and each subsequent E/M code.

Example: Patient is seen in the dermatology clinic in the morning and the orthopedic clinic in the afternoon. A level III clinic visit is performed at both visits. The hospital would report 99213 with 99213–27.

CMS has instructed hospitals to assign E/M codes for facility billing based on their own system, which reflects the facility's resources to give care to the patient.

32 Mandated Services: Modifier 32 can be reported by physicians when an entity such as a third-party payer or a quality improvement organization mandates a service. Most often, this modifier is reported with the consultation codes.

57 Decision for Surgery: Modifier 57 can be reported by physicians along with the appropriate E/M services code when an E/M service was the result of an initial decision to perform surgery on a patient. Modifier 57 is appropriate with procedures that Medicare designates as major, which typically are those with a 90-day global fee period assigned. Generally, it is not required when the decision for surgery occurs at a time earlier than the day of or before surgery. Some insurance plans include consultation and/or visit codes where the decision is made in the global fee for surgery and do not provide separate payment.

Example: An office visit is provided to a Medicare patient complaining of acute right, upper-quadrant pain and tenderness referred to the right scapula, nausea and vomiting, and anorexia. A low-grade fever and an elevated white blood cell count are noted. An ultrasound confirms the diagnosis of acute cholecystitis with cholelithiasis. The physician recommends that surgery be performed later that day. The physician can report the appropriate office visit code along with modifier 57 to identify that, during this office visit, it was decided to perform a cholecystectomy.

Exercise 7.5 Evaluation and Management

Unless otherwise noted, all answers can be found in appendix D of this book. Answers to selected exercises are located in the Instructor's Guide and available only to faculty of educational programs.

Circle the correct answer for each of the following statements.

1. The AMA and CMS developed documentation guidelines for use with the CPT codebook.

   True False

2. All seven of the following are considered key components in selecting an E/M level of service: history, examination, medical decision making, coordination of care, counseling, nature of presenting problem, and time.

   True False

3. CMS mandates use of the E/M documentation guidelines.

   True False

4. The review of systems is a chronological description of the development of the patient's presenting symptoms.

   True False

5. The element of time is never considered a factor in selecting an E/M level of service.

   True False

Exercise 7.5 (Continued)

Based on 1995 documentation guidelines, write the answer to each of the following questions in the spaces provided.

6. An 86-year-old patient presents with a CC of vomiting and dizziness. Yesterday, she became dizzy while getting ready to go to church. In addition, she vomited bile several times and complained of deafness in her left ear at the start of the dizziness. Based on this information, is this history of present illness (HPI) brief or extended?

   ____

   ____

7. The CC is chest pain. The examination determined: respiration quiet and unlabored; skin with good color, warm and dry, and no rashes; mucous membranes moist; ears and throat clear; lungs with good breath sounds in all fields; rare expiratory wheeze, no rales, no rhonchi; heart regular rate and rhythm with normal heart sounds, no murmur; abdomen soft with no liver or spleen enlargement; and bowel sounds active. Based on this information, what is the level of examination?

   ____

   ____

8. New patient presents to the office with a CC of nasal congestion and headache. ROS: Denies shortness of breath or fever, stiffness of neck, or visual disturbances. Past history: No drug allergies or other allergies were noted, nor any history of TB, COPD, or asthma. Last physical examination 1 year ago was unremarkable. Based on this information, is this past, family, and/or social history pertinent or complete?

   ____

   ____

Categories of E/M Services

E/M services are divided into many different types of services as listed previously.

Office or Other Outpatient Services (99201–99215)

The office or other outpatient services category may be used to describe services provided in the physician's office, the outpatient clinic, or some other ambulatory facility. This category is divided into two subcategories: new patient and established patient. It is important to remember that the basic difference between a new and established patient is whether the patient received professional services within the past three years from the same physician or another physician within the same group practice. Whereas the new patient level of services requires meeting all three of the key components prior to assigning a code, the established patient level of services requires meeting only two of the three key components.

Reporting an office visit code is inappropriate if, during the course of events within a specific encounter, the physician admits the patient to the hospital as an inpatient or observation patient or to a nursing care facility. Only the resulting admission service should be reported in such a situation, which should incorporate the level of care provided in the office. There may be a rare circumstance where the patient receives office services early in the day and then returns later and must be admitted to the hospital from the office. Such a situation would merit use of modifier 25 to show that the services were separately identifiable.

Hospital Observation Services (99217–99220, 99224–99226) and Hospital Observation or Inpatient Care Services (99234–99236)

The hospital observation services category identifies patients who are admitted to a hospital or are placed in observation status in a hospital and the services span more than one calendar date. For observation and inpatient care where admission and discharge occur on the same date, codes 99234 through 99236 would be used.

Consulting physicians providing services while patients are in observation status would use either outpatient consultation (99241–99245) or inpatient consultation codes (99251–99255), depending on the patient's status at the time of service. Only attending physicians should use the observation codes. When a patient is admitted to the hospital (and not discharged on the same date), the initial hospital or inpatient consultation codes will be used, as appropriate.

The initial encounter with a patient in observation status is reported with a code from 99218 to 99220. Coding professionals should note that all three key components must be met to assign a particular level of service. In the rare circumstance that a patient remains in observation status after the date of admission, but is removed before the date of discharge, codes 99211–99215 may be used to report a physician visit on the intervening dates between removal from observation status and discharge.

Code 99217 (Observation care discharge services) is used to describe the services provided to a patient on discharge from observation status, but only if the discharge was not on the same date as the initial care. These services include a final examination of the patient, discussion of the hospital stay, instructions for continuing care, and completion of the health record.

Hospital Inpatient Services (99221–99239)

The hospital inpatient services category includes codes for initial hospital care (99221–99223), subsequent hospital care (99231–99233), and hospital discharge services (99238–99239). These codes also may be used to describe services provided to patients in a so-called partial hospital setting. Partial hospitalization is used for crisis stabilization, intensive short-term daily treatment, or intermediate-term treatment of psychiatric disorders.

The initial hospital care codes (99221–99223) are used to report the physician's first inpatient hospital visit with a new or established patient. Coding professionals should note that all three of the key components must be met to assign a particular level of service.

Codes 99231–99233 are reported for subsequent hospital services provided by the physician. Changes in the patient's medical status and the related documentation in the health record allow the physician to report various levels of service for the subsequent hospital care. It should be noted that only two of the three key components must be met to assign a specific level of service for subsequent hospital care services.

Codes 99238–99239 are used to report the services related to discharging a patient from the hospital. This reflects the added work the physician must perform, such as final examination of patient, discussion of hospital stay, instructions for home care, and completion of the health record. Code selection is based on time. For example, code 99238 describes discharge services requiring 30 minutes or less, and code 99239 identifies those services requiring more than 30 minutes.

Patients receiving inpatient or observation services when admission and discharge occur on the same date are reported using codes 99234 through 99236.

Consultations (99241–99255)

The CPT codebook defines a consultation as a type of service provided by a physician at the request of another physician or appropriate source to either recommend care for a specific condition/problem or to determine whether to accept responsibility for ongoing management of the patient's entire care or for the care of a specific condition or problem. Although consulting physicians may initiate diagnostic and/or therapeutic services, they cannot assume responsibility for any portion of that patient's care. If responsibility is assumed, the service is no longer considered a consultation and the appropriate code should be assigned for hospital care or office or other outpatient services.

Documentation to support a consultation is essential and should include the request and need for a consultation, the opinion of the consultant, and any services ordered and/or performed. All this information should be documented in the health record and communicated by written report to the requesting physician or other appropriate source.

When a consultation is requested by the patient and/or his or her family, but not by another physician or other appropriate source (for example, physician assistant, nurse practitioner), the physician should report the service using the office visit, home services, or domiciliary/rest home care codes.

Effective January 1, 2010, CMS stopped making payments for consultation services. For Medicare/Medicaid claims, inpatient consultation codes (99251–99255) will be reported with the 99221–99233 inpatient initial admission service codes. In the office setting, the consultation codes (99241–99245) should be reported with codes for the 99201–99205 series for new patients and the E/M codes 99212–99215 for established patients.

Introductory language for consultation codes in CPT is provided preceding code 99241. Although CMS no longer recognizes consultation codes, other private payers may accept these codes.

Office or Other Outpatient Consultations (99241–99245)

Codes 99241–99245 describe office or other outpatient consultation services provided to new or established patients. These services may be provided in an office, outpatient or other ambulatory facility, hospital observation services program, home services program, domiciliary, rest home, custodial care program, or emergency department. Subsequent visits to the consulting physician's office are reported using the office visit codes for established patient (99211–99215). All three key components must be met in the selection of a level of service code from 99241 to 99245.

Inpatient Consultations (99251–99255)

Inpatient consultation codes (99251–99255) are used to report consulting services provided to hospital inpatients, residents of nursing facilities, or patients in a partial hospital setting. All three key components must be met in the selection of a level of service code from 99251 to 99255. In addition, a consultant can report only one consultation code per admission.

Emergency Department Services (99281–99288)

Emergency department services category codes are used to report E/M services that a physician provides when treating a patient in the emergency department. The CPT codebook defines the emergency department as an organized hospital-based facility for the provision of unscheduled episodic services to patients who present for immediate medical attention. Moreover, the facility must be available 24 hours a day. All three of the key components, as stated within each level, must be met prior to selection of an emergency services code.

Special attention should be given to the description of code 99285, "which requires these three key components within the constraints imposed by the urgency of the patient's clinical condition and mental status." This description allows the code to be assigned, even when not all the documentation meets the criteria so stated. For example, when the patient is unconscious, it may be impossible to document a comprehensive history.

Again, code selection by physicians rather than coding or billing professionals is important because a physician is the only one in a position to determine clinical condition and mental status. Nonphysicians may verify compliance of the code selection to the current guidelines, but the provider of service best determines the level of code selection.

When a patient receives critical care services in the emergency department, codes 99291 and 99292 may be reported for these services, provided the requirements for critical care are met.

Critical Care Services (99291–99292)

The critical care services category involves the care of critically ill patients in a medical emergency that requires the constant attention of the physician. However, the physician's constant attendance/monitoring does not have to be continuous on a given date. Types of medical emergencies can include cardiac arrest, shock, bleeding, respiratory failure, and postoperative complications. Although usually provided in critical care areas such as a coronary care unit, intensive care unit (ICU), or emergency department, this type of care may be offered in other settings as well.

Critical care provided to neonatal and pediatric inpatients is reported with codes 99468 through 99480.

Critical care services include the following procedures, which should not be reported separately:

- Interpretation of cardiac output measurements (93561, 93562)
- Chest x-rays (71010, 71015, 71020)
- Pulse oximetry (94760, 94761, 94762)
- Blood gases and information data stored in computers (99090)
- Gastric intubation (43752, 43753)
- Temporary transcutaneous pacing (92953)
- Ventilator management (94002–94004, 94660, 94662)
- Vascular access procedures (36000, 36400, 36410, 36415, 36600)

Other services performed that are not included in the preceding list may be reported separately.

Time is a key factor when selecting a critical care code. Code 99291 is reported for the first 30 to 74 minutes of critical care on a given date and may be reported only once per date. Code 99292 is reported for each additional 30 minutes of care beyond the first 74 minutes. As mentioned previously, coding professionals should note that the constant attention the physician provides need not be continuous on a given date. Critical care of less than 30 minutes on a given date should be reported with an appropriate E/M services code, such as subsequent hospital inpatient services, rather than a critical care code. A comprehensive explanation of time as an element in code selection can be found in the note under the critical care services subcategory.

Nursing Facility Services (99304–99310)

The codes in the nursing facility services category are used to report services in the following facilities:

- Skilled nursing facilities (SNFs), including hospital-based skilled care or swing beds in rural hospitals
- Intermediate care facilities
- Long-term care facilities

Nursing facilities (NFs) are required by law to perform a comprehensive assessment of each resident's functional capacity upon admission. Additional assessments must be conducted immediately after significant changes in a resident's condition, or at least every 12 months. The assessments are documented in a form called the resident assessment instrument (RAI), which is composed of a uniform Minimum Data Set (MDS) and resident assessment protocols (RAPs). The MDS includes a minimum set of assessment elements to evaluate SNF and NF residents. SNFs and NFs are responsible for completing the RAI, although specific portions of the form must be completed by a physician only.

CPT recognizes two types of NF services: initial nursing facility care and subsequent nursing facility care. Both subcategories apply to new or established patients. All three of the key components must be met in initial visits before code selection. The CPT descriptions include time to assist physicians in selecting the most appropriate level of service. The Coding Tip (before code 99304) outlines the guidelines for specific application of "time" in the coding selections.

Subsequent NF care (99307–99310) includes reviewing the health record, noting changes in the resident's status since the last visit, and reviewing and signing orders. Subsequent NF care requires that only two of the three key components be met before assigning a specific level of service code. The time designation for these codes specifies that the physician must be at the bedside and on the patient's facility floor or unit.

NF discharge day management codes are used to report the total duration of time spent by a physician for the final NF discharge of a patient. These include final examination of the patient and discussion of the NF stay, even when the time spent on that date is not continuous. Instructions are given for continuing care to all relevant caregivers and for preparation of discharge records, prescriptions, and referral forms. These codes are 99315 for services of 30 minutes or less and 99316 for services of more than 30 minutes.

Domiciliary, Rest Home, or Custodial Care Services (99324–99337)

Physician visits to patients being provided room, board, and other personal assistance services (usually on a long-term basis) are reported using codes 99324–99337. A medical component is not part of the facility's services. Such facilities may include group homes, assisted-living, or correctional facilities. All three key components, as defined in the levels of service, must be met before code assignment in the new patient subcategory (99324–99328). However, only two of the three key components must be met in the established patient subcategory (99334–99337).

Domiciliary, Rest Home (e.g. Assisted Living Facility), or Home Care Plan Oversight Services (99339–99340)

These codes identify physician's time in care-plan development and oversight for patients cared for in assisted living. Physicians report 15 minutes or more within a calendar month of care-plan oversight for patients not enrolled in a home healthcare agency or a hospital and not in a nursing facility. Codes 99339 and 99340 report development of complex and multidisciplinary care modalities and/or revision of care plans, review of subsequent reports of patient status, review of related laboratory and other studies, communication (including telephone calls) for purposes of assessment or care decisions with healthcare professional(s), family member(s), surrogate decision maker(s) (such as a legal guardian), and /or key caregiver(s) involved in the patient's care, integration of new information into the medical treatment plan, and/or adjustment of medical therapy.

Home Services (99341–99350)

Home services codes 99341–99350 are used to report E/M services provided in a private residence. As stated in the levels of service, all three key components are required prior to code assignment in the new patient subcategory (99341–99345). However, only two of the three key components must be met in the established patient subcategory (99347–99350).

Prolonged Services (99354–99359) and Physician Standby Services (99360)

The first set of codes (99354–99357) is used when a physician (or other qualified health care professional) provides prolonged service involving direct contact with the patient that is beyond the usual service in either the inpatient or outpatient setting. Direct patient contact is face-to-face and includes additional non-face-to-face services on the patient's floor or unit in the hospital during the same session. The time the physician spends providing prolonged service on a given date need not be continuous. Coding professionals should note that these codes may be reported in addition to other services, including E/M services at any level. Moreover, other procedures or supplies provided during the same encounter should be reported according to payer directions or guidelines. Coders should review the complete set of instructions with a reference table (before code 99354) before attempting to assign codes in this area.

The codes are further subdivided to identify prolonged services provided in the outpatient setting (99354–99355) and the inpatient or observation setting (99356–99357). Codes 99354 and 99356 describe the first hour of prolonged service and should be reported only once per any given date. Codes 99355 and 99357 describe each additional 30 minutes of prolonged service. Coding professionals should note that prolonged service of less than 30 minutes should not be reported separately.

Codes 99358–99359 describe prolonged physician service without direct or face-to-face contact with the patient that is beyond the usual non-face-to-face component of physician service time. These codes may be reported along with other services, including E/M services at any level. Code 99358 is used to report the first hour of prolonged service (reported only once per date) regardless of the place of service, and code 99359 describes each additional 30 minutes of service. Prolonged service of less than 30 minutes should not be reported separately.

Code 99360 is used to report physician standby services requested by another physician that require prolonged physician attendance without direct or face-to-face contact. This type of service may involve a physician who stands by for assistance in surgery or high-risk delivery for care of a newborn. Code 99360 may be reported for each full 30-minute period the physician stands by. Less than 30 minutes of standby service may not be reported separately.

Coding professionals should reference the detailed instructions and illustration provided before code 99354 for additional guidance.

Case Management Services (99363–99368)

The case management services category includes services when a physician (or another qualified healthcare professional) is responsible for providing direct care for a patient, as well as coordinating and controlling access to other healthcare services or initiating and/or supervising them. This category includes two subcategories, Anticoagulant Management and Medical Team Conferences.

Anticoagulant Management

Anticoagulant management codes (99363–99364) describe the outpatient services provided to manage warfarin therapy. The codes include services such as ordering, reviewing, and interpreting International Normalized Ratio (INR) testing. Coding professionals should carefully review the CPT notes pertaining to the use of these codes, which appear after the heading.

Medical Team Conferences

Codes 99366 through 99368 describe a team conference that includes a physician, an interdisciplinary health team, or representatives of community agencies for the purpose of coordinating the activities of the patient. The two codes differentiate between direct (face-to-face) contact or without direct contact with patient and/or family.

Care Plan Oversight Services (99374–99380)

The care plan oversight services category describes the services a physician provides when supervising and coordinating the patient's care within a 30-day period, but not actually seeing the patient face-to-face. These codes are appropriate when a physician provides recurrent supervision of therapy for patients in NFs, home health agencies, or hospice beds. Care plan oversight services for patients in home, domiciliary, or rest home (for example, assisted living facility) are assigned codes in the 99339–99340 range.

Code 99374 (home health), code 99377 (hospice), or code 99379 (NF) is reported for services lasting between 15 and 29 minutes, whereas codes 99375, 99378, and 99380 cover services lasting longer than 30 minutes. Only one physician may report this type of service within a 30-day period. Work involved in providing very low-intensity services or infrequent supervision is included in the preencounter and postencounter work for the home, office/outpatient, and NF or domiciliary visit codes and should not be reported with care plan oversight codes.

Preventive Medicine Services (99381–99429)

The preventive medicine services category codes are used to report the preventive medicine evaluation and management of infants, children, adolescents, and adults. When an abnormality is discovered or a preexisting condition is addressed during this service, the appropriate office visit code also should be reported if the condition/abnormality proves significant enough to require additional workup. Moreover, modifier 25 should be added to the office visit code to indicate that the same physician provided a significant and separate E/M service on the same date as the preventive medicine service. Any insignificant conditions/abnormalities discovered during the preventive medicine services that do not require additional workup should not be reported separately.

Ancillary procedures (such as laboratory or radiologic procedures), screening tests identified with a specific CPT code, and immunizations provided during the preventive medicine encounter should be coded and reported separately.

The subcategories of preventive medicine services distinguish between new and established patients, with the individual codes identifying specified age ranges. Codes 99401 through 99412 are used to report services provided to individuals at a separate encounter for the purpose of promoting health and preventing illness or injury. Counseling and/or risk factor reduction intervention vary with age and should address issues such as family problems, diet and exercise, substance abuse, sexual practices, injury prevention, dental health, and diagnostic and laboratory test results available at the time of visit.

A separate code is not needed for counseling (99401–99412) when provided as part of preventive medicine services (99381–99397) or during an E/M service. The preventive medicine codes (99381–99397) include counseling, anticipatory guidance, and risk factor reductions in the service provided. An additional code is not required to identify them. The E/M services codes also include counseling in the care provided.

Non-Face-to-Face Physician Services (99441–99444)

Certain services provided by physicians, such as telephone services and online medical evaluations, do not require face-to-face contact with the patient. CPT guidelines are provided to direct the coding of these services.

Telephone Services

Codes 99441 through 99443 describe E/M services provided by the physician via the telephone. The codes are differentiated by time (for example, 5 to 10 minutes for code 99441). The detailed guidelines outline the use of these codes, such as:

- Care initiated by established patient (or guardian of patient)
- If the telephone call ends with a decision to see the patient within 24 hours (or soonest available appointment), then this code is not reported.
- If the call refers to an E/M service performed and reported by the physician within the previous seven days (for example, postoperative follow-up) then these telephone services are considered part of that previous E/M service or procedure.

Online Medical Evaluations

Guidelines for online medical evaluations (99444) are similar to those for telephone services, but these services are provided via the Internet. Documentation guidelines state that the patient's inquiry and physician's response must be maintained in permanent storage (electronic or hard copy).

Special E/M Services (99450–99456)

The special evaluation and management services category codes were developed to report services that can be performed in the office setting or other setting to establish baseline information before life or disability insurance certificates are issued. Coding professionals should note that no active management of the patient's problem is performed during this visit. If other E/M services and/or procedures are performed on the same date, the appropriate E/M services codes also should be reported, with modifier 25 appending them.

Newborn Care (99460–99463)

The newborn care codes are used to report services provided to normal newborns in different settings. Codes are applicable from the initial first days after birth (per day) until home discharge. Codes differentiate between initial and subsequent days of service. Reporting of these codes reflect services such as newborn history, physician exam, ordering tests, treatments, meeting with family, and preparation of hospital records.

Delivery/Birthing Room Attendance (99464–99465)

Code 99464 is used to report attendance at a delivery at the request of the delivering physician for initial stabilization of the newborn. Newborn resuscitative services are reported with code 99465, which includes the provision of positive pressure ventilation and/or chest compressions in the presence of acute inadequate ventilation and/or cardiac output. Code 99464 cannot be reported with 99465. When other procedures are performed in addition to the resuscitative services, additional codes should be reported.

Inpatient Neonatal Intensive Care Services and Pediatric and Neonatal Critical Care Services (99466–99480)

Pediatric Critical Care Patient Transport (99466–99467)

The first two codes in this subsection (99466–99467) are used to report face-to-face critical care services delivered by a physician during the interfacility transport of a critically ill or injured pediatric patient, 24 months of age or younger.

Code 99466 is used to report the first 30 to 74 minutes, and code 99467 is an add-on code for each additional 30 minutes. Transport time less than 30 minutes should be reported with the appropriate E/M code.

Inpatient Neonatal and Pediatric Critical Care (99468–99476)

These codes are used to report services performed by a physician to direct the care of a critically ill neonate or infant. Code 99468 should be assigned for the initial critical care services provided to a neonatal patient (birth through 28 days of age), and code 99469 should be assigned for subsequent critical care. Code 99471 should be assigned for the initial critical care services provided to a pediatric patient (29 days to 24 months of age), and code 99472 should be assigned for subsequent critical care. The last set of codes (initial and subsequent) identifies patients that are 2 years of age through 5 years of age.

Coding guidelines dictate that these codes may be reported only once by a single physician per patient per day. It is important to note that the CPT book provides detailed coding guidelines before code 99468.

Initial and Continuing Intensive Care Services (99477–99480)

CPT code 99477 is provided to report initial services for the neonate requiring intensive observation, frequent interventions, and other intensive care services.

Codes (99478–99480) are used by physicians to report intensive (noncritical) care given to infants with low birth weights. Subsequent intensive care visits (per day) can be distinguished by body weight: 99478 (body weight of less than 1,500 grams), 99479 (body weight of 1,500–2,500 grams), and 99480 (body weight of 2,501–5,000 grams).

Other E/M Services (99499)

The other E/M services category code is used to report an unlisted E/M service that does not fit into the previous categories.

Exercise 7.6 Chapter 7 Review

Unless otherwise noted, all answers can be found in appendix D of this book. Answers to selected exercises are located in the Instructor's Guide and available only to faculty of educational programs.

Assign only the appropriate E/M services code(s) for the following cases.

1. An established patient with hypertension visits a physician's office for a blood pressure check. The nurse performs the service under the physician's supervision.

   ____

2. A new patient was seen in the physician's office for abdominal pain. The physician performs a detailed history and comprehensive examination. Medical decision making is of moderate complexity.

   ____

3. A patient with rectal bleeding was seen in the office of a gastroenterologist. The patient's primary care physician requested that the gastroenterologist provide advice about this case. The specialist conducted a comprehensive history and examination, and medical decision making was high. The consultant documented his findings and communicated them via written report to the primary care physician.

   ____

4. A new patient is seen in the physician's office for a cough, sore throat, and fever. The physician performs an expanded problem-focused history and a detailed examination, and medical decision making was of low complexity.

   ____

5. Dr. Jones provides critical care services in the emergency department for a patient in respiratory failure and with congestive heart failure. Ventilator management is initiated. Dr. Jones spends 1 hour and 10 minutes providing critical care for this patient.

   ____

Note: Answers to exercises 6 through 11 do not appear in appendix D of this text. They are located in the Instructor's Guide and available to faculty of educational programs.

6. Dr. Michaels provides E/M services for a patient in acute hysteria who has been admitted to the emergency department. After performing a problem-focused history and examination with straightforward medical decision making, he determines that the patient is suffering from acute grief reaction secondary to the death of her granddaughter due to sudden infant death syndrome (SIDS). At discharge, the patient is in complete control of her actions and is referred to a SIDS organization.

   ____

7. Dr. Gerald provides preventive medicine services to an established 45-year-old patient who is in good health and has no complaints. Dr. Gerald obtains a comprehensive history, performs a comprehensive examination, and counsels the patient on proper diet and exercise.

   ____

Exercise 7.6 (Continued)

8. Dr. Hawthorne sees an established patient in his office for evaluation of Type I diabetes mellitus with nephropathy. In addition to a problem-focused history, he performs an expanded problem-focused examination that includes a limited examination of the genitourinary, immunologic, skin, and musculoskeletal systems, and documents all positive and negative findings. The patient's status does not seem to have changed, and medical decision making is of low complexity. Dr. Hawthorne discusses the patient's insulin dosage, diet, and exercise, and plans to see the patient in 6 months.

    ____

9. An established patient sees Dr. Ryan in his office with complaints of chest pain. Dr. Ryan decides to admit the patient to Central Hospital on March 2 under observation status. He obtains a comprehensive history that includes a complete review of body systems and complete past, family, and social histories. The patient reveals that he has been under emotional stress the past month due to his recent divorce and that this is the first time he has experienced chest pain. Dr. Ryan performs a comprehensive examination that includes a complete evaluation of the respiratory and cardiovascular systems. Pertinent diagnostic tests reveal no coronary artery disease. Dr. Ryan performs medical decision making of moderate complexity and determines the origin of the pain to be musculoskeletal secondary to stress. He discharges the patient on March 2 and recommends that he join a stress management group.

    ____

10. In her office, Dr. Childers sees an established patient who complains of abdominal pain. She provides a problem-focused history and examination, which reveals the onset of abdominal pain beginning early that morning and characterized by a sharp, crampy feeling with some radiation to the back. Nausea and dry heaves are present, but no vomiting. The patient had a normal bowel movement in the morning. No fever or chills are noted, and bowel sounds are active. A rectal examination reveals hard stool in the rectal vault, guaiac negative. An x-ray of the abdomen is negative except for extensive gas. Dr. Childers tells the patient to take an enema and return if the pain is not relieved. A change in diet would involve increasing the intake of fiber. The impression is that the patient's pain is the result of impacted feces.

    ____

11. A new patient sees Dr. Reynolds in his office complaining of diarrhea and watery stool the previous night, as well as nausea, vomiting, and crampy, lower abdominal pain. Dr. Reynolds provides a detailed history and examination, and medical decision making of moderate complexity.

    ____

Chapter 8

Medicine

The medicine section of the CPT codebook comprises a wide variety of specialty services and procedures such as psychiatric therapy, chemotherapy, rehabilitation, and immunization. The modifiers that apply to medicine codes were discussed extensively in earlier chapters of this workbook.

The medicine section includes the following subsections:

Subsection	Code Range
Immunoglobulins	90281–90399
Immunization Administration for Vaccines/Toxoids	90460–90474
Vaccines and Toxoids	90476–90749
Psychiatry	90801–90899
Biofeedback	90901–90911
Dialysis	90935–90999
Gastroenterology	91010–91299
Ophthalmology	92002–92499
Special Otorhinolaryngologic Services	92502–92700
Cardiovascular	92950–93799
Noninvasive Vascular Diagnostic Studies	93880–93998
Pulmonary	94002–94799
Allergy and Clinical Immunology	95004–95199
Endocrinology	95250–95251
Neurology and Neuromuscular Procedures	95800–96020
Medical Genetics and Genetic Counseling Services	96040
Central Nervous System Assessments/Tests	96101–96125
Health and Behavior Assessment/Intervention	96150–96155
Hydration, Therapeutic, Prophylactic, Diagnostic Injections and Infusions, and Chemotherapy and other Highly Complex Drug or Highly Complex Biologic Agent Administration	96360–96549
Photodynamic Therapy	96567–96571
Special Dermatological Procedures	96900–96999

Physical Medicine and Rehabilitation	97001–97799
Medical Nutrition Therapy	97802–97804
Acupuncture	97810–97814
Osteopathic Manipulative Therapy	98925–98929
Chiropractic Manipulative Treatment	98940–98943
Education and Training for Patient Self-Management	98960–98962
Non-Face-to-Face Nonphysician Services	98966–98969
Special Services, Procedures, and Reports	99000–99091
Qualifying Circumstances for Anesthesia	99100–99140
Moderate (Conscious) Sedation	99143–99150
Other Services and Procedures	99170–99199
Home Health Procedures/Services	99500–99602
Medication Therapy Management Services	99605–99607

Specific subsections are discussed later in this chapter. In some cases, the services listed in the medicine section may be performed in conjunction with services or procedures listed elsewhere in the CPT codebook. It may be appropriate to use multiple codes from different sections of the codebook to identify the particular circumstances.

Example: An established patient was seen in the physician's office for DTP immunization injection. In addition to the immunization, the physician provides documentation for a minimal-level office visit. The following codes are reported: 90701, 90471, and 99211–25 (E/M code).

Immunization Injections

Separate codes exist for the administration (immunization procedure) of vaccines and toxoids and for the toxoid products themselves. Codes 90460–90474 are used to report the administration of a toxoid substance, and a code or codes from the 90476–90749 range identify the type of immunization or vaccine (measles, polio, DTP, and so on). The immunization administration codes are selected based on how the immunization was administered (intranasal/oral [codes 90473–90474] or other routes [intramuscular]), number of vaccines (single vs. multiple), age of patient, and whether counseling is performed by the physician or other qualified healthcare professional. Note the following differences between the code selections:

90460	Immunization administration (any route) *through 18 years of age* with counseling; first vaccine/toxoid component
+90461	each additional vaccine (add-on code)
90471	Immunization (no face-to-face counseling) *over age of 18;* 1 vaccine
+90472	each additional vaccine

When a significant, separately identifiable E/M service (for example, office or other outpatient services or preventive medicine services) is performed, the appropriate E/M services code appended with modifier 25 should be reported in addition to the immunization administration and toxoid substance codes. For some health plans, other types of injections, including immunization administration, are bundled with E/M services and not reported separately.

Exercise 8.1 Immunizations

Unless otherwise noted, all answers can be found in appendix D of this book. Answers to selected exercises are located in the Instructor's Guide and available only to faculty of educational programs.

Assign the appropriate CPT code(s) for each of the following procedures/services.

1. A 5-year-old patient receives immunization injection for measles, mumps, rubella, and varicella vaccine (MMRV). Pediatrician counsels mother about potential side effects.

   ____

2. A 25-year-old patient receives a scheduled, routine IM injection for tetanus

   ____

3. 50-year-old man traveling abroad requires IM injection for hepatitis A; IM flu shot also administered during this encounter

   ____

4. A 19-year-old female receives IM injection for HPV virus (bivalent, 3 dose schedule)

   ____

5. IM injection of hepatitis B and *Haemophilus influenzae* B vaccine

   ____

Psychiatry

The psychiatric services included in codes 90801 through 90899 may be provided in an outpatient or inpatient setting or in a partial hospital setting. The Centers for Medicare and Medicaid Services (CMS) defines psychiatric facility partial hospitalization as a facility for the diagnosis and treatment of mental illness that provides a planned therapeutic program for patients who do not require full-time hospitalization, but who need broader programs than are possible from outpatient visits in a hospital-based or hospital-affiliated facility. Partial hospitalization may be used for crisis stabilization, intensive short-term daily treatment, or intermediate-term treatment of psychiatric disorders.

When E/M services such as hospital or office visits are provided along with services from the psychiatry subsection, a code from the E/M section and a code from the psychiatry subsection are usually reported. However, some codes in the psychiatry subsection combine the psychiatric services and the E/M services into one code. In this situation, only the code from the psychiatry subsection is reported.

Example #1: A psychiatrist provided psychoanalysis along with E/M services to an established patient in the office setting. The office visit included an expanded, problem-focused history and an examination and medical decision making of low complexity. The following codes should be reported: 90845 and 99213–25.

Example #2: A patient in a clinic receives individual insight-oriented psychotherapy for more than 25 minutes. The physician also provides E/M services that include a problem-focused history, a problem-focused examination, and a straightforward level of medical decision making. Code 90805 should be reported.

Note that some third-party payers do not reimburse for an E/M service and psychotherapy when both are performed on the same day.

The psychiatry subsection is further divided to identify consultative and therapeutic services such as psychotherapy, electroconvulsive therapy, and hypnotherapy.

General Diagnostic and Evaluative Interview Procedures

Code 90801, Psychiatric diagnostic interview examination, typically is reported during the initial phases of psychiatric treatment. This service includes a complete medical and psychiatric history, which may be obtained from the patient and/or the patient's family, and a complete mental status examination that focuses on the patient's condition at the time of the examination. When this service is provided in an inpatient hospital setting, it may be reported only once during the hospital stay.

Psychiatric Therapeutic Procedures

Codes 90804 through 90899 describe specific psychotherapeutic procedures in the treatment of mental disorders and behavioral disturbances, including interactive psychotherapy, supportive psychotherapy, psychoanalysis, narcosynthesis, electroconvulsive therapy, and so on. Interactive psychotherapy (90810–90815 and 90823–90829) uses physical aids and nonverbal communication as a way for physicians to communicate with patients who are unable to interact verbally. Narcosynthesis (90865) involves the administration of a medication that frees patients of their inhibitions and allows them to reveal information they might otherwise have found difficult to discuss.

It should be noted that some psychotherapy codes factor in the amount of time spent with the patient. When the amount of time spent with a patient is less or greater than the time specified in the code description, modifier 22, Increased Procedural Services, or 52, Reduced Services, may be reported to reflect the actual situation.

Exercise 8.2 Psychiatry

Unless otherwise noted, all answers can be found in appendix D of this book. Answers to selected exercises are located in the Instructor's Guide and available only to faculty of educational programs.

Assign the appropriate CPT code(s) for each of the following procedures/services.

1. Psychiatric evaluation of patient's health records, psychiatric reports, and tests in order to make a diagnosis

   ____

2. Psychotherapy involving patient and family members

   ____

3. Individual behavior modification and insight-oriented psychotherapy in office for 45 minutes

   ____

Dialysis

The CPT code selections are divided into four subcategories: Hemodialysis, Miscellaneous Dialysis Procedures, End-Stage Renal Disease (ESRD) Services, and Other Dialysis Procedures. Each subcategory begins with a notes paragraph for coding guidance. Table 8.1 outlines each of the subcategories and differentiates between the codes.

End-Stage Renal Disease (ESRD)

Two methods are used to treat patients with end-stage renal disease: hemodialysis and peritoneal dialysis. Hemodialysis can be defined as the process of removing metabolic waste products, toxins, and excess fluid from the blood. Codes 90951–90970 identify services for patients with ESRD. The codes in the first range (90951–90962) are used for services provided in an outpatient setting and are based on the number of face-to-face visits per month. In addition, the levels of services are distinguished by the age of the patient. The codes in the second range (90963–90966) identify services provided in the home setting, per month. Again, age is a determining factor for code selection. If the services provided are less than a full month, codes are selected from the range of 90967–90970. Codes describing development of a shunt, cannula, or fistula for hemodialysis are categorized in the surgery section of the CPT codebook.

Peritoneal dialysis involves the insertion of a catheter into the abdominal cavity and infusion of a fluid (dialysate) into the peritoneum that allows for diffusion between the dialyzing fluid and the body fluids containing the waste products. The fluid containing the waste products then is removed from the peritoneum through the catheter. These services are reported using code 90945 or 90947 based on the physician's evaluation.

Table 8.1. Dialysis

Subcategory	CPT Code Range	Characteristics
Hemodialysis	90935–90940	• Used for inpatient ESRD and non-ESRD procedures or outpatient non-ESRD dialysis services
Miscellaneous Dialysis Procedures	90945–90947	• Identifies dialysis procedures *other than* hemodialysis
End-Stage Renal Disease Services	90951–90970	Codes differentiate between: • Outpatient setting vs. home • Age of patient • Number of visits
Other Dialysis Procedures	90989–90999	Training, Hemoperfusion, and unlisted code

Exercise 8.3 Dialysis

Unless otherwise noted, all answers can be found in appendix D of this book. Answers to selected exercises are located in the Instructor's Guide and available only to faculty of educational programs.

Assign the appropriate CPT code(s) for each of the following physician procedures/services.

1. A 50-year-old patient with end-stage renal disease treated in the outpatient dialysis unit for the past month. The physician documents one face-to-face visit during that time period.

   ____

2. Peritoneal dialysis with a single physician evaluation

   ____

3. A 19-year-old patient was diagnosed with ESRD. During the first week of service for the month, the patient was treated twice before being transferred to Cleveland Clinic for further treatment.

   ____

Gastroenterology

This subsection contains many types of tests and nonsurgical treatments performed on the esophagus, stomach, and intestine.

Ophthalmology

The ophthalmology subsection includes codes (92002–92499) describing ophthalmologic medical services provided to both new and established patients. The definitions for new and established patient are the same as those mentioned for E/M services:

- A new patient is one who has not received any professional services (face-to-face) within the past three years from the physician or another physician of the same specialty who belongs to the same group practice.
- An established patient is one who has received professional services (face-to-face) within the past three years from the physician or another physician of the same specialty who belongs to the same group practice.

Complete definitions and examples for intermediate and comprehensive ophthalmologic services are provided in the CPT codebook. Briefly, the two types of service can be described as follows:

- *Intermediate services* involve the evaluation of a new or existing condition complicated with a new diagnostic or management problem and include a history, general medical observation, external ocular and adnexal examination, and other diagnostic procedures as indicated.
- *Comprehensive services* involve a general evaluation of the complete visual system and include a history, general medical observation, an external and ophthalmoscopic

examination, gross visual fields, and a basic sensorimotor examination. Initiation of diagnostic and treatment programs is always part of a comprehensive service.

An ophthalmologic examination and evaluation performed under general anesthesia is reported with code 92018 or 92019.

The prescription of contact lenses is not part of the general ophthalmologic service and should be reported separately with a code from the series 92310 through 92326. When supplying contact lenses is part of the service of fitting them (92310–92317), a separate code should not be reported.

The prescription of glasses is considered part of a general ophthalmologic service and thus should not be reported separately. Because the actual fitting of the glasses is considered a separate procedure, the fitting should be reported with a code from the series 92340 through 92371.

Exercise 8.4 Ophthalmology

Unless otherwise noted, all answers can be found in appendix D of this book. Answers to selected exercises are located in the Instructor's Guide and available only to faculty of educational programs.

Assign the appropriate CPT code(s) for each of the following procedures/services.

1. Gonioscopy is performed under general anesthesia.

   ____

2. New patient has a comprehensive ophthalmologic examination and evaluation.

   ____

Otorhinolaryngologic Services

Special otorhinolaryngologic services include the diagnostic and therapeutic services usually provided by ear, nose, and throat specialists. Vestibular function tests and audiologic function tests are found in this section. No specific coding guidelines apply to these codes other than to use modifier 52, Reduced Services, for audiological function tests when a test is applied to only one ear.

Cardiovascular Services

The cardiovascular subsection includes codes describing diagnostic and therapeutic services such as electrocardiography, cardiac catheterization, atrial septostomy, and percutaneous transluminal coronary atherectomy. The first series of codes in this subsection (92950–92998) describes therapeutic services such as cardiopulmonary resuscitation, percutaneous transluminal coronary angioplasty (PTCA), percutaneous valvuloplasty, and coronary thrombolysis.

Stent Placement

Code 92980 is reported for transcatheter stenting of a single coronary vessel. This code is only reported once per vessel even when multiple stents are placed. Code 92981 is an add-on code that can be used for stenting of additional vessels. These codes include PTCA and/or atherectomy in the same vessel.

Example: Physician performs stenting of the right coronary artery, and angioplasty and stenting of the left circumflex artery. Report the following codes: 92980–RC (stenting of right coronary artery), 92981–LC (stenting of left circumflex artery). Note that the angioplasty is not separately coded.

Drug-eluting stents coated with medication are used to prevent build-up of new tissue that would reclog the artery. Physicians report code 92980 or 92981 for placement of the drug-eluting stents. Hospitals report HCPCS Level II codes for placement of drug-eluting stents, as follows:

- G0290 Transcatheter placement of a drug-eluting intracoronary stent(s), percutaneous, with or without other therapeutic intervention, any method; single vessel
- G0291 Each additional vessel

Atherectomy

Percutaneous transluminal coronary atherectomy is reported with 92995 (for first vessel treated) and 92996 (for each additional vessel). This procedure debulks atherosclerotic plaque from coronary arteries. These CPT codes include any angioplasty performed in the same vessel.

Percutaneous Transluminal Coronary Angioplasty

Percutaneous transluminal coronary angioplasties (PTCAs) are reported with 92982 (for the first vessel) and 92984 (for each additional vessel). These codes should be assigned per vessel even when multiple strictures are treated within the same vessel. Angioplasty procedures performed with a cutting balloon are reported by assigning a PTCA procedure code (not an atherectomy code).

Thrombectomy

Code 92973 should be reported when a percutaneous transluminal coronary thrombectomy (for example, with Angiojet catheter) is performed in conjunction with stenting or angioplasty. Code 92973 is considered an add-on code.

Brachytherapy

Code 92974 should be reported for a transcatheter placement of a radiation delivery device for intravascular brachytherapy. This procedure is used to prevent repeat stenosing of the cardiac arteries. Code 92974 is an add-on code and does not include the radiation oncology service for brachytherapy.

It should be noted that the codes describing PTCA procedures (92982–92984), athrectomies (92995–92996), and transcatheter placements of stent(s) (92980–92981) require the assignment of additional codes when more than one vessel is involved, as follows:

Procedure	Single Vessel	Each Additional Vessel
Stent placement	92980	92981
Coronary angioplasty	92982	92984
Coronary atherectomy	92995	92996

Example: Percutaneous transluminal coronary balloon angioplasty involving three vessels. The following codes should be reported: 92982 (first vessel), 92984 (second vessel), and 92984 (third vessel).

Codes 92995 and 92996 describe percutaneous transluminal coronary atherectomy that may or may not be accompanied by balloon angioplasty of the same vessel.

When percutaneous coronary atherectomy and balloon angioplasty are performed during the same episode on different vessels, the two treatment modes should be reported with multiple codes to describe them.

Example: Percutaneous transluminal coronary balloon angioplasty of the left anterior descending artery and percutaneous transluminal coronary atherectomy of the right anterior descending artery. The following codes should be reported: 92995 and 92982.

Cardiography

The next two series of codes involve diagnostic cardiography (93000–93278), which includes electrocardiograms (EKGs) and stress tests, and echocardiography (93303–93350), which includes echocardiograms (ultrasounds of the heart).

Cardiovascular Monitoring Services

The coding selection in this section identifies cardiovascular services using both in-person and remote technology. The Notes section preceding code 93279 is extensive and provides definitions and instructions for use of the implantable and wearable code device evaluations codes. In addition to the specific description of the device and frequency of reporting, the codes can be differentiated by "in-person" and "remote." Table 8.2 provides an example of the coding format for pacemaker monitoring in this section.

Cardiac Catheterization

Cardiac catheterization (93451–93461) is a diagnostic procedure that can identify diseases in the coronary arteries. (See figure 8.1.) For a routine cardiac catheterization, only one code is required because the combination code includes associated procedures such as placement, intraprocedural injections for coronary angiography, and imaging (supervision and interpretation). According to the CPT definition, a cardiac catheterization includes the following procedures and services:

- Introduction, positioning, and repositioning of catheter(s)
- Recording of intracardiac and intravascular pressure
- Obtaining blood samples for measurement of blood gases or dilution curves
- Cardiac output measurements (Fick or other method) with or without electrode catheter placement
- Final evaluation and report of procedure

Table 8.2. Implantable and wearable cardiac device evaluations

CPT Code	In Person	Frequency Described in Code
93279	Programming device evaluation with iterative adjustment of the implantable device to test the function of the device and select optimal permanent programmed values with physician analysis, review, and report; *single lead* pacemaker system	—
93280	(same as above) with *dual lead* pacemaker system	—
93281	(same as above) with *multiple lead* pacemaker system	—
93288	Interrogation device evaluation with physician analysis, review, and report, includes connection, recording, and disconnection per patient encounter; single, dual, or multiple lead pacemaker system	Per patient encounter
	Remote	
93294	Interrogation device evaluation(s) (remote), up to 90 days; single, dual, or multiple lead pacemaker system with interim physician analysis, review(s) and report(s)	Report once per 90 days *(Do not report if the monitoring period is less than 30 days)*
93296	Interrogation device evaluation(s) (remote), up to 90 days; single, dual, or multiple lead pacemaker system or implantable cardioverter-defibrillator system, remote data acquisition(s), receipt of transmissions and technical review, technical support, and distribution of results	Report once per 90 days *(Do not report if the monitoring period is less than 30 days)*

Figure 8.1. Cardiac catheterization

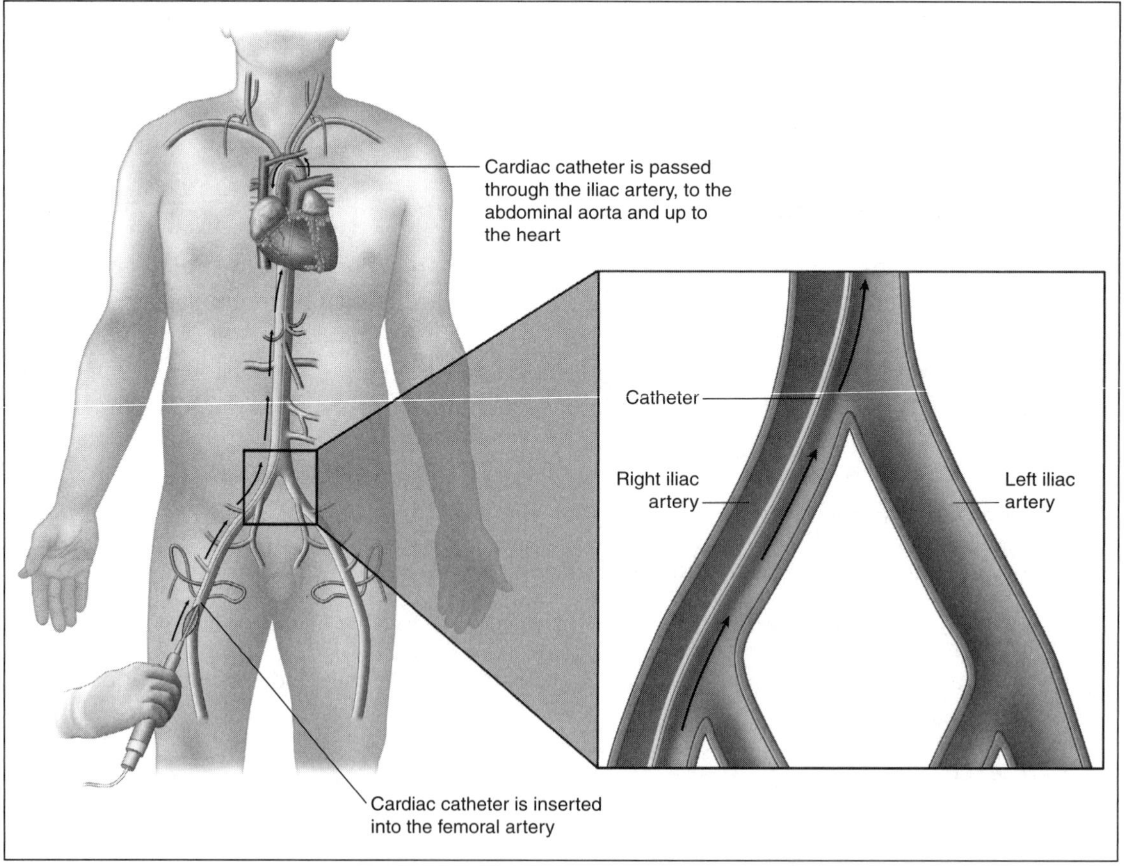

The following cardiac catheterization procedures are the most common procedures:

- *Right-heart catheterization (93451):* The thin hollow tube (catheter) is inserted through a vein, typically in the neck or groin. With radiological guidance, the physician threads the catheter along the vein, through the heart and into the blood vessels going to the lungs. During the procedure, the physician can check blood pressure in the chambers of the heart. In addition, the oxygen levels of the blood can be measured.
- *Left-heart catheterization (93452):* The catheter is introduced into the artery in the groin and threaded into the heart's left ventricle. The physician can test the strength of the heart muscles, check blood pressure inside the heart, and examine the valves.
- *Combined right and left (93453):* This single code describes a procedure that is both a right-heart catheterization and a retrograde left-heart catheterization.

Example: Physician performs percutanenous left cardiac catheterization with injection of contrast for selective left ventricular and coronary angiography. From the Medicine section, the facility would assign the following codes:

93452 Left heart catheterization

Note that there are other codes for unusual techniques, including direct ventricular puncture and puncture of the septum between the left and right atrium.

A family of injection procedure codes (93563–93568) is available for reporting "other" types of injections for right ventricular, right atrial, aortic, or pulmonary angiography performed during cardiac catheterization.

Example: Physician performs a left cardiac catheterization with left ventriculography and supravalvular ascending aortography. The facility would report the following codes:

93452 Left heart catheterization
93567 Supravalvular ascending aortography

Swan-Ganz Catheterization

Swan-Ganz catheterization is the passing of a thin tube (catheter) into the right side of the heart. The procedure is done to see blood movement through the heart and to monitor the heart's function. Code 93503 is assigned to report placement of a Swan-Ganz catheter for monitoring purposes. This procedure is typically performed on patients who are critically ill or undergoing major surgery.

Infusion during Cardiac Catheterization Procedure

Physicians often infuse medications such as nitroglycerine during cardiac catheterization procedures. The January 1998 issue of *CPT Assistant* states that infusion of medications should be considered an intrinsic part of the catheterization procedure.

Intracardiac Electrophysiological Procedures and Studies

Electrophysiological testing is performed on patients with cardiac arrhythmias that result in palpitations, near syncope, or syncope with cardiac arrest. Intracardiac electrophysiological procedures, which may be diagnostic or therapeutic, are reported with codes from the range 93600 through 93662. The services described in codes 93600 through 93652 include the insertion and repositioning of catheters.

Codes 93600 through 93612 include diagnostic electrophysiological procedures that provide only recording and pacing from a single site. Codes 93619 through 93622 describe a comprehensive electrophysiological evaluation that may be reported when recording and pacing are performed from multiple sites.

Exercise 8.5 Cardiovascular Services

Unless otherwise noted, all answers can be found in appendix D of this book. Answers to selected exercises are located in the Instructor's Guide and available only to faculty of educational programs.

Assign the appropriate CPT code(s) for each of the following procedures/services.

1. Patient with ventricular arrhythmia undergoes a microvolt T-wave alternans test.

   ____

2. Left-heart catheterization with intraprocedural injection for left ventriculography

   ____

3. Coronary thrombolysis by IV infusion

   ____

4. Cardiac stress test via treadmill performed under physician supervision with interpretation and report

   ____

5. Laser (percutaneous) atherectomy of left circumflex and left anterior descending coronary arteries and angioplasty of left anterior descending (assign Level II modifiers)

   ____

6. PTCA of two branches of the left anterior descending artery; PTCA of the right coronary artery (assign Level II modifiers)

   ____

7. Physician performs a telephonic rhythm strip pacemaker evaluation of a dual lead pacemaker system (monitoring period of 45 days)

   ____

Pulmonary Services

Pulmonologists and hospitals use codes from the pulmonary subsection for pulmonary testing. When E/M services are provided separately, a code from the E/M section also should be assigned. Codes 94010 through 94799 include the performance of laboratory procedures and the interpretation of the test results.

Exercise 8.6 Pulmonary Services

Unless otherwise noted, all answers can be found in appendix D of this book. Answers to selected exercises are located in the Instructor's Guide and available only to faculty of educational programs.

Assign the appropriate CPT codes for the following procedures/services.

1. Spirometry for bronchodilator response evaluation

 ____

2. Continuous positive airway pressure (CPAP)

 ____

3. Hypoxia response curve

 ____

Allergy and Clinical Immunology

The allergy and clinical immunology subsection includes the categories of allergy testing and allergen immunotherapy. The codes for allergy sensitivity tests include the performance and evaluation of selective skin and mucus tests in association with the patient's history and physical examination. Immunotherapy (desensitization, hyposensitization) involves the parenteral administration of allergenic extracts as antigens at periodic intervals, usually on a higher dosage than a maintenance dosage. The CPT codebook provides more complete definitions.

Codes from the E/M services section should be used to report visits with the patient involving the use of mechanical and electronic devices such as air conditioners, air filters, and humidifiers; climatotherapy; and physical, occupational, and recreational therapy.

Allergy testing (95004–95075) is further divided by type of test: percutaneous, intracutaneous, patch or application, and so on. For most of the codes in this series, the number of tests performed should be reported on the CMS-1500 form under item 24G.

> **Example:** Ten percutaneous tests with allergenic extracts were performed. The following should be reported: 95004 with 10 (to identify the number of tests) in item 24G of the CMS-1500 form.

Allergen immunotherapy (95115–95199), more commonly referred to as allergy shots, includes the professional services related to the immunotherapy. A separate office visit code(s) should not be reported unless some other identifiable service was provided during the visit.

Exercise 8.7 Allergy and Clinical Immunology

Unless otherwise noted, all answers can be found in appendix D of this book. Answers to selected exercises are located in the Instructor's Guide and available only to faculty of educational programs.

Assign the appropriate CPT code(s) for each of the following procedures/services.

1. Scratch test performed to determine allergy to bees, wasps, and yellowjackets

   ____

2. Allergy shot for grass pollen (includes extract)

   ____

Neurology and Neuromuscular Procedures and Central Nervous System Assessments and Tests

Consulting neurologists and hospitals generally use the range of codes in the subsections classifying neurology and neuromuscular procedures and central nervous system tests to report such procedures, assessments, and tests. Sleep testing, nerve conduction studies, and developmental testing are classified to this area of the medicine section of the CPT codebook.

Health and Behavior Assessment and Intervention

The focus of health and behavior assessments and interventions (codes 96150–96155) is not on mental health, but on the biopsychosocial factors affecting physical health problems and treatments (that is, patients with chronic illnesses). The codes can be reported by clinical social workers, advanced practice nurses, psychologists, and other healthcare professionals who have training in health and behavior assessment and intervention procedures. Physicians performing these services are directed to report E/M or preventive medicine codes.

Hydration, Therapeutic, Prophylactic, Diagnostic Injections and Infusions, and Chemotherapy and Other Highly Complex Drug or Highly Complex Biologic Agent Administration

It is important for coding professionals to carefully read the detailed guidelines preceding each of the coding subsections/subcategories. For example, the Notes section preceding the Injection/Infusion codes differentiates between reporting requirements for *physicians* and *facilities.* CPT provides the following guidance for reporting these codes:

For physicians: The initial code that best describes the key or primary reason for the encounter should always be reported, irrespective of the order in which the infusions or injections occur.

For facility reporting: Instructions include the following hierarchy:

- Chemotherapy infusions
- Chemotherapy injections
- Therapeutic (nonchemotherapy) infusions

- Therapeutic (nonchemotherapy) injections
- Hydration infusions

Facility Example: Patient seen in the Emergency Department for severe dehydration. An IV infusion of fluids is ordered for hydration. Forty minutes later, the patient reports that she is experiencing nausea and is given an IV push of Phenergan. The following codes would be reported:

96374 Therapeutic (IV push)
96360 IV infusion, hydration; initial, 31 minutes–1 hour

Note that the following services are included if performed to facilitate the infusion or injection:

- Use of local anesthesia
- IV start
- Access to indwelling IV, subcutaneous catheter or port
- Flush at conclusion of infusion
- Standard tubing, syringes, and supplies

If it is elected during the patient encounter to administer multiple infusions, injections, or combinations, only one "initial" service code should be reported, unless medical protocol requires that two separate IV sites be used. This section of coding is complex and requires close examination of payers' guidelines. For Medicare guidelines, coders are encouraged to review Chapter 4, section 230.2 of the *Medicare Claims Manual.*

Hydration (96360–96361)

Two codes are provided for hydration IV infusion: code 96360 for the initial (31 minutes to 1 hour) infusion and 96361 for each additional hour. Hydration codes are to be submitted when reporting hydration IV infusion that consists of a prepackaged fluid and/or electrolyte solutions (for example, normal saline, D5-1/2 normal saline+30mEq KC1/L) but are not to be used to report infusion of drugs or other substances.

Example: Patient with severe gastroenteritis is seen in the emergency department. Physician orders IV infusion for hydration (total of 1 hour, 45 minutes). Code assignment would be:

96360 Intravenous infusion, hydration; initial, 31 minutes to 1 hour
+96361 each additional hour

CPT Notes guide the coding professional to report 96361 for hydration if provided as a secondary or subsequent service after a different initial service (96360, 96365, 96374, 96409, 96413) is administered through the same IV access.

Therapeutic, Prophylactic, and Diagnostic Injections and Infusions (Excluding Chemotherapy and Other Highly Complex Drug or Highly Complex Biologic Agent Administration) (96365–96379)

CPT codes from this section are used to describe administration of substances and/or drugs. The fluid used to administer the drug(s) is incidental hydration and is not reported with a separate CPT code.

The codes are differentiated according to the route of administration, such as IV, and the injection status (initial, sequential, concurrent).

The specific substance injected must be reported with another code. For Medicare cases, a Level II HCPCS code (J series) is reported with the identification of the specific substance or drug; for non-Medicare cases, code 99070 may be reported. (HCPCS Level II codes [J codes] are discussed in chapter 10 of this workbook.) This series of codes is not to be used for allergy injections or immunizations; specific CPT codes are available for these services.

The payment policies of individual payers (including Medicare) differ and should be reviewed carefully to ensure appropriate payment.

Example: Patient with a wound infection undergoes a one-hour infusion of Vancomycin HCl 1000 mg. The correct code assignment would be:

96365	Intravenous infusion, for therapy, prophylaxis, or diagnosis (specify drug); initial, up to 1 hour
J3370 × 2	Vancomycin 500 mg

Chemotherapy and Other Highly Complex Drug or Highly Complex Biologic Agent Administration (96401–96549)

The administration of chemotherapy is reported with codes 96401 through 96549. The codes further identify the mode of administration: subcutaneous or intramuscular, intralesional, intravenous, or intra-arterial. The codes describing intravenous and intra-arterial administration are further subdivided to identify the technique—infusion or push—and length of time. Codes 96440 through 96450 describe the administration of chemotherapy to specific body sites: pleural or peritoneal cavity, or central nervous system. Codes 96521 and 96522 describe the maintenance and refilling of portable or implantable pumps or reservoirs.

Although preparation of the chemotherapy agent is included in the administration, provision of the chemotherapy drug is not. For Medicare claims, a code from the J series of the Level II HCPCS should be reported to identify the specific drug administered. (The CMS Web site provides chemotherapy coding guidelines.) The individual payer should be contacted for further directions. Codes describing the placement of pumps, catheters, or reservoirs can be found in the surgery section of the CPT codebook.

Example: Patient with lung cancer is seen in the hospital outpatient department for chemotherapy treatment. The patient receives Cisplatin 80 mg IV for one hour. The following should be reported:

96413	Chemotherapy administration, infusion, first hour
J9060	Cisplatin, per 10 mg (bill would reflect 8 units because 80 mg was administered).

When additional services are provided on the same day as the chemotherapy and are independent of the chemotherapy, the physician may bill the additional services separately (for example, an E/M office visit).

Exercise 8.8 Injections and Infusions

Unless otherwise noted, all answers can be found in appendix D of this book. Answers to selected exercises are located in the Instructor's Guide and available only to faculty of educational programs.

Assign the appropriate CPT code(s) for each of the following procedures/services.

1. Intramuscular vitamin B_{12} injection

 ____

2. IV infusion hydration for one hour

 ____

3. IV infusion of Cisplatin (chemotherapy) administered for two hours

 ____

4. Intra-arterial chemotherapy administration, IV push

 ____

Special Dermatological Procedures

Services such as actinotherapy and photochemotherapy are found in the special dermatological procedures subsection of CPT. Generally, these codes are used by consulting dermatologists.

Physical Medicine and Rehabilitation

The number of physical medicine and rehabilitation services available to patients continues to expand as new modalities and therapeutic procedures are developed. The CPT codes for these services (97001–97799) are used by the physiatrists and physical therapists who provide physical therapy services to patients recovering from injuries, strokes, and other debilitating conditions. Test and measurement codes can be reported to document the use of prosthetic devices and physical performance testing apparatus. No special coding guidelines apply to this section. Physiatrists use the E/M section for professional service billing.

Active Wound Care Management

Active wound care management (97597–97606) codes are also provided in this subsection. These codes are to be assigned to report active wound care performed by nonphysician healthcare professionals (for example, nurses, physician assistants, physical therapists, and occupational therapists).

According to CPT coding guidelines, the wound care management codes should not be reported in addition to the debridement codes (11040–11044) included in the integumentary system subsection of the Surgery section. The debridement codes (11040–11044) are considered surgical debridement, whereas wound care management codes are considered nonsurgical.

The nonsurgical debridement can be described as either selective or nonselective. Codes 97597 and 97598 are assigned for the selective technique, which includes the use of scalpels, scissors, and forceps to cut and remove the necrotic tissue. Other selective debridement includes the use of high-pressure water jets, enzyme applications, and autolysis. Code 97602 is assigned for nonselective techniques, which include the gradual removal of loosely adherent areas of necrotic tissue achieved by irrigating the wound and hydrotherapy.

Codes 97605 and 97606 are used to report negative pressure wound therapy, which is often described as a vacuum-assisted closure. This system encourages wound closure by applying localized negative pressure to the surface and margins of the wound. Negative pressure therapy is applied to a special dressing positioned in the wound cavity or over a flap or graft. The pressure-distributing wound dressing helps drain fluids from the wound.

Exercise 8.9 Physical Medicine and Rehabilitation

Unless otherwise noted, all answers can be found in appendix D of this book. Answers to selected exercises are located in the Instructor's Guide and available only to faculty of educational programs.

Assign the appropriate CPT code(s) for each of the following procedures/services.

1. TENS unit applied by therapist for patient with low back pain, 30 minutes

   ____

2. Thirty minutes of water aerobics with therapist for treatment of arthritis

   ____

3. Physician orders a reevaluation of a knee injury following a course of athletic training

   ____

4. Physical therapist provides whirlpool therapy to promote healing of a necrotic wound

   ____

Manipulative Treatment

Osteopathic physicians and chiropractic physicians as well as other physicians trained in manipulation techniques use the codes found in the osteopathic manipulative treatment and chiropractic manipulative treatment subsections. E/M service codes are to be reported separately only when the services are significant and separate from the manipulative treatments. In these cases, modifier 25, Significant, Separately Identifiable Evaluation and Management Service by the Same Physician on the Same Day of the Procedure or Other Service, may be appended to the E/M code to communicate the circumstances on a claim form.

Non-Face-to-Face Nonphysician Services

There are two subcategories for assessment and management of patient services via the telephone or with Internet communication. The selection of codes 98966–98969 is designated for use by qualified healthcare professionals (physicians are to use codes 99441–99444). Guidelines are summarized below:

- Initiated by established patient (or guardian)
- If the telephone call ends with the decision to see the patient within 24 hours (or next available urgent appointment), then the code is not reported.

- If call refers to a service performed within previous seven days or within the postoperative period, then the telephone services are considered part of the previous service or procedure; therefore ***not*** reported

The above guidelines also pertain to the Internet services. The online communication must be maintained in permanent storage, either electronically or in hard copy.

Special Services, Procedures, and Reports

The special services and reports subsection (99000–99091) of the CPT Medicine section describes certain procedures and services or reports that the physician may add to other basic services. Codes 99050 through 99060 describe special services provided to a patient beyond the basic service, such as those requested between 10 p.m. and 8 a.m. (code 99052). Because a third-party payer may or may not reimburse these services, a review of each payer's policies might be informative. However, coded information is also used in many activities unrelated to reimbursement, and so assigning the codes for nonreimbursable services may be desirable from a data management perspective.

CPT code 99070 may be reported when the physician submits claims for supplies and other materials to an insurance plan that does not recognize Level II HCPCS codes. For Medicare claims, coding professionals should remember that, in most cases, a more specific code describing a particular supply may exist in Level II of HCPCS, and routine supplies associated with professional services are not reimbursed separately.

Qualifying Circumstances for Anesthesia

Four CPT codes (99100–99140) may be used to report qualifying circumstances or additional information on patients undergoing anesthesia who show greater risk of complications. For example, codes describing patients of extreme age (elderly or newborn), with total body hypothermia or controlled hypotension, or with possible emergency conditions, may need to be reported in addition to the code describing the anesthesia service.

Moderate (Conscious) Sedation

The moderate sedation codes are available to report moderate (conscious) sedation, a technique used during a number of endoscopic and other procedures. The use of these codes requires the presence of an independent, trained observer to assist the operating physician in monitoring the patient's level of consciousness and physiological status. The codes represent performance and documentation of presedation and postsedation evaluations of the patient, administration of the sedation, and monitoring of cardiorespiratory functions.

Other Services and Procedures

The Medicine section of CPT also provides codes for several miscellaneous procedures that are performed by physicians but do not fit into the other sections of CPT. One example is hyperbaric oxygen therapy supervision. Another is the administration of ipecac and observation of the patient until the stomach is emptied of poison. Such codes are located in the other services and procedures subsection.

Home Health Procedures and Services

Codes from the section on home health procedures and services (99500–99512) are used by nonphysician healthcare professionals who provide medical services in the homes of patients. Physicians use codes from the E/M section for coding the home health services they provide. Healthcare professionals who are authorized to use E/M home visit codes (99341–99350) may report codes from the range 99500 through 99512 with the E/M code when a patient's condition requires significant evaluation and management services beyond the home health service or procedure. In such cases, modifier 25 may be appended to the E/M code.

Home Infusion Procedures/Services

Codes from the home infusion procedures section (99601 and 99602) include a code for home visits by nonphysician healthcare professionals and a code for all the necessary solutions, equipment, and supplies required to deliver a therapeutic service in one visit. Drugs are excluded from this code and should be reported separately.

Medication Therapy Management Services

CPT codes 99605–99607 are codes to report for face-to-face medication therapy management services (MTMS) by a pharmacist. The code selection is based on new versus established patient and time. Guidelines specify that MTMS documentation include the following:

- Review of pertinent patient history, medication profile
- Recommendations for improving health outcomes
- Treatment compliance

Exercise 8.10 Chapter 8 Review

Unless otherwise noted, all answers can be found in appendix D of this book. Answers to selected exercises are located in the Instructor's Guide and available only to faculty of educational programs.

Assign the appropriate code(s) from the CPT Medicine section as well as modifiers, when appropriate, for each of the following non-Medicare cases.

1. Patient (42 years old) diagnosed with ESRD requires home dialysis for the month of April.

   ____

2. A 50-year-old male is given an IM injection of Diphtheria toxoid (immunization) by the nurse practitioner.

   ____

3. Routine EKG with 15 leads, with the physician providing only the interpretation and report of the test

   ____

4. IV chemotherapy lasting three hours

   ____

5. Bundle of His electrography recording performed to evaluate patient with syncope

   ____

6. Speech audiometry with threshold and recognition, both ears

   ____

7. Intramuscular steroid injection

   ____

8. Individual interactive psychotherapy for 45 minutes provided in the outpatient setting

   ____

9. Percutaneous transluminal coronary atherectomy with balloon angioplasty of left posterior descending and left obtuse marginal arteries

   ____

10. Comprehensive ophthalmologic services provided to an established patient with extended color vision examination

    ____

Note: Answers to exercises 11 through 21 do not appear in appendix D of this text. They are located in the Instructor's Guide and available to faculty of educational programs.

11. Percutaneous angioplasty and thrombectomy of right coronary artery; angioplasty and placement of drug-eluting stent, left circumflex

    ____

(Continued on next page)

Exercise 8.10 (Continued)

12. Leg prosthetic training for 45 minutes by a physical therapist

____

13. In addition to E/M services, a physician provided a medical service on July 4 to fulfill a patient's request for the service

____

14. Complete duplex scan of the lower extremity arteries

____

15. EMG of three extremities and related paraspinal areas

____

16. Physician treats plaque psoriasis of arms and legs with use of laser (200 sq cm)

____

17. Osteopathic manipulation; head, cervical, thoracic, and lumbar spine

____

18. Pharmacist spends 30 minutes providing medication therapy management services to a new patient.

____

19. Nurse makes a home visit for newborn care and assessment

____

20. MDI (metered dose inhaler) treatment for patient with asthma

____

21. Sleep study including EKG, recordings of breathing, and O_2 saturation, performed by a technician

____

Chapter 9

Anesthesia

CPT codes in this section can be reported under the condition that the procedures/services were performed by, or under the responsible supervision of, a physician or a certified registered nurse anesthetist (CRNA). Coding professionals should keep in mind that they are selecting an anesthesia code based on the surgical procedure performed. The anesthesia section of the CPT codebook includes codes that describe general and regional anesthesia services, and supplementation of local anesthesia or other supportive services. These services should be reported by the physician who provides or supervises the anesthesia. The anesthesia services (00100–01999) in this section include:

- Usual preoperative and postoperative visits
- Anesthesia provided during the procedure
- Administration of fluids and/or blood
- Usual monitoring services, such as EKG, temperature, blood pressure, oximetry, capnography, and mass spectrometry. (Unusual monitoring, such as intra-arterial, central venous, or Swan-Ganz, is not included and should be reported separately.)

The codes in the Anesthesia section are arranged first by body site and then by specific surgical procedure performed (except for Radiological Procedures and Other Procedures at the end of the chapter). They may be found in the alphabetic index of the CPT codebook by referencing the main entries of Anesthesia or Analgesia.

For anesthesia services, it is important to review third-party payer rules and regulations before submitting CPT codes.

Types of Anesthesia

There are several methods of administering anesthesia.

- *Local anesthesia:* This method involves an injection of a numbing agent directly into the area of the body, which will block pain in minor procedures.
- *Regional anesthesia:* This method involves an injection, but the anesthetic is applied to a larger area of body surface. For example, a peripheral nerve block injected near a

specific nerve will block the sensation for a group of nerves supplied by the injected nerve. This type of technique is often used for procedures on hands, feet, arms, and legs. Another example of a regional anesthesia is an epidural or spinal block.

- *General anesthesia:* This method requires that the anesthetic be administered intravenously or by inhalation. The patient is unconscious during the surgery.

CPT Format

The anesthesia section is primarily organized by anatomic site (with a few exceptions). Closer examination of the code descriptions will reveal that several procedures may be assigned to one anesthesia code. For example:

00770	Anesthesia for all procedures on major abdominal blood vessels

Note the following format for anesthesia codes:

Anatomic site → **Knee and Popliteal Area**

01380	Anesthesia for all closed procedures on knee joint
01382	Anesthesia for diagnostic arthroscopic procedures of knee joint

Coding Procedure

Using the surgical procedure, diagnostic arthroscopy of the knee, apply the following procedure for correct coding assignment.

1. In the alphabetic index of CPT, locate the main term **Anesthesia.**
2. Refer to the subterm **Arthroscopic Procedures** and scan for **Knee.**
3. Note the code selection of 01382, 01400.
4. Refer to both codes and you will determine that the best CPT code is 01382.

To illustrate another method of locating the correct code, locate the main term **Anesthesia** and refer to subterm **Knee.** There is a large range of codes to reference and the coding process will take significantly longer but the correct code is among this range.

Conscious Sedation

Conscious sedation produces a level of consciousness that retains the patient's ability to independently and continuously maintain an airway and respond appropriately to physical stimulation or verbal command. CPT codes 99143–99145 are used to report moderate conscious sedation provided by a physician who is also performing the procedure. Additional code selections are available for a physician other than the healthcare professional performing the diagnostic or therapeutic service that the conscious sedation supports (99148–99150).

Time Reporting

Time may be reported for reimbursement of services, if preferred by the local carrier. Counting anesthesia time should begin with preparation of the patient by the anesthesiologist for induction of anesthesia (usually in the operating room) and end when the anesthesiologist no longer is in attendance.

Anesthesia Modifiers

When reporting anesthesia services, a physical status modifier code should be used to distinguish between various levels of complexity of the anesthesia service provided. The anesthesiologist usually provides physical status modifiers on the anesthesia record. The ranking of patient physical status by the American Society of Anesthesiologists (ASA) is consistent with the following modifiers:

P1 A normal, healthy patient
P2 A patient with mild systemic disease
P3 A patient with severe systemic disease
P4 A patient with severe systemic disease that is a constant threat to life
P5 A moribund patient who is not expected to survive without the operation
P6 A declared brain-dead patient whose organs are being removed for donor purposes

Under certain circumstances, other modifiers may be assigned. The following modifiers are commonly used with codes from the anesthesia section.

22 Increased Procedural Services: Modifier 22 may be reported to identify that the service provided was greater than that usually required for a particular service. Supportive documentation may need to be submitted to the third-party payer to justify use of modifier 22.

23 Unusual Anesthesia: Modifier 23 may be reported when anesthesia is administered for a procedure that usually requires local anesthesia or none at all. This modifier would be reported along with the appropriate code describing the anesthesia service.

51 Multiple Procedures: Modifier 51 may be reported to identify that multiple anesthesia services were provided on the same day or during the same operative episode. The first procedure listed should identify the major or most resource-intensive service provided. Subsequent or secondary services should be appended with modifier 51.

53 Discontinued Procedure: Modifier 53 is appropriate for circumstances when the physician elects to terminate or discontinue a procedure, usually because of risk to the patient's well-being. However, this modifier is not meant to report the elective cancellation of a procedure before the patient's surgical preparation or induction of anesthesia. Also, the appropriate ICD-9-CM code should be assigned to identify the reason for the procedure's termination or discontinuation.

59 Distinct Procedural Service: Modifier 59 may be used to identify that a procedure/service was distinct or independent from other services provided on the same day.

Modifier 47, Anesthesia by Surgeon, is never used as a modifier for the anesthesia procedures in the CPT codebook (00100–01999).

HCPCS Level II Modifiers

The following National Code modifiers are applicable to anesthesia services:

AA Anesthesia services performed personally by anesthesiologist

AD Medical supervision by a physician: more than four concurrent anesthesia procedures

G8 Monitored anesthesia care (MAC) for deep complex, complicated or markedly invasive surgical procedures

G9 Monitored anesthesia care for a patient who has a history of a severe cardiopulmonary condition

QK Medical direction of two, three, or four concurrent anesthesia procedures involving qualified individuals

QS Monitored anesthesia care service

QX CRNA service; with medical direction by a physician

QY Medical direction of one certified registered nurse anesthetist (CRNA) by an anesthesiologist

QZ CRNA service; without medical direction by a physician

The assignment of modifier QK indicates that the anesthesiologist provided medical direction to at least two, but not more than four, certified nurse anesthetists.

Qualifying Circumstances

When anesthesia services are provided under difficult circumstances because of the patient's condition, operative conditions, or unusual risk factors, an additional code may be reported along with the code describing the basic anesthesia service. Codes 99100 through 99140 can never be reported alone. Located in the medicine section of the CPT codebook, these codes (99100–99140) are described as follows:

- 99100, Anesthesia for patient of extreme age, under 1 year and over 70 years
- 99116, Anesthesia complicated by utilization of total body hypothermia
- 99135, Anesthesia complicated by utilization of controlled hypotension
- 99140, Anesthesia complicated by emergency conditions

When code 99140 is reported, a separate report must be submitted describing the type of emergency. According to the CPT codebook, an emergency exists when delay in treatment of the patient would significantly increase the threat to life or body part.

Application of Anesthesia Codes in the Hospital Setting

Because the anesthesia codes were developed to represent the professional services provided by anesthesiologists, the anesthesia codes cannot be reported by hospitals unless the hospitals perform billing services for the anesthesiologists.

Exercise 9.1 Chapter 9 Review

Unless otherwise noted, all answers can be found in appendix D of this book. Answers to selected exercises are located in the Instructor's Guide and available only to faculty of educational programs.

Assign the appropriate codes and physical status modifiers to describe the anesthesia services for the following Medicare claims. The anesthesia codes should be assigned from the Anesthesia section.

1. Anesthesia services for radical mastectomy with internal mammary node dissection; patient has diabetes mellitus well controlled with American Dietetic Association (ADA) diet

   ____

2. Anesthesia services for closed treatment of fracture of humerus, patient is 85 years old but healthy

   ____

3. Anesthesia services for CABG surgery of five vessels with pump oxygenator; patient has severe coronary artery disease as well as hypertensive end-stage renal disease requiring hemodialysis

   ____

4. Anesthesia services for left lobectomy due to lung carcinoma; patient also has severe chronic obstructive pulmonary disease and emphysema treated with bronchodilators

   ____

5. Anesthesia services for left carotid endarterectomy; patient is otherwise healthy

   ____

Note: Answers to exercises 6 through 10 do not appear in appendix D of this text. They are located in the Instructor's Guide and available to faculty of educational programs.

6. Anesthesia services for partial nephrectomy in a patient with renal cell carcinoma; 45-year-old patient also has mild coronary artery disease and hypertension treated with medication

   ____

7. Anesthesia services for heart transplant secondary to congenital heart defect; patient is 3 weeks old and requires a transplant to survive

   ____

8. Anesthesia services for carotid thromboendarterectomy with patch graft for severe carotid artery stenosis; patient is 75 years old and has had recurrent carotid artery stenosis; patient also has a pacemaker for control of atrial fibrillation

   ____

9. Anesthesia services for vaginal hysterectomy; patient is 45 years old and in good health

   ____

10. Anesthesia services for blepharoplasty; patient is in good health

   ____

Chapter 10

HCPCS Level II

Developed by the Centers for Medicare and Medicaid Services (CMS), Level II HCPCS also is referred to as the National Codes. The National Codes were designed to report physician and nonphysician services such as drugs, chiropractic services, dental procedures, durable medical equipment, and other selected procedures.

Although the National Codes were developed for Medicare, they also are used by commercial payers. Coding professionals should note that some Medicare carriers mandate the use of Level II codes rather than specific CPT codes. For example, there is a CPT code for removal of impacted cerumen (69210), but CMS will deny payment for this code. HCPCS Level II code G0268 should be reported for the earwax removal procedure. Bulletins from Medicare carriers announce such mandates. Some Medicaid programs and private insurance carriers also may accept or mandate the use of National Codes.

The American Hospital Association (AHA) and the Centers for Medicare and Medicaid Services (CMS) have joined together in establishing the AHA clearinghouse to handle coding questions on established HCPCS usage. The American Health Information Management Association (AHIMA) also provides input through the Editorial Advisory Board. In addition to publishing a *Coding Clinic* for ICD-9-CM, AHA also publishes a *Coding Clinic* specifically for HCPCS.

As mentioned in chapter 1 of this workbook, a listing of these codes may be purchased from the U.S. Government Printing Office or any local Medicare carrier (which provides them as a computer-generated list). In addition, several publishing firms offer the National Codes in book format, which can offer better indexing and cross-references. Finally, a file containing the most current versions of the HCPCS Level II codes can be found at the following CMS Web site: http://www.cms.hhs.gov/HCPCSReleaseCodeSets. The HCPCS Level II codes included in this publication are current as of October 1, 2011.

Structure of the HCPCS Level II Codes

Level II HCPCS consists of five-digit alphanumeric codes beginning with an alphabetic character (A through V, excluding S) followed by four numbers.

Example:	A4625	Tracheostomy care kit for new tracheostomy
	G0426	Telehealth Consultation
	J2360	Injection, orphenadrine, citrate, up to 60 mg
	V2500	Contact lens, PMMA, spherical, per lens

The National Codes are divided into the following sections:

Codes	Section
A codes	Transportation Services, Including Ambulance Medical and Surgical Supplies Administrative, Miscellaneous, and Investigational
B codes	Enteral and Parenteral Therapy
C codes	Temporary Codes for Use with Outpatient PPS
D codes	Dental Procedures
E codes	Durable Medical Equipment (DME)
G codes	Procedures/Professional Services (Temporary)
H codes	Alcohol and Drug Abuse Treatment Services
J codes	Drugs Administered, Other Than Oral Method, Chemotherapy Drugs
K codes	Temporary (Assigned to Durable Medical Equipment Regional Carriers [DMERC])
L codes	Orthotic Procedures, Prosthetic Procedures
M codes	Medical Services
P codes	Pathology and Laboratory Services
Q codes	Miscellaneous Services (Temporary Codes)
R codes	Diagnostic Radiology Services
S codes	Temporary National Codes (Non-Medicare)
T codes	Established for State Medicaid Agencies
V codes	Vision Services, Hearing Services

General Guidelines for HCPCS Level II Coding

The HCPCS coding guidelines, like the CPT coding guidelines, establish a four-step coding process:

1. Never code directly from the index.
2. Search for main terms and any applicable subterms.
3. Note the reference codes as given in the index.
4. Verify the codes by reading the entire description.

Exercise 10.1 HCPCS Level II Codes

Unless otherwise noted, all answers can be found in appendix D of this book. Answers to selected exercises are located in the Instructor's Guide and available only to faculty of educational programs.

Using the HCPCS Level II code book or Excel file of HCPCS codes (downloaded from CMS Web site (http://www.cms.hhs.gov/HCPCSReleaseCodeSets), assign HCPCS Level II codes for the following. If using the Excel file, click "Edit" and use the "Find" function to locate the correct codes.

1. Battery, heavy duty, replacement for patient-owned ventilator

   ____

2. Healthcare professional conducts a (non-medical) family planning session

   ____

3. Capecitabine, oral 150 mg

   ____

4. Prolotherapy

   ____

5. Pinworm examination

   ____

Table of Drugs

The HCPCS National Codes describe drugs that have been administered with codes that begin with the capital letter J. J codes describe drugs using their generic names, amounts, and routes of administration. The following abbreviations are used to designate the route of administration:

IA	Intra-arterial
IT	Intrathecal
IV	Intravenous
IM	Intramuscular
SC	Subcutaneous
INH	Inhalant solution
VAR	Various routes
ORAL	Oral
OTH	Other routes

The abbreviation VAR is used for drugs that are commonly administered into cavities, joints, or tissues, or as topical applications. OTH refers to other administration methods such as suppositories or catheter injections.

The following is an excerpt from HCPCS Table of Drugs:

Alatrofloxacin mesylate, injection	100 mg IV	J0200
Albuterol	0.5 mg INH	J7620
Albuterol, concentrated form	per mg INH	J7611
Albuterol, unit dose form	per mg INH	J7613

HCPCS Level II Modifiers

The modifiers used in HCPCS Level II were developed to serve the same purpose that modifiers serve in the CPT codebook. The assignment of a modifier may indicate that a service or procedure was modified in some way, but with no change to its basic definition. HCPCS modifiers can be used to indicate the following types of information:

- The service was supervised by an anesthesiologist.
- The service was performed by a healthcare professional other than a physician, such as a clinical psychologist, a nurse practitioner, or a physician assistant.
- The service was provided as part of a specific government program.
- The service was provided to a specific site of the body.
- Equipment was purchased or rented.
- Single or multiple patients were seen during nursing home visits.

In the coding of Medicare claims, HCPCS Level II modifiers may be used with the National Codes or with CPT Category I codes.

The HCPCS modifiers consist of one or two characters and are appended to the appropriate HCPCS Level II or CPT Category I codes. The following are examples of HCPCS Level II modifiers (a complete list of modifiers can be located on the CMS Web site):

AA	Anesthesia services personally furnished by the anesthesiologist
AH	Clinical psychologist
AJ	Clinical social worker
AM	Physician, team member service
AS	Physician assistant, nurse practitioner, or clinical nurse specialist services for assistant at surgery
GA	Waiver of liability statement on file

Example: A patient is recovering at home after having surgery for a hip fracture. The DME (durable medical equipment) provider rents the patient a rigid adjustable-height walker for 30 days. The DME provider would report the following HCPCS Level II code and modifier:

E0130-RR (The HCPCS Level II modifier RR is for rental.)

Exercise 10.2 Chapter 10 Review

Unless otherwise noted, all answers can be found in appendix D of this book. Answers to selected exercises are located in the Instructor's Guide and available only to faculty of educational programs.

Use the HCPCS Level II codebook to answer the following questions.

1. What is the code for a gel mattress?

   ____

2. What code would be assigned if the surgeon provided a surgical tray for a procedure?

   ____

Exercise 10.2 (Continued)

3. If a patient was given a vitamin B_{12} injection in the office, what HCPCS code would be assigned for the actual substance?

 ____

4. What Level II code would indicate that the patient received an above-the-knee surgical stocking?

 ____

5. If a patient was given an IM injection of 30 mg of hydrocortisone sodium phosphate, what HCPCS code would be assigned for this drug?

 ____

Note: Answers to exercises 6 through 10 do not appear in appendix D of this text. They are located in the Instructor's Guide and available to faculty of educational programs.

Assign HCPCS Level I (CPT) code(s) and HCPCS Level II code(s) to the following procedures.

6. The physician inserted a temporary indwelling Foley catheter

 CPT code for procedure: ______________________________

 HCPCS code for catheter supply: ______________________________

7. Patient was treated for a sprained ankle; strapping was applied, and the patient was given crutches (a pair of adjustable, underarm wood crutches with pads, tips, and handgrips).

 CPT code for procedure: ______________________________

 HCPCS code for crutches: ______________________________

In addition to HCPCS Level I (CPT) codes, assign HCPCS Level II modifiers for the following procedures, if applicable.

8. Patient is seen in the emergency department for a 1.5-cm laceration of the lower right eyelid. Physician performs a simple wound repair.

 ____

9. Avulsion of nail bed of left great toe and left second toe

 ____

10. Release of trigger finger, right ring finger

 ____

Chapter 11

Reimbursement in the Ambulatory Setting

The purpose of this chapter is to provide an overview of reimbursement systems in ambulatory care settings. Coding professionals must be aware of, and apply skills to, the reimbursement systems used by government payers and other health plans. Because these systems utilize codes as the basis for calculating payment amounts, complete and accurate coding is a key element in the financial performance of healthcare organizations. Thus, coding professionals must understand the coding guidelines currently in use and how to apply them to ensure that their facilities receive appropriate reimbursement for their services.

Although all the reimbursement systems use codes, the ways in which payments to healthcare facilities are determined can vary greatly. For example, guidelines for reimbursement for ambulatory services provided to Medicare patients changed with implementation of ambulatory payment classifications (APCs), which divide outpatient services into fixed-payment groups. Fees for services provided to Medicare patients by physicians are determined by a fee schedule based on the resource-based relative value scale (RBRVS), designed to provide a systematic and more equitable approach to compensation.

Managed care organizations often contract with physicians and facilities for a fee schedule that lists CPT codes with the corresponding amount of payment. When they participate in these plans, physicians and/or healthcare facilities agree that they will not expect or require more than this amount in compensation for the services provided to patients covered by the plan. Paying attention to reporting requirements for codes, as well as to rules on bundling of services, is essential for optimizing reimbursement in a managed care environment or within a government-mandated prospective payment system (PPS).

Reimbursement for Ambulatory Services Provided to Medicare Patients

Reimbursement for ambulatory services provided to Medicare patients changed significantly in 2000 with implementation of APCs in hospital settings.

Hospital Outpatient Prospective Payment System

In 2000, the Centers for Medicare and Medicaid Services (CMS) issued its final rule on an outpatient prospective payment system (OPPS). This payment system is based on groups of services, APCs, which divide outpatient services into fixed-payment groups. Each APC may include multiple CPT/HCPCS codes but is clinically similar and requires comparable resources. National payment rates were established with an adjustment for geographical factors. Table 11.1

is an excerpt from the *Federal Register* that shows APCs 0001 through 0004 with the associated HCPCS codes, descriptions, status indicators, relative weights, and payments.

Case Study

Using APC 0004 from table 11.1 as a reference, follow this simulated case study. Assume a patient with Medicare insurance was seen in the hospital outpatient surgery suite for a puncture aspiration of a cyst of the breast. CPT code 19000 was assigned for the procedure. Note that from the reference above, CPT code 19000 is assigned to APC 0004. According to table 11.1, the hospital will be reimbursed $319.03 for providing the services applicable to this procedure. The APC payment will include packaged items such as room charges, medical–surgical equipment, surgical dressings and supplies, and pharmaceuticals. The APC payment methodology is only applicable to the hospital services; the physician will be reimbursed under another method.

Now look at the status indicators in table 11.2. Every APC has a status indicator code. Code T for APC 0004 designates that the APC payment is subject to payment reduction when multiple procedures are performed during the same visit. In the above case study, there were no additional procedures so the status indicator does not affect payment. A complete list of status indicators is found in table 11.2.

Some outpatient facility services are not paid under OPPS. Medicare has a variety of payment methods for a range of outpatient services. Every HCPCS code is assigned a status indicator, as shown in table 11.2. The indicator shows how each service is to be reimbursed. For example, ambulance services are reimbursed by the ambulance fee schedule.

Drug and Device Pass-Through Payments

Under the APC system, additional reimbursement may be made for certain drugs and devices. Certain high-cost drugs are not packaged into the APC groups. Additional information can be found on the CMS Web site at www.cms.hhs.gov.

Reimbursement for Ambulatory Surgery Centers

An ambulatory surgery center (ASC) is a state-licensed supplier of surgical healthcare services. It is a separate entity from any other facility, such as a hospital. Since 2008, ambulatory surgery centers have been paid under a revised APC payment system that aligns payment rates to those rates for similar services in the OPPS. The revised ASC payment rates are being phased in over four years. Calendar year 2011 was the final year of this transition plan. Although there are a few exceptions, payment is based on a percentage for the same services under OPPS. The fixed payment will cover the costs of nursing services, supplies, equipment, and use of the facility.

Table 11.1. Excerpt from the APC file

APC	HCPCS	APC Title	HCPCS Short Description	Status Indicator	Relative Weight	Payment Rate
0001	96900	Level I photochemotherapy	Ultraviolet light therapy	S	0.5025	$34.88
0003	38220	Bone marrow biopsy/aspiration	Bone marrow aspiration	T	3.9075	$271.26
0003	38221	Biopsy marrow biopsy/aspiration	Bone marrow biopsy	T	3.9075	$271.26
0004	19000	Level I needle biopsy/aspiration except bone marrow	Drainage of breast lesion	T	4.5956	$319.03

Table 11.2. Addendum D1—APC status

Indicator	Item/Code/Service	OPPS Payment Status
A	Services furnished to a hospital outpatient that are paid under a fee schedule or payment system other than OPPS, for exampIe: • Ambulance Services • Clinical Diagnostic Laboratory Services • Nonimplantable Prosthetic and Orthotic Devices • EPO for ESRD Patients • Physical, Occupational, and Speech Therapy • Routine Dialysis Services for ESRD Patients Provided in a Certified Dialysis Unit of a Hospital • Diagnostic Mammography • Screening Mammography	Not paid under OPPS. Paid by fiscal intermediaries under a fee schedule or payment system other than OPPS.
B	Codes that are not recognized by OPPS when submitted on an outpatient hospital Part B bill type (12x and 13x).	Not paid under OPPS. • May be paid by intermediaries when submitted on a different bill type, for example, 75x (CORF), but not paid under OPPS. • An alternate code that is recognized by OPPS when submitted on an outpatient hospital Part B bill type (12x and 13x) may be available.
C	Inpatient Procedures	Not paid under OPPS. Admit patient. Bill as inpatient.
D	Discontinued Codes	Not paid under OPPS or any other Medicare payment system.
E	Items, Codes, and Services: • That are not covered by Medicare based on statutory exclusion. • That are not covered by Medicare for reasons other than statutory exclusion. • That are not recognized by Medicare but for which an alternate code for the same item or service may be available. • For which separate payment is not provided by Medicare.	Not paid under OPPS or any other Medicare payment system.
F	Corneal Tissue Acquisition; Certain CRNA Services and Hepatitis B Vaccines	Not paid under OPPS. Paid at reasonable cost.
G	Pass-Through Drugs and Biologicals	Paid under OPPS; Separate APC payment includes pass-through amount.
H	Pass-Through Devise Categories	Separate cost-based pass-through payment. Not subject to coinsurance.
K	(1) Non-Pass-Through Drugs and Biologicals	Paid under OPPS. Separate APC payment.
	(2) Therapeutic Radiopharmaceuticals	Paid under OPPS. Separate APC payment.
	(3) Brachytherapy Services	Paid under OPPS. Separate APC payment.
	(4) Blood and Blood Products	Paid under OPPS. Separate APC payment.
L	Influenza Vaccine; Pneumococcal Pneumonia Vaccine	Not paid under OPPS. Paid at reasonable cost; Not subject to deductible or coinsurance.
M	Items and Services Not Billable to the Fiscal Intermediary	Not paid under OPPS.
N	Items and Services Packaged into APC Rates	Paid under OPPS; payment is packaged into payment for other services, including outliers. Therefore, there is no separate APC payment.
P	Partial Hospitalization	Paid under OPPS; per diem APC payment.
Q	Packaged Services Subject to Separate Payment Under OPPS Payment Criteria	Paid under OPPS; addendum B displays APC assignments when services are separately payable. (1) Separate APC payment based on OPPS payment criteria. (2) If criteria are not met, payment is packaged into payment for other services, including outliers. Therefore, there is no separate APC payment.
S	Significant Procedure, Not Discounted when Multiple	Paid under OPPS; separate APC payment.
T	Significant Procedure, Multiple Reduction Applies	Paid under OPPS; separate APC payment.
V	Clinic or Emergency Department Visit	Paid under OPPS; separate APC payment.
Y	Nonimplantable Durable Medical Equipment	Not paid under OPPS. All institutional providers other than home health agencies bill to DMERC.
X	Ancillary Services	Paid under OPPS; separate APC payment.

Note that the physician's fee for performing the procedure is reported separately. More information about this payment methodology can be found at the CMS Web site.

Payment and Quality Measures

CMS has been reviewing methods to align payment incentives for high-quality care. One initiative called Hospital Outpatient Quality Data Reporting Program (HOP QDRP) requires hospitals to report data associated with specific quality measures. For example, one measure titled "Timing of Antibiotic Prophylaxis" requires that a prophylactic antibiotic be initiated within one hour prior to surgical incision. Data elements associated with this measure would be reported to CMS. CMS reduces payments for hospitals that fail to successfully report required quality measures. The complete set of quality measures can be located on the CMS Web site.

Reimbursement for Physician Services Provided to Medicare Patients

In 1985, the Health Care Financing Administration (now the CMS) awarded a contract to W. C. Hsiao and his colleagues at the Harvard School of Public Health to develop a resource-based relative value scale (RBRVS) for application in a reimbursement system for physician services. The goals of the project were:

- To provide a systematic, rational approach to establishing physician payments for services provided to Medicare beneficiaries
- To establish a fair and equitable approach to compensating physicians
- To eliminate distortions in current fees
- To enhance cost-effective medical care

In September 1990, the *Federal Register* published the initial RBRVS values. With payment reforms implemented through the Omnibus Reconciliation Acts of 1989 and 1990, the RBRVS fee schedule was phased in over a five-year period. RBRVS was implemented on January 1, 1992, along with the newly developed E/M services codes in the CPT codebook. Before this time, physicians were paid for Medicare claims on the basis of customary, prevailing, and reasonable charges.

The standard relative values per procedure include the following elements:

- *Physician work:* Technical skill, physical and mental effort; level of risk; and related stress
- *Practice expense:* The cost of supplies and equipment, wages for employees, and other overhead expenses, such as rent and utilities (there are currently values for facility and nonfacility physician practice expenses in the RBRVS system; services rendered at a facility have a lower RVU associated with them than nonfacility or office-based services)
- *Malpractice expense:* The average cost of malpractice insurance

For determining payment, the geographic practice cost index value considers similar factors:

- *Physician work:* Percentage of difference between the physician's work effort in a geographic area and the national average for the work effort

- *Practice expense:* Relative cost of the mix of goods and services in a geographic area
- *Malpractice expense:* Relative cost of malpractice insurance in a geographic area

The following formula is used to determine the RBRVS for a specific CPT code:

$$(\text{RVU}w \times \text{GPCI}w) + (\text{RVU}pe \times \text{GPCI}pe) + (\text{RVU}m \times \text{GPCI}m) = \text{RBRVS}$$
$$\text{Total RBRVs} \times \text{CF} = \text{fee}$$

In the preceding equation, RVU stands for the relative value unit of the procedure; *w* stands for physician work; GPCI stands for geographic practice cost index value; *pe* stands for practice expense; *m* stands for malpractice expense; and CF stands for conversion factor (a variable).

The RVUs for CPT codes are updated every year, as reported in the *Federal Register.* Payment files can be located on the CMS Web site: www.cms.hhs.gov/physicians. For example, the RVU for CPT code 19000 in 2011 was calculated using .84 for the physician's work, 2.14 for the physician's practice expense, and 0.11 for the physician's malpractice expense.

Then, assuming a simulated geographic practice expense of 0.961 (Ohio), a malpractice expense of 1.230, work of 1.0, and a conversion factor (CF) of $33.9764, one can calculate the payment for this procedure as follows:

$(.84 \times 1.0) + (2.14 \times .961) + (0.11 \times 1.230 = 3.03184$	$3.03184 \times \$33.9764 = \$103.01$
$(\text{RVU}w \times \text{GPCI}w) + (\text{RVU}pe \times \text{GPCI}pe) + (\text{RVU}m \times \text{GPCI}m) = \text{RBRVS}$	$\text{RBRVs} \times \text{CF} = \text{fee}$

You may recall in an earlier case study that the APC payment rate for the hospital (for the same procedure) was calculated as $319.03.

Medicare Outpatient Code Editor

CMS carefully evaluates the procedural and diagnostic data submitted with ambulatory claims. The agency requires Medicare Administrative Contractors (MACs) (organizations that process Medicare claims under contracts with the CMS) to use a tool known as the Medicare Outpatient Code Editor (OCE). The goal is to weed out incomplete or incorrect claims. With CMS's emphasis on detecting potential cases of fraud and abuse, coding professionals are expected to exhibit a high degree of competency in CPT coding. CMS also is particularly interested in the correct application of coding guidelines.

Since implementation of the Medicare OPPS, the functionality of the OCE has been greatly expanded. The OCE performs four basic functions:

- Editing the data on the claim for accuracy
- Specifying the action the MAC should take when specific edits occur
- Assigning APCs to the claim (for hospital outpatient services)
- Determining payment-related conditions that require direct reference to HCPCS codes or modifiers

Routine edits for age and sex inconsistencies are performed on all claim forms. In addition to editing HCPCS codes, the hospital billing form (UB-04) is checked for revenue codes, modifier use, and service units. All claims are subject to National Correct Coding Initiative (NCCI) edits. The NCCI edits identify combinations of procedures that are mutually exclusive. If an NCCI edit occurs, payment for the component code is denied. When an OCE edit occurs, the MAC may take one of six different actions:

- *Claim rejection:* When a claim is rejected, the provider may correct and resubmit the claim, but it cannot appeal the MAC's decision.
- *Claim denial:* The provider cannot resubmit the claim, but it may appeal the MAC's decision.
- *Claim returned to provider (RTP):* The provider may correct and resubmit the claim.
- *Claim suspension:* Payment is delayed for MAC determination; the MAC may need additional information before it can make a decision.
- *Line item rejection:* The claim is paid, but one of the line items is rejected; the provider may correct and resubmit the claim, but the MAC's decision cannot be appealed.
- *Line item denial:* The claim is paid, but some line items are denied; the provider cannot resubmit the claim, but the MAC's decision can be appealed.

Reimbursement and record-processing efficiency are seriously compromised when incomplete or error-ridden claims are returned to the provider for correction and resubmission. Most insurance carriers accept only "clean claims," that is, claims that have passed OCE scrutiny.

Office of Inspector General

The mission of the Office of Inspector General (OIG), as mandated by Public Law 95-452 (as amended), is to protect the integrity of Department of Health and Human Services (HHS) programs, as well as the health and welfare of the beneficiaries of those programs. This mandate includes investigating cases of healthcare fraud. The OIG's yearly Work Plan often includes a focus on coding issues, such as:

- *Upcoding*—practice of purposely assigning a code to receive additional or increased payment
- *Unbundling*—practice of using multiple codes when the services should be represented with a single code

Some of the areas of focus for the 2012 Work Plan include:

- Hospital readmissions
- Hospital reporting for adverse events
- Observation services during outpatient visits
- Trends in coding of E/M services
- Use of modifiers during global surgery period

The complete Work Plan can be found on the Web site of the Office of the Inspector General.

Quality Controls

Every healthcare facility, clinic, hospital, physician practice, and ambulatory service should implement quality controls to limit coding and claim errors so as to ensure that no fraudulent or abusive coding practices occur. ICD-9-CM and CPT codebooks must be updated annually to ensure that the most current and complete codes are available for reporting purposes. Coding professionals should receive routine training to promote skill development and increase knowledge of new payment guidelines and rules. A regular coding review is a key element in any Medicare compliance program.

Updated CPT codebooks are available late in the year (usually in October), and the updated codes go into effect sometime after January 1. The actual implementation dates vary among third-party payers. The updated ICD-9-CM codebooks are available in late summer or early fall, and changes take effect on October 1 every year.

Exercise 11.1 Chapter 11 Review and Optional ICD-10-CM Coding Exercise

Unless otherwise noted, all answers can be found in appendix D of this book. Answers to selected exercises are located in the Instructor's Guide and available only to faculty of educational programs.

Review the following scenarios and the codes suggested for reporting the services on the CMS-1500 billing form. Determine whether the CPT codes are correct or incorrect, and circle your answer. For those codes that are incorrect, identify the coding error. The ICD-9-CM codes are provided for reference only.

Optional Activity: To begin the transition from ICD-9-CM to ICD-10-CM for diagnosis coding, you may elect to assign ICD-10-CM codes for each of the following scenarios. The following link will provide access to the electronic files for ICD-10-CM: http://www.cdc.gov/nchs/icd/icd10cm.htm.

For example in Case #1, In ICD-10-CM, the initial encounter for a patient with a laceration of the forehead would be assigned code S01.81xA. In the Alphabetic Index for ICD-10–CM, refer to the key term "Laceration" and subterm "forehead" to obtain the code to verify in the Tabular list.

1. The patient was seen in the emergency department for facial lacerations. Simple repairs were performed on a 3.0-cm laceration on the forehead, a 2.8-cm laceration of the left upper eyelid, and a 1.0-cm laceration of the right upper eyelid.

   Correct (Incorrect)

Comments: 12014, add them all together

ICD-10-CM code(s): ______________________ *(optional activity)*

21. DIAGNOSIS OR NATURE OF ILLNESS OR INJURY (Relate Items 1, 2, 3 or 4 to Item 24E by Line)
1. 873.42
2. 870.0
3. ___ . ___
4. ___ . ___

22. MEDICAID RESUBMISSION CODE — ORIGINAL REF. NO.

23. PRIOR AUTHORIZATION NUMBER

	24. A. DATE(S) OF SERVICE From MM	DD	YY	To MM	DD	YY	B. PLACE OF SERVICE	C. EMG	D. PROCEDURES, SERVICES, OR SUPPLIES (Explain Unusual Circumstances) CPT/HCPCS	MODIFIER	E. DIAGNOSIS POINTER	F. $ CHARGES	G. DAYS OR UNITS	H. EPSDT Family Plan	I. ID. QUAL.	J. RENDERING PROVIDER ID. #
1	01	19							12013		1				NPI	
2	01	19							12013	LT	2				NPI	
3	01	19							12011	RT	2				NPI	
4															NPI	
5															NPI	
6															NPI	

(Continued on next page)

Exercise 11.1 (Continued)

2. The patient was seen in the dermatologist's office, where seven skin tags were removed from the neck.

   Correct ~~Incorrect~~ (Incorrect circled)

Comments: 11200

ICD-10-CM code(s): ______________________ *(optional activity)*

21. DIAGNOSIS OR NATURE OF ILLNESS OR INJURY (Relate Items 1, 2, 3 or 4 to Item 24E by Line)	22. MEDICAID RESUBMISSION CODE / ORIGINAL REF. NO.
1. 701.9 3. ___ . ___	23. PRIOR AUTHORIZATION NUMBER
2. ___ . ___ 4. ___ . ___	

	24. A. DATE(S) OF SERVICE From MM	DD	YY	To MM	DD	YY	B. PLACE OF SERVICE	C. EMG	D. PROCEDURES, SERVICES, OR SUPPLIES (Explain Unusual Circumstances) CPT/HCPCS	MODIFIER	E. DIAGNOSIS POINTER	F. $ CHARGES	G. DAYS OR UNITS	H. EPSDT Family Plan	I. ID. QUAL.	J. RENDERING PROVIDER ID. #
1	01	19							17000		1				NPI	
2	01	19							17003		1				NPI	
3															NPI	
4															NPI	
5															NPI	
6															NPI	

3. The patient underwent a diagnostic colonoscopy to determine the etiology of intestinal bleeding. Using the snare technique, the physician removed a benign polyp of the cecum.

   Correct Incorrect (Incorrect circled)

Comments: 45385, diagnostic is included in surgical

ICD-10-CM code(s): ______________________ *(optional activity)*

21. DIAGNOSIS OR NATURE OF ILLNESS OR INJURY (Relate Items 1, 2, 3 or 4 to Item 24E by Line)	22. MEDICAID RESUBMISSION CODE / ORIGINAL REF. NO.
1. 211.3 3. ___ . ___	23. PRIOR AUTHORIZATION NUMBER
2. ___ . ___ 4. ___ . ___	

	24. A. DATE(S) OF SERVICE From MM	DD	YY	To MM	DD	YY	B. PLACE OF SERVICE	C. EMG	D. PROCEDURES, SERVICES, OR SUPPLIES (Explain Unusual Circumstances) CPT/HCPCS	MODIFIER	E. DIAGNOSIS POINTER	F. $ CHARGES	G. DAYS OR UNITS	H. EPSDT Family Plan	I. ID. QUAL.	J. RENDERING PROVIDER ID. #
1	01	19							45378		1				NPI	
2	01	19							45385		1				NPI	
3															NPI	
4															NPI	
5															NPI	
6															NPI	

Exercise 11.1 (Continued)

4. The patient's chief complaint was dysuria. The physician performed a cystourethroscopy, ureteroscopy, and fulguration of ureteral polyp.

   Correct ~~~ **(Incorrect)** (circled)

Comments: 52354

ICD-10-CM code(s): ______________________________ *(optional activity)*

21. DIAGNOSIS OR NATURE OF ILLNESS OR INJURY (Relate Items 1, 2, 3 or 4 to Item 24E by Line)
1. 593.89
2. ___ . ___
3. ___ . ___
4. ___ . ___

22. MEDICAID RESUBMISSION CODE | ORIGINAL REF. NO.

23. PRIOR AUTHORIZATION NUMBER

	24. A. DATE(S) OF SERVICE From MM DD YY	To MM DD YY	B. PLACE OF SERVICE	C. EMG	D. PROCEDURES, SERVICES, OR SUPPLIES (Explain Unusual Circumstances) CPT/HCPCS	MODIFIER	E. DIAGNOSIS POINTER	F. $ CHARGES	G. DAYS OR UNITS	H. EPSDT Family Plan	I. ID. QUAL.	J. RENDERING PROVIDER ID. #
1	01 19				52214		1				NPI	
2											NPI	
3											NPI	
4											NPI	
5											NPI	
6											NPI	

5. A gynecologist performed a total abdominal hysterectomy with bilateral salpingo-oophorectomy. The pathological diagnosis was submucous leiomyoma of the uterus.

   Correct ~~~ **(Incorrect)** (circled)

Comments: 58150, unbundling

ICD-10-CM code(s): ______________________________ *(optional activity)*

21. DIAGNOSIS OR NATURE OF ILLNESS OR INJURY (Relate Items 1, 2, 3 or 4 to Item 24E by Line)
1. 218.0
2. ___ . ___
3. ___ . ___
4. ___ . ___

22. MEDICAID RESUBMISSION CODE | ORIGINAL REF. NO.

23. PRIOR AUTHORIZATION NUMBER

	24. A. DATE(S) OF SERVICE From MM DD YY	To MM DD YY	B. PLACE OF SERVICE	C. EMG	D. PROCEDURES, SERVICES, OR SUPPLIES (Explain Unusual Circumstances) CPT/HCPCS	MODIFIER	E. DIAGNOSIS POINTER	F. $ CHARGES	G. DAYS OR UNITS	H. EPSDT Family Plan	I. ID. QUAL.	J. RENDERING PROVIDER ID. #
1	01 19				58150		1				NPI	
2	01 19				58720		1				NPI	
3											NPI	
4											NPI	
5											NPI	
6											NPI	

(Continued on next page)

Exercise 11.1 (Continued)

Note: Answers to exercises 6 through 10 do not appear in appendix D of this text. They are located in the Instructor's Guide and available to faculty of educational programs.

6. A laboratory performed a hepatic function test, including albumin, total bilirubin, direct bilirubin, alkaline phosphatase, and SGOT for a patient with jaundice.

   Correct (Incorrect)

Comments: 82040, 82247, 82248, 84075, 84450

ICD-10-CM code(s): ______________________ *(optional activity)*

21. DIAGNOSIS OR NATURE OF ILLNESS OR INJURY (Relate Items 1, 2, 3 or 4 to Item 24E by Line)
1. 782.4   2. ___   3. ___   4. ___

22. MEDICAID RESUBMISSION CODE   ORIGINAL REF. NO.

23. PRIOR AUTHORIZATION NUMBER

	24. A. DATE(S) OF SERVICE From MM	DD	YY	To MM	DD	YY	B. PLACE OF SERVICE	C. EMG	D. PROCEDURES, SERVICES, OR SUPPLIES (Explain Unusual Circumstances) CPT/HCPCS	MODIFIER	E. DIAGNOSIS POINTER	F. $ CHARGES	G. DAYS OR UNITS	H. EPSDT Family Plan	I. ID. QUAL.	J. RENDERING PROVIDER ID. #
1	01	19							80076		1				NPI	
2															NPI	
3															NPI	
4															NPI	
5															NPI	
6															NPI	

7. A gynecologist performed a hysteroscopy with biopsy and dilation and curettage for a patient with dysfunctional uterine bleeding.

   Correct (Incorrect)

Comments: 58558, unbundling

ICD-10-CM code(s): ______________________ *(optional activity)*

21. DIAGNOSIS OR NATURE OF ILLNESS OR INJURY (Relate Items 1, 2, 3 or 4 to Item 24E by Line)
1. 626.8   2. ___   3. ___   4. ___

22. MEDICAID RESUBMISSION CODE   ORIGINAL REF. NO.

23. PRIOR AUTHORIZATION NUMBER

	24. A. DATE(S) OF SERVICE From MM	DD	YY	To MM	DD	YY	B. PLACE OF SERVICE	C. EMG	D. PROCEDURES, SERVICES, OR SUPPLIES (Explain Unusual Circumstances) CPT/HCPCS	MODIFIER	E. DIAGNOSIS POINTER	F. $ CHARGES	G. DAYS OR UNITS	H. EPSDT Family Plan	I. ID. QUAL.	J. RENDERING PROVIDER ID. #
1	01	09							58558		1				NPI	
2	01	09							58120		1				NPI	
3															NPI	
4															NPI	
5															NPI	
6															NPI	

Exercise 11.1 (Continued)

8. A physician performed an excision of left breast mass.

   (Correct) Incorrect

Comments: ____________________

ICD-10-CM code(s): ____________________ *(optional activity)*

21. DIAGNOSIS OR NATURE OF ILLNESS OR INJURY (Relate Items 1, 2, 3 or 4 to Item 24E by Line)
1. 611.72
2. ___ . ___
3. ___ . ___
4. ___ . ___

22. MEDICAID RESUBMISSION CODE | ORIGINAL REF. NO.

23. PRIOR AUTHORIZATION NUMBER

	24. A. DATE(S) OF SERVICE From MM DD YY	To MM DD YY	B. PLACE OF SERVICE	C. EMG	D. PROCEDURES, SERVICES, OR SUPPLIES (Explain Unusual Circumstances) CPT/HCPCS	MODIFIER	E. DIAGNOSIS POINTER	F. $ CHARGES	G. DAYS OR UNITS	H. EPSDT Family Plan	I. ID. QUAL.	J. RENDERING PROVIDER ID. #
1	01 09				19120	LT	1				NPI	
2											NPI	
3											NPI	
4											NPI	
5											NPI	
6											NPI	

9. A surgeon reported that he removed a 1.0-cm lesion of the chin with 0.5-cm margins around the diameter. Pathology report revealed basal cell carcinoma.

   Correct (Incorrect)

Comments: 11642, malignant not benign

ICD-10-CM code(s): ____________________ *(optional activity)*

21. DIAGNOSIS OR NATURE OF ILLNESS OR INJURY (Relate Items 1, 2, 3 or 4 to Item 24E by Line)
1. 173.3
2. ___ . ___
3. ___ . ___
4. ___ . ___

22. MEDICAID RESUBMISSION CODE | ORIGINAL REF. NO.

23. PRIOR AUTHORIZATION NUMBER

	24. A. DATE(S) OF SERVICE From MM DD YY	To MM DD YY	B. PLACE OF SERVICE	C. EMG	D. PROCEDURES, SERVICES, OR SUPPLIES (Explain Unusual Circumstances) CPT/HCPCS	MODIFIER	E. DIAGNOSIS POINTER	F. $ CHARGES	G. DAYS OR UNITS	H. EPSDT Family Plan	I. ID. QUAL.	J. RENDERING PROVIDER ID. #
1	01 09				11442		1				NPI	
2											NPI	
3											NPI	
4											NPI	
5											NPI	
6											NPI	

(Continued on next page)

Exercise 11.1 (Continued)

10. A surgeon performed a flexible bronchoscopy with cell washings and brushings for a patient with acute bronchitis.

Correct Incorrect

Comments: 31623, unbundling

ICD-10-CM code(s): ______________________ *(optional activity)*

21. DIAGNOSIS OR NATURE OF ILLNESS OR INJURY (Relate Items 1, 2, 3 or 4 to Item 24E by Line)

1. 466.0
2. ___
3. ___
4. ___

22. MEDICAID RESUBMISSION CODE — ORIGINAL REF. NO.

23. PRIOR AUTHORIZATION NUMBER

	24. A. DATE(S) OF SERVICE From MM	DD	YY	To MM	DD	YY	B. PLACE OF SERVICE	C. EMG	D. PROCEDURES, SERVICES, OR SUPPLIES (Explain Unusual Circumstances) CPT/HCPCS	MODIFIER	E. DIAGNOSIS POINTER	F. $ CHARGES	G. DAYS OR UNITS	H. EPSDT Family Plan	I. ID. QUAL.	J. RENDERING PROVIDER ID. #
1	01	09							31622		1				NPI	
2	01	09							31623		1				NPI	
3															NPI	
4															NPI	
5															NPI	
6															NPI	

Appendix A

References, Bibliography, and Web Resources

References and Bibliography

American Health Information Management Association. 1990–2011. Coding Notes and Clinical Notes. *Journal of AHIMA.* Chicago: AHIMA.

American Medical Association. 2011. *Current Procedural Terminology 2011.* Chicago: AMA.

American Medical Association. 1989–2011 *CPT Assistant.* Chicago: AMA.

Ingenix. 2011. *HCPCS Level II Expert.* Salt Lake City, Utah: Ingenix.

Ingenix. 2011. *Coder's Desk Reference for Procedures.* Salt Lake City, Utah: Ingenix.

Schraffenberger, L.A. 2012. *Basic ICD-10/PCS and ICD-9-CM Coding, 2012 ed.* Chicago: AHIMA.

Society of Cardiovascular and Interventional Radiology, et al. 2009. *Interventional Radiology Coding User's Guide,* 5th ed. Fairfax, VA: Society of Cardiovascular and Interventional Radiology, American College of Radiology, Radiology Business Management Association, American Health Radiology Administrators.

Web Resources

Aetna IntelliHealth: http://www.intelihealth.com
Aetna IntelliHealth is a partnership between Harvard Medical School and Aetna. It includes search tests/procedures, a medical dictionary, lists of drugs, and so on. It also is simple to navigate.

American Academy of Dermatology: http://www.aad.org
Click on "Public Resources" for links to sites about diseases of skin.

American Academy of Facial Plastic and Reconstructive Surgery: http://www.aafprs.org
Click on "Procedures" for links. A glossary and a page featuring common surgeries are included.

American Academy of Family Physicians: http://www.aafp.org
This Web resource includes articles on documentation guidelines.

American Academy of Orthopaedic Surgeons: http://www.aaos.org
Click on "Patient Information" to find fact sheets on many diseases and procedures.

American College of Cardiology: http://www.acc.org
Click on "Payer Advocacy" for information about CPT.

American College of Gastroenterology: http://www.acg.gi.org
Click on "Patient Information" for links of interest.

American College of Obstetricians and Gynecologists: http://www.acog.org
This site has information on patient education and provides links to coding/nomenclature.

American Gastroenterological Association: http://www.gastro.org
Click "Patient Center" and procedures for explanation of common gastroenterological procedures

American Health Information Management Association: http://www.ahima.org
This site provides coding products and an educational forum for coders called Communities of Practice (members only).

American Medical Association: http://www.ama-assn.org
This site contains information about coding products, CPT Assistant, and CPT updates and errata.

American Society of Plastic Surgery: http://www.plasticsurgery.org
Click on "Procedures."

Anatomy: http://www.innerbody.com
This site contains diagrams and definitions.

Anatomy: http://www.medtropolis.com
This site uses audio and visual effects to explain basic human anatomy. Visit the "Virtual Body."

Cancer: http://www.cancer.gov
Click on "Cancer Information" and then choose from the various types.

Cardiology: http://www.hgcardio.com
This site offers diagrams and descriptions of cardiac procedures.

Centers for Medicare and Medicaid Services (CMS): http://www.cms.hhs.gov

Discovery Health: http://health.discovery.com
This site has numerous links and has search features.

Encyclopedia of Medicine: http://findarticles.com
Clink on "Health" for a variety of links to health information articles.

Health Central: http://www.healthcentral.com
Health Central is a consumer-friendly site and is easy to navigate.

Healthfinder: http://www.healthfinder.gov
This consumer-friendly site offers a free guide for health and human services.

Heart Center: http://www.heartcenteronline.com
Click on "Patients" on this consumer-friendly site for quizzes and descriptions of cardiac procedures.

How Stuff Works: http://www.howstuffworks.com
Click on "Health."

MayoClinic: http://www.mayoclinic.com
This site provides consumer-oriented information about illnesses.

MedLearn: http://www.medlearn.com
MedLearn sells coding products, including a guide for interventional radiology coding.

MEDLINEplus: http://www.nlm.nih.gov/medlineplus/
Operated by the U.S. National Library of Medicine, MEDLINEplus includes encyclopedic background on all diseases, definitions of medical terms, and referrals to other organizations that deal with specific illnesses.
 Surgery Videos: http://www.nlm.nih.gov/medlineplus/surgeryvideos.html
 Interactive Tutorials: http://www.nlm.nih.gov/medlineplus/tutorial.html

National Library of Medicine: http://www.nlm.nih.gov
This site offers numerous resources.

Stanford Health Library: http://healthlibrary.stanford.edu/index.html
This site offers links providing information on diseases, disorders, and treatment.

WebMD: http://www.webmd.com
WebMD provides basic facts on any condition. The site guides you from general topics to more specific facts.

Appendix B

Evaluation and Management Documentation Guidelines

The following information was excerpted from the 1997 document developed by CMS and the AMA. A complete copy of this document and up-to-date information on the status of revised guidelines can be found on the CMS Web site at www.cms.gov.

To qualify for a given level of multisystem examination, the following content and documentation requirements should be met:

- A problem-focused examination should include performance and documentation of one to five elements identified by a bullet (•) in one or more organ system(s) or body area(s).
- An expanded problem-focused examination should include performance and documentation of at least six elements identified by a bullet (•) in one or more organ system(s) or body area(s).
- A detailed examination should include at least six organ systems or body areas. For each system/area selected, performance and documentation of at least two elements identified by a bullet (•) are expected. Alternatively, a detailed examination may include performance and documentation of at least 12 elements identified by a bullet (•) in two or more organ systems or body areas.
- A comprehensive examination should include at least nine organ systems or body areas. For each system/area selected, all elements of the examination identified by a bullet (•) should be performed, unless specific directions limit the content of the examination. For each area/system, documentation of at least two elements identified by a bullet is expected.

Examination Documentation Guidelines

- Specific abnormal and relevant negative findings of the examination of the affected or symptomatic body area(s) or organ system(s) should be documented. A notation of "abnormal" without elaboration is insufficient.
- Abnormal or unexpected findings of the examination of any asymptomatic body area(s) or organ system(s) should be described.
- A brief statement or notation indicating "negative" or "normal" is sufficient to document normal findings related to unaffected area(s) or asymptomatic organ system(s).

Content and Documentation Requirements

General Multisystem Examination

System/Body Area	Elements of Examination
Constitutional	• Measurement of *any three of the following seven vital signs:* (1) sitting or standing blood pressure; (2) supine blood pressure; (3) pulse rate and regularity; (4) respiration; (5) temperature; (6) height; and (7) weight (may be measured and recorded by ancillary staff) • General appearance of patient (for example, development, nutrition, body habitus, deformities, attention to grooming)
Eyes	• Inspection of conjunctivae and lids • Examination of pupils and irises (for example, reaction to light and accommodation, size, and symmetry) • Ophthalmoscopic examination of optic discs (for example, size, C/D ratio, appearance) and posterior segments (for example, vessel changes, exudates, hemorrhages)
Ears, Nose, Mouth, and Throat	• External inspection of ears and nose (for example, overall appearance, scars, lesions, masses) • Otoscopic examination of external auditory canals and tympanic membranes • Assessment of hearing (for example, whispered voice, finger rub, tuning fork) • Inspection of nasal mucosa, septum, and turbinates • Inspection of lips, teeth, and gums • Examination of oropharynx: oral mucosa, salivary glands, hard and soft palates, tongue, tonsils, and posterior pharynx
Neck	• Examination of neck (for example, masses, overall appearance, symmetry, tracheal position, crepitus) • Examination of thyroid (for example, enlargement, tenderness, mass)
Respiratory	• Assessment of respiratory effort (for example, intercostal retractions, use of accessory muscles, diaphragmatic movement) • Percussion of chest (for example, dullness, flatness, hyperresonance) • Palpation of chest (for example, tactile fremitus) • Auscultation of lungs (for example, breath sounds, adventitious sounds, rubs)
Cardiovascular	• Palpation of heart (for example, location, size, thrills) • Auscultation of heart with notation of abnormal sounds and murmurs Examination of: • Carotid arteries (for example, pulse amplitude, bruits) • Abdominal aorta (for example, size, bruits) • Femoral arteries (for example, pulse amplitude, bruits) • Pedal pulses (for example, pulse amplitude) • Extremities for edema and/or varicosities
Chest (Breasts)	• Inspection of breasts (for example, symmetry, nipple discharge) • Palpation of breasts and axillae (for example, masses or lumps, tenderness)
Gastrointestinal (Abdomen)	• Examination of abdomen with notation of presence of masses or tenderness • Examination of liver and spleen • Examination for presence or absence of hernia • Examination of anus, perineum, and rectum, including sphincter tone, presence of hemorrhoids, rectal masses • Obtain stool sample for occult blood test when indicated

System/Body Area	Elements of Examination
Genitourinary	*Male:* • Examination of the scrotal contents (for example, hydrocele, spermatocele, tenderness of cord, testicular mass) • Examination of the penis • Digital rectal examination of prostate gland (for example, size, symmetry, nodularity, tenderness) *Female:* Pelvic examination (with or without specimen collection for smears and cultures), including: • Examination of the external genitalia (for example, general appearance, hair distribution, lesions) and vagina (for example, general appearance, estrogen effect, discharge, lesions, pelvic support, cystocele, rectocele) • Examination of urethra (for example, masses, tenderness, scarring) • Examination of bladder (for example, fullness, masses, tenderness) • Cervix (for example, general appearance, lesions, discharge) • Uterus (for example, size, contour, position, mobility, tenderness, consistency, descent, or support) • Adnexa/parametria (for example, masses, tenderness, organomegaly, nodularity)
Lymphatic	Palpitation of lymph nodes in two or more areas: • Neck • Axillae • Groin • Other
Musculoskeletal	• Examination of gait and station • Inspection and/or palpation of digits and nails (for example, clubbing, cyanosis, inflammatory conditions, petechiae, ischemia, infections, nodes) Examination of joints, bones, and muscles of **one or more of the following six areas:** (1) head and neck; (2) spine, ribs, and pelvis; (3) right upper extremity; (4) left upper extremity; (5) right lower extremity; and (6) left lower extremity. The examination of a given area includes: • Inspection and/or palpation with notation of presence of any misalignment, asymmetry, crepitation, defects, tenderness, masses, or effusions • Assessment of range of motion with notation of any pain, crepitation, or contracture • Assessment of stability with notation of any dislocation (luxation), subluxation, or laxity • Assessment of muscle strength and tone (for example, flaccid, cog wheel, spastic) with notation of any atrophy or abnormal movements
Skin	• Inspection of skin and subcutaneous tissue (for example, rashes, lesions, ulcers) • Palpation of skin and subcutaneous tissue (for example, induration, subcutaneous nodules, tightening)
Neurologic	• Test cranial nerves with notation of any deficits • Examination of deep tendon reflexes with notation of pathological reflexes (for example, Babinski) • Examination of sensation (for example, touch, pin, vibration, proprioception)
Psychiatric	• Description of patient's judgment and insight Brief assessment of mental status, including: • Orientation to time, place, and person • Recent and remote memory • Mood and affect (for example, depression, anxiety, agitation)

(Continued on next page)

Content and Documentation Requirements

Level of Examination	Perform and Document:
Problem-focused	**One to five** elements identified by a bullet
Expanded problem-focused	**At least six** elements identified by a bullet
Detailed	**At least two** elements identified by a bullet **from each of 6 areas/systems** *or* **at least 12** elements identified by a bullet **in two or more areas/systems**
Comprehensive	Perform **all elements** identified by a bullet in **at least nine** organ systems or body areas and document **at least two** elements identified by a bullet **from each of nine areas/systems**

Appendix C

Additional Practice Exercises

The following surgical cases were performed in an ambulatory setting of Central Hospital. Determine the appropriate CPT code(s) for each case so that the hospital can receive the correct reimbursement. It is important to practice using the CPT index and to note how, in many instances, the codes may be found using more than one index entry. The appropriate modifiers should be assigned, when applicable, and the index entry(s) used to locate the code(s) should be noted.

If you wish to practice assigning codes by body system, the following reference will help.

Practice Exercises Indexed by Surgical Section

Integumentary System
- Case #17
- Case #25
- Case #26
- Case #27
- Case #33
- Case #39
- Case #43
- Case #50
- Case #54
- Case #57

Musculoskeletal System
- Case #4
- Case #10
- Case #12
- Case #20
- Case #42
- Case #44
- Case #45
- Case #47
- Case #60
- Case #62

Respiratory System
- Case #6
- Case #13 (also Digestive System)
- Case #18
- Case #41
- Case #55

Cardiovascular System
- Case #15
- Case #31
- Case #48
- Case #52

Hemic and Lymphatic Systems
- Case #38

Digestive System
- Case #1
- Case #3
- Case #11
- Case #13 (also Respiratory System)
- Case #14
- Case #19
- Case #21
- Case #22
- Case #23
- Case #24
- Case #30
- Case #32
- Case #53
- Case #56

Urinary System
- Case #2
- Case #9
- Case #51
- Case #59

Male/Female Genital System
- Case #7
- Case #8
- Case #16
- Case #28
- Case #29
- Case #36
- Case #63

Nervous System
- Case #35
- Case #37
- Case #58
- Case #61

Eye and Ocular Adnexa
- Case #5
- Case #34
- Case #40
- Case #46
- Case #49

Surgical Case #1

Operative Report

Procedure: Tonsillectomy

Diagnosis: Recurrent tonsillitis

Indications: This 10-year-old patient was found to have recurrent tonsillitis, and a tonsillectomy was planned.

Technique: The patient was placed in the supine position, and general endotracheal anesthesia was begun. The nasopharynx was inspected, revealing only a very small amount of adenoid, which was not removed. The tonsils were noted to be very large and obstructive, and were removed by dissection and snare technique. The bleeders were electrocoagulated. The inferior cuff was suture ligated with 2-0 plain catgut. The patient tolerated the procedure well and was brought to the recovery room in satisfactory condition.

Assign appropriate CPT code(s) for the preceding procedures and indicate the index entries that were used to identify the codes. Assign only CPT codes (no E/M codes) and append any applicable modifiers.

Code(s):____________________________________

Index entries:

____

____

Surgical Case #2

Operative Report

Procedure: Extracorporeal shock wave lithotripsy of right kidney stone

Diagnosis: Right kidney stone

Anesthesia: IV sedation

Technique: Under IV sedation, the patient was placed in the supine position. The stone in the upper right kidney was positioned at F2. The extracorporeal lithotripsy was started at 19 KV, which subsequently was increased to a maximum of 26 KV at 1,600 shocks. The stone was revisualized, and repositioning was done considering the transverse colon passing right anterior to the stone. Because the stone appeared to be in the same place after the repositioning, shocks were delivered. Apparent adequate fragmentation was obtained after a total of 2,400 shocks had been administered. The patient tolerated the procedure quite well.

Assign appropriate CPT code(s) for the preceding procedures and indicate the index entries that were used to identify the codes. Assign only CPT codes (no E/M codes) and append any applicable modifiers.

Code(s):____________________________________

Index entries:

____

____

Surgical Case #3

Operative Report

Procedure: Esophagogastroduodenoscopy with biopsy

Diagnosis: Gastritis and duodenitis

Technique: The patient was premedicated and brought to the endoscopy suite where his throat was anesthetized with Cetacaine spray. He then was placed in the left lateral position and given 2 mg Versed, IV.

An Olympus gastroscope was advanced into the esophagus, which was well visualized with no significant segmental spasms. Subsequently, the scope was advanced into the distal esophagus, which was essentially normal. Then the scope was advanced into the stomach, which showed evidence of erythema and gastritis. The pylorus was intubated and the duodenal bulb visualized. The duodenal bulb showed severe erythema, suggestive of duodenitis. Multiple biopsies were taken. The scope was withdrawn, and the patient tolerated the procedure well.

Assign appropriate CPT code(s) for the preceding procedures and indicate the index entries that were used to identify the codes. Assign only CPT codes (no E/M codes) and append any applicable modifiers.

Code(s):____

Index entries:

____

____

Surgical Case #4

Emergency Department Record

Chief Complaint:	Right shoulder dislocation
History of Present Illness:	The patient is a 53-year-old man who has dislocated his right shoulder three previous episodes. Today, he was kayaking and dislocated his shoulder while paddling.
Past Medical History:	Previous right shoulder dislocation
Medications:	Vitamins
Allergies:	Sulfa
Physical Examination:	Alert male in no acute distress
Right Upper Extremity:	He has obvious deformity with loss of the right shoulder prominence with a palpable anterior dislocation of the humeral head. He has good distal pulses with the remainder of his arm being nontender.
Emergency Department Course:	X-ray of his right shoulder shows an anterior dislocation.
Procedure:	Reduction of the shoulder dislocation. The patient was placed on a monitor with continuous pulse oximetry. He was given Demerol and Phenergan IV for pain control. In-line traction and reduction was accomplished after three attempts. Reduction films showed good position of the shoulder. He had good distal neurovascular status after reduction. He tolerated the procedure well.
Diagnosis:	Anterior dislocation, right shoulder
Disposition and Plan:	Sling and swathe for two to three days. Vicodin #30. Follow up with Dr. Smith in one to two days or call for an orthopedic referral. The patient states he has been avoiding any potential surgery at this point and would prefer to avoid it. I explained to him that he should follow up with Dr. Smith or an orthopedist. He should not use the shoulder in the next several days until reevaluation.

Assign appropriate CPT code(s) for the preceding procedures and indicate the index entries that were used to identify the codes. Assign only CPT codes (no E/M codes) and append any applicable modifiers.

Code(s):______________________________

Index entries:

____

____

Surgical Case #5

Operative Report

Procedure: Extracapsular cataract extraction with intraocular lens implantation, right eye

Diagnosis: Cataract of the right eye

Technique: The patient was given a retrobulbar injection of 2.5 to 3.0 cc of a mixture of equal parts of 2% lidocaine with epinephrine and 0.75% Marcaine with Wydase. The area around the right eye was infiltrated with an additional 6 to 7 cc of this mixture in a modified Van Lint technique. A self-maintaining pressure device was applied to the eye, and a short time later, the patient was taken to the OR.

The patient was properly positioned on the operating table, and the area around the right eye was prepped and draped in the usual fashion. A self-retaining eyelid speculum was positioned and 4-0 silk suture passed through the tendon of the superior rectus muscle, thereby deviating the eye inferiorly. A 160° fornix-based conjunctival flap was created followed by a 150° corneoscleral groove with a #64 Beaver blade. Hemostasis was maintained throughout with gentle cautery. A 6-0 silk suture was introduced to cross this groove at the 12 o'clock position and looped out of the operative field. The anterior chamber was then entered superiorly temporally, and after injecting Occucoat, an anterior capsulotomy was performed without difficulty. The nucleus was easily brought forward into the anterior chamber. The corneoscleral section was opened with scissors to the left and the nucleus delivered with irrigation and gentle lens loop manipulation. Interrupted 10-0 nylon sutures were placed at both the nasal and lateral extent of the incision. A manual irrigating aspirating setup then was used to remove remaining cortical material from both the anterior and posterior chambers.

At this point, a modified C-loop posterior chamber lens was removed from its package and irrigated and inspected. It then was positioned into the inferior capsular bag without difficulty, and the superior haptic was placed behind the iris at the 12 o'clock location. The lens was rotated to a horizontal orientation in an attempt to better enhance capsular fixation. Miochol was used to constrict the pupil, and a peripheral iridectomy was performed in the superior nasal quadrant. In addition, three or four interrupted 10-0 nylon sutures were used to close the corneal scleral section. The silk sutures were removed, and the conjunctiva advanced back into its normal location and was secured with cautery burns at the 3 and 9 o'clock positions. Approximately 20 to 30 mg of both Gentamicin and Kenalog were injected into the inferior cul-de-sac in a subconjunctival and sub-Tenon fashion. After instillation of 2% Pilocarpine and Maxitrol ophthalmic solution, the eyelid speculum was removed and the eye dressed in a sterile fashion. The patient was discharged to the recovery room in good condition.

Assign appropriate CPT code(s) for the preceding procedures and indicate the index entries that were used to identify the codes. Assign only CPT codes (no E/M codes) and append any applicable modifiers.

Code(s): ______________________________

Index entries:

____

____

Surgical Case #6

Operative Report

Procedure: Fiberoptic bronchoscopy

Diagnosis: Hemoptysis with easily bruisable mucosa and bronchiectasis

Technique: The patient was brought to the endoscopy suite and placed on a stretcher. Oxygen was given via nasal cannula at 3 L/min. Local anesthetic lidocaine was given to anesthetize the upper airway. Because the nostrils had considerable blockage secondary to trauma, the oral route was used for the bronchoscopy. Following placement of a bite block and application of Cetacaine to the posterior pharynx, the fiberoptic bronchoscope was placed without difficulty into the upper airway.

The epiglottis appeared somewhat prominent, but normal. In addition, the vocal cords appeared normal. The bronchoscope was passed easily through the cords into the trachea, which also appeared normal, although somewhat easily bruisable. The carina appeared normal. The right side was entered first. The right upper lobe and its subsegments were seen very clearly, and there appeared to be bronchiectasis. The 6-mm bronchoscope would go very easily into the subsegments. No mass lesions were seen. The bronchus intermedius, right middle lobe, lower lobe, and its subsegments also were entered; and, again, bronchiectasis was noted. There appeared to be no abnormal mucosal lesions and no abnormal secretions; however, the bronchial tree was easily bruisable. The bronchoscope then was withdrawn to the carina and the left side entered.

The left main bronchus, upper lobe, lower lobe, and its subsegments were seen. There appeared to be an extrinsic compression of a subsegment of the left lower lobe; however, no mucosal lesions were seen and this area appeared pulsatile, which suggested extrinsic compression from the descending aorta. Once again, easy bruisability of the mucosa was noted. The bronchoscope was withdrawn. There were no apparent complications.

Assign appropriate CPT code(s) for the preceding procedures and indicate the index entries that were used to identify the codes. Assign only CPT codes (no E/M codes) and append any applicable modifiers.

Code(s):____

Index entries:

____

____

Surgical Case #7

Operative Report

Procedure:	Colposcopy
Diagnosis:	Class II Pap; cervicitis
History of Present Illness:	The patient is a 27-year-old woman who had previously undergone a Pap smear showing class II Pap. She is admitted today for a colposcopy.
Technique:	The patient was placed in the lithotomy position. Her vagina and cervix were examined and a speculum inserted; dyeing was done with acetic acid followed by gram iodine and methylene blue. Cervical biopsies were performed at indicated areas, with Monsel solution applied for cautery. There were no complications, and the patient tolerated the procedure well.
Plan:	The patient is to call the office within one week for her biopsy report.

Assign appropriate CPT code(s) for the preceding procedures and indicate the index entries that were used to identify the codes. Assign only CPT codes (no E/M codes) and append any applicable modifiers.

Code(s):________________________________

Index entries:

____

____

Surgical Case #8

Operative Report

Procedure:	Laparoscopic tubal ligation with application of Falope rings; dilatation and curettage (D&C) and removal of intrauterine device
Diagnosis:	Multiparity, voluntary sterilization; removal of retained intrauterine device
Anesthesia:	General
Technique:	Placed in the supine lithotomy position, the patient was prepped and draped in the usual manner for a laparoscopic and D&C procedure. A D&C was performed to gain access to a deeply embedded IUD. This was curetted up and eventually removed with some difficulty. Both the IUD and the curetted endometrial tissue were submitted to pathology. A two-puncture laparoscopy was performed in the usual manner of insufflation through a Veress needle inserted infraumbilically. Through a first puncture, a trocar insertion infraumbilically was followed by the laparoscope and a second trocar insertion suprapubically in the midline was followed by, first, a probe and, then, a Falope ring applicator. Both tubes were ligated in their midsegment. On the right side, two rings were applied because of the round position of the Falope ring director. The left tube was ligated singly. The procedure was performed with no complications. After the operation, the trocar sites were closed with subcuticular sutures of 2-0 Vicryl, and the patient was transferred to the recovery room in satisfactory condition.

Assign appropriate CPT code(s) for the preceding procedures and indicate the index entries that were used to identify the codes. Assign only CPT codes (no E/M codes) and append any applicable modifiers.

Code(s):________________________________

Index entries:

____

____

Surgical Case #9

Operative Report

Procedure: Transurethral resection of the prostate

Diagnosis: Bladder outlet obstruction; benign prostatic hypertrophy

Anesthesia: General

Technique: The patient was placed under general anesthesia and in the dorsolithotomy position. Two grams of Claforan parenterally were used. The Iglesias resectoscope was introduced through the obturator, and this was followed by the working element connected to the Olympus video camera. The obstructive prostatic tissue was appreciated mainly anteriorly and to the left lateral lobe. Resection was started at the bladder neck down to the level of the verumontanum and toward the capsule, as necessary, in all directions. Bleeders were fulgurated, with satisfactory patency with coagulation having been secured. Dissected tissues were removed using the Ellik evacuator. A size 24 three-way Foley catheter was retained with a 30-cc balloon inflation. Minimal blood loss was appreciated. The patient tolerated the procedure well and was transferred to the recovery room in stable condition.

Assign appropriate CPT code(s) for the preceding procedures and indicate the index entries that were used to identify the codes. Assign only CPT codes (no E/M codes) and append any applicable modifiers.

Code(s):____

Index entries:

____

____

Surgical Case #10

Operative Report

Procedure: Open reduction of left zygomatic arch fracture

Diagnosis: Left zygomatic arch fracture

Anesthesia: General

Technique: The patient was placed on the operating table in the supine position and administered general endotracheal anesthesia. He was prepped and draped in the usual fashion. A small incision was made in the temporal scalp area and carried down through the superficial temporal fascia until the deep temporal fascia was identified. This was incised, and an elevator was passed beneath the deep fascia until it was below the zygomatic arch. The arch was reduced manually and elevated back into its anatomical position noted by palpation. The wound was irrigated, and hemostasis was obtained with cautery.

The superficial temporal fascia was reapproximated using interrupted 4-0 Monocryl sutures. The skin was closed with interrupted 4-0 nylon sutures, and a sterile dressing was applied along with a metal cup to protect the zygomatic arch. The patient was extubated and transferred to the recovery room in stable condition.

Assign appropriate CPT code(s) for the preceding procedures and indicate the index entries that were used to identify the codes. Assign only CPT codes (no E/M codes) and append any applicable modifiers.

Code(s):____

Index entries:

____

____

Surgical Case #11

Operative Report

Procedure: Lateral lobe parotidectomy with facial nerve preservation

Diagnosis: Warthin's tumor of the parotid gland

Anesthesia: General

Findings: The patient has a long history of a right parotid mass that apparently has grown and fluctuated in size. An office examination revealed the nose, nasopharynx, larynx, and neck to be normal. She is status post thyroidectomy with a well-healed thyroidectomy incision. The parotid mass is overlying the mandible approximately 2 to 2.5 × 3 cm in diameter, and there is a possibility of another mass or lymphadenopathy in the lower aspect of the parotid gland. Facial nerve functions are normal.

Technique: Placed in the supine position, the patient was given general endotracheal anesthesia. Her neck was positioned, and the whole right side of her face and neck was prepped and draped in the usual manner.

The modified Blair type of incision was made in the preauricular area vertically and then curved behind and below the earlobe and extended as a curved submandibular incision. The bleeders were electrocoagulated and the dissection deepened in the lower part to the platysma. The dissection and front of the tragus were done by both sharp and blunt dissection until the external ear canal cartilage was identified and palpated. The dissection was pushed through this and inferiorly, identifying the anterior border of the sternocleidomastoid muscle, mastoid process, and, subsequently, the main trunk of the facial nerve, which was preserved from trauma. The major lower and inferior subdivisions were followed, identifying the cervical, mandibular, and buccal branches, as well as the upper division.

The cystic mass was bluish in color. The lateral lobe of the parotid gland was removed and given for frozen section, and this was reported as a benign cystic mass. No lobe was encountered with suspicion of malignancy, and no other masses were in the deep lobe. Hemostasis was obtained by electrocautery on the superficial oozing points and ligature of the small vessels. The wound was washed, and afterward the main trunk and subdivisions of the facial nerve again were identified and verified to be intact.

The lower Hemovac drain was placed. The wound was closed with 3-0 chromic catgut, interrupted, involving both the subcutaneous tissue and the platysma muscle with continuous and interrupted mattress sutures using 5-0 silk. The wound was cleaned, Bacitracin ointment was applied, and a dry sterile occlusive dressing was placed over it. After the procedure was terminated, the patient was extubated and brought to the recovery room in good condition.

Assign appropriate CPT code(s) for the preceding procedures and indicate the index entries that were used to identify the codes. Assign only CPT codes (no E/M codes) and append any applicable modifiers.

Code(s):______________________________

Index entries:

____

____

Surgical Case #12

Operative Report

Procedure: Arthroscopic partial medial meniscectomy

Diagnosis: Torn left medial meniscus

Anesthesia: General

Technique: After induction with general anesthesia, a standard three-portal approach of the knee was evaluated. Mild synovitic changes were noted in the suprapatellar pouch. No chondromalacia changes were noted in all three compartments. The anterior cruciate ligament was intact, as was the lateral meniscus; and there were only slight synovitic changes in the anterior compartment. The anterior portion of the medial meniscus had a flap tear, which was débrided with an aggressive resector.

After all instruments were withdrawn, 4-0 nylon horizontal mattress stitches were used to close the wound, and pressure dressings were applied. The patient was awakened and removed to the recovery room in good condition.

Assign appropriate CPT code(s) for the preceding procedures and indicate the index entries that were used to identify the codes. Assign only CPT codes (no E/M codes) and append any applicable modifiers.

Code(s):______________________________

Index entries:

____

____

Surgical Case #13

Operative Report

Preoperative Diagnosis: Bilateral vocal cord neoplasm

Postoperative Diagnosis: The same, with right postprocedural pharyngeal bleed

Procedures:
1. Laryngoscopy with bilateral vocal cord stripping with use of operating microscope
2. Control of oral pharyngeal hemorrhage, less than 20 cc

Indications for Surgery: This 65-year-old woman presented to the ENT service with a two-year history of hoarseness. Upon evaluation, she was noted to have bilateral vocal cord neoplasms. The patient also has a history of smoking. A decision for the above-stated procedures was made for definitive diagnosis.

Procedure: The patient was brought to the operating suite, given a general anesthetic, and properly prepared and draped. It was noted that her teeth were not in good repair, and that the lateral incisor was already loose on the right side. However, teeth guards were put into place. The Jako laryngoscope was carefully introduced into the oral cavity with attention not to injure the lips, gums, or teeth. The base of the tongue, vallecula, epiglottis, paraform sinuses, and false and true vocal cords all were visualized. The laryngoscope was fixed into place with microsuspension. The vocal cords were well visualized. There were polypoid-type neoplasms bilaterally. These were grasped anteriorly, stripped to the posterior bilaterally, and sent to pathology. Hemostasis was obtained with an adrenaline cotton ball and silver nitrate. After good hemostasis was obtained, the scope was removed. However, upon removal, she was noted to have a pooling of blood in the posterior pharynx and that the blood was coming from the right tonsillar fossa. Apparently, this had been abraded with the laryngoscope upon insertion. Therefore, a self-retaining mouth gag was carefully introduced into the oral cavity. The patient did not have good extension of the mandible, but after this was visualized, the right pharyngeal wall was noted to have oozing and some irritation. This was controlled with the help of silver nitrate and suction cautery. After good hemostasis was obtained, the oral cavity was irrigated with a saline solution. When the patient exhibited good hemostasis, she was taken out of anesthetic and transferred to the recovery room in stable condition.

Assign appropriate CPT code(s) for the preceding procedures and indicate the index entries that were used to identify the codes. Assign only CPT codes (no E/M codes) and append any applicable modifiers.

Code(s):______________________________

Index entries:

____

____

Surgical Case #14

Operative Report

Procedure: Percutaneous endoscopic gastrostomy (PEG) tube placement

Diagnosis: Old cerebrovascular accident with inanition and need for supplemental nutritional support with no contraindication to enteral access

Technique: After anesthetization of the gag reflex, the gastroscope was introduced. There was no abnormality of the esophagus, stomach, pylorus, or duodenum. The abdomen had been prepped and draped as a sterile field. The light was found to transilluminate in the left upper quadrant. The skin was anesthetized with 1% Xylocaine. A blunt needle was used to access the stomach percutaneously and a guide wire inserted. The guide wire was grasped with a snare and brought through the mouth, along with the gastroscope. The feeding tube was threaded over the guide wire and brought through the abdominal wall with a small stab incision made along the guide wire. The gastroscope was reinserted and the PEG tube photo-documented. There was no evidence of bleeding or undue tension as a result of tube placement. Air was suctioned from the stomach, and the gastroscope was removed with no other findings. The Silastic fastener was placed on the PEG tube near the skin entrance. The PEG tube then was connected to dependent drainage. The patient tolerated the procedure well and was taken to the recovery area with stable vital signs.

Assign appropriate CPT code(s) for the preceding procedures and indicate thc index entries that were used to identify the codes. Assign only CPT codes (no E/M codes) and append any applicable modifiers.

Code(s):______________________________

Index entries:

____

____

Surgical Case #15

Operative Report

Procedure: Right carotid thromboendarterectomy and vein patch angioplasty

Diagnosis: Right carotid artery stenosis with hemorrhagic plaque

Anesthesia: General

Technique: Under general anesthesia, the right side of the patient's neck was prepared and draped in a sterile fashion. An incision was made along the sternocleidomastoid muscle, and a sharp dissection was carried down to expose the common internal and external carotid arteries. Care was taken to avoid injury to the hypoglossal, vagus, and ansa cervicalis nerves. The vessels were inserted with elastic tapes. The patient was heparinized, and an arteriotomy was made. A very high-grade stenosis estimated at 1.5-mm opening was present at the origin of the internal carotid artery, and there was evidence of significant hemorrhage and degeneration in the plaque. A shunt was placed for cerebral perfusion, and then the endarterectomy was done in the usual fashion. The vessel was picked free of any debris or other plaque and then closed with a patch angioplasty using saphenous vein from the left groin. This was sutured in place with 6-0 Prolene. Flow was first directed into the external carotid to allow any possible air or debris to escape and then restored to the internal carotid. The wound was packed open until the end of the procedure and after the heparin was reversed. Then the wound was closed with 3-0 Vicryl in the subcutaneous and platysma muscle and 4-0 Vicryl for a subcuticular skin closure. The patient left the operating room in satisfactory condition.

Assign appropriate CPT code(s) for the preceding procedures and indicate the index entries that were used to identify the codes. Assign only CPT codes (no E/M codes) and append any applicable modifiers.

Code(s):________________________________

Index entries:

____

____

Surgical Case #16

Operative Report

Procedure:	McDonald's cerclage placement
Diagnosis:	Intrauterine pregnancy at 12 weeks, history of cervical incompetence
Anesthesia:	Epidural
History:	The patient is a 36-year-old gravida 3 para 2 with a last menstrual period (LMP) on January 28. Positive HCG was noted on March 1. Intrauterine pregnancy was determined to be at 12 weeks by time of LMP and at first trimester by ultrasound. She has a history of cervical incompetence in a previous pregnancy that was brought to term with a cerclage. She also has a history of diethylstilbestrol exposure and of cerclage placement times 2, D&C times 2, and umbilical herniorrhaphy.
Findings and Technique:	Preoperatively, her internal os was approximately 1 cm dilated. The posterior cervix was approximately 2 cm long, and the interior cervix was approximately 1 cm long. At the end of the procedure, the knot could be felt at the 12 o'clock position and the internal os was closed to digital examination. The patient was in the dorsal lithotomy position. She had internal and external perineal preps and was draped for the procedure. A Mersilene band on two needles was used with one needle placed in at the 6 o'clock position and brought out at 3 o'clock, and replaced at the same position and brought out at 12 o'clock. The other needle was taken in at 3 o'clock and brought out at 9 o'clock, and then replaced and brought out at 12 o'clock. The Mersilene band then was tied at the 12 o'clock position until the internal os was closed. It was palpable at the end of the procedure, and the two ends were cut long. The patient received perioperative antibiotics, and her heart tones were Dopplerable before the procedure. The procedure was without complications, and the patient was taken to the recovery room in stable condition.

Assign appropriate CPT code(s) for the preceding procedures and indicate the index entries that were used to identify the codes. Assign only CPT codes (no E/M codes) and append any applicable modifiers.

Code(s):____

Index entries:

____

____

Surgical Case #17

Operative Report

Procedure: Modified radical mastectomy

Diagnosis: Infiltrating ductal carcinoma, left breast

Indications: The patient is a 79-year-old woman who recently noticed a left breast mass. A subsequent mammogram revealed a spiculated suspicious lesion. On examination, she had a 2.5 to 3 cm palpable mass with no obvious axillary adenopathy. After an outpatient breast biopsy performed a week ago showed the mass was positive for carcinoma, she was admitted for a mastectomy.

Technique: Under general anesthesia, the patient's left breast was prepped. A transverse elliptical incision, including the nipple, areolar complex, and the previous biopsy site were utilized. Flaps were elevated medially to the sternum, superiorly to the clavicle, laterally to the latissimus, and inferiorly to the rectus. The depressed and anteropectoral fascia were dissected from medial to lateral with cautery dissection. The axilla was entered and the axillary vein identified. The venous tributaries were clipped inferiorly and divided. The long thoracic and thoracodorsal nerves were identified and traced to their insertions; the axillary contents were swept inferiorly and laterally out with the breast specimen.

Hemostasis was obtained with a Bovie knife in addition to clips and sutures. Two Jackson Pratt drains were placed. The subcutaneous tissue was reapproximated with interrupted 3-0 Vicryl, and the skin was closed with clips. Some of the skin flaps were trimmed to make the closure more acceptable cosmetically. The patient tolerated the procedure well and was returned to the recovery area in satisfactory condition.

Assign appropriate CPT code(s) for the preceding procedures and indicate the index entries that were used to identify the codes. Assign only CPT codes (no E/M codes) and append any applicable modifiers.

Code(s):____________________________________

Index entries:

____

____

Surgical Case #18

Operative Report

Procedure: Direct microlaryngoscopy under general anesthesia

Diagnosis: Dysphonia

Technique: A 40-year-old patient was taken to the OR where, under general anesthesia, the Jako laryngoscope was inserted with the operating microscope to perform a laryngoscopy. The vocal cords were found to be totally normal on both sides with no evidence of nodules or granuloma formation. The entire endolarynx was well visualized. Moreover, there was no evidence of subglottic stenosis; and as the patient was awakening, vocal cord mobility appeared to be normal. The procedure was terminated, and the patient awakened and was taken to the recovery room in good condition with stable vital signs.

Recommendation: Speech therapy

Assign appropriate CPT code(s) for the preceding procedures and indicate the index entries that were used to identify the codes. Assign only CPT codes (no E/M codes) and append any applicable modifiers.

Code(s):____

Index entries:

____

____

Surgical Case #19

Operative Report

Procedure: Colonoscopy

History and Indications: The patient is a 30-year-old woman who has had complaints of abdominal pain, altered bowel habits, and a 2- to 3-g documented decline in her hemoglobin level. Her stools have been heme negative, but there is significant suspicion that she may have pathology in the colon.

Technique: The patient was sedated with 1.5 mg Versed and received antibiotics prior to the procedure per the recommendations of the cardiology service. She is status post heart transplant with significant cardiac complications.

In the endoscopy suite with appropriate monitoring of pulse, oxygenation, temperature, blood pressure, and other vital signs, a digital rectal examination was performed. Following the examination, the Pentax video colonoscope was inserted through the anus and advanced to the cecum. There was no evidence of malignancy. The scope was withdrawn.

Assign appropriate CPT code(s) for the preceding procedures and indicate the index entries that were used to identify the codes. Assign only CPT codes (no E/M codes) and append any applicable modifiers.

Code(s):____

Index entries:

____

____

Surgical Case #20

Operative Report

Preoperative Diagnosis:	Sebaceous cyst, right posterior neck
Postoperative Diagnosis:	Lipomatous lesion, approximately 1.5 cm, right posterior neck, intramuscular
Procedure:	Excision of lipoma, right posterior neck
Technique:	The patient was brought to the operating suite and was placed in the prone position on the operating table. The patient's right neck was then prepped and draped in a sterile fashion. At this point, we suspected the patient to have a cyst. We subsequently decided to do a circumferential incision around what was thought to be the puncta. The incision was marked, and the area was prepped and draped with a local anesthetic. A skin incision was made. The incision was carried down to the subcutaneous tissue. At this point, we realized that it was not a cyst but, rather, a lipoma, which was actually deep into the muscle area. We excised the skin, dissected down through the capsule of the lipoma, and then were able to harvest this from its capsule within the muscle fibers. This was done with sharp dissection. Bleeding was controlled with cautery. The wound was closed with 3-0 Vicryl subcutaneous sutures, and a 4-0 Vicryl subcuticular stitch was placed. The wound edges were painted with Benzoin and Steri-Strips applied. The patient tolerated the procedure well and was taken to the recovery area in stable condition.

Assign appropriate CPT code(s) for the preceding procedures and indicate the index entries that were used to identify the codes. Assign only CPT codes (no E/M codes) and append any applicable modifiers.

Code(s):____

Index entries:

____

____

Surgical Case #21

Operative Report

Procedure:	Colonoscopy
Indications for Procedure:	This is a 65-year-old woman with a family history of colonic malignancy who is being evaluated for altered bowel function. When evaluated in my office prior to the procedure, her vital signs, cardiac status, pulmonary status, and mental status were stable and adequate for conscious sedation.
Description of Procedure:	The patient was given Demerol 50 mg IV and Versed 3 mg IV, and the CF100I video colonoscope was inserted and passed without difficulty to the cecum. Its position was confirmed by the ileocecal valve. Diverticulosis was observed in the left colon. A 5- to 7-mm circular, semipedunculated polyp was observed in the cecal area. It was secured with the snare and recovered. The patient tolerated the procedure well.
Impression:	She has a small cecal polyp, which has been removed. She has diverticulosis and will need reevaluation in three years.
Clinical Diagnosis:	Polyp, cecum
Pathological Diagnosis:	Polyp, cecum: Villotubular adenoma

Assign appropriate CPT code(s) for the preceding procedures and indicate the index entries that were used to identify the codes. Assign only CPT codes (no E/M codes) and append any applicable modifiers.

Code(s):________________________________

Index entries:

____

____

Surgical Case #22

Operative Report

Preoperative Diagnosis:	Cholecystitis with cholelithiasis
Postoperative Diagnosis:	Cholecystitis with cholelithiasis
Procedure Performed:	Laparoscopic cholecystectomy with operative cholangiogram
Anesthesia:	General
Bleeding:	None
Complications:	None
Description of Procedure:	The patient was brought to the OR, placed in the supine position, and given general anesthesia. The skin over the abdomen was prepped with DuraPrep and draped in the sterile fashion. A 1-cm incision was made above the umbilicus, and the Veress needle was introduced into the abdominal cavity obtaining pneumoperitoneum. A 10-mm trocar was inserted and a laparoscope introduced. The patient had significant cholecystitis. Direct exploration of the abdomen was normal. Other trocars were inserted into the subcostal space under direct vision. Lysis of adhesions was performed. Exposure to the gallbladder bed was obtained, and the cystic artery and the cystic duct were isolated. The common duct was of normal size. The cystic duct was ligated distally and proximally and was opened. We inserted the biliary catheter and obtained a cholangiogram that showed a normal biliary tree. The catheter was removed and the cystic duct double ligated with hemoclips and divided. The gallbladder was removed through the upper trocar and dissected with electrocautery. The area was irrigated with saline solution. The trocars were removed under vision and pneumoperitoneum decompressed. The skin was closed with subcuticular #4-0 Vicryl, and a sterile dressing was applied. The patient tolerated the procedure well.

Assign appropriate CPT code(s) for the preceding procedures and indicate the index entries that were used to identify the codes. Assign only CPT codes (no E/M codes) and append any applicable modifiers.

Code(s):______________________________

Index entries:

____

____

Surgical Case #23

Operative Report

Procedure:	Endoscopy
Preoperative Diagnosis:	Abdominal pain, possible peptic ulcer disease Patient has upper abdominal pain, unresponsive to H2 blockers.
Postoperative Diagnosis:	1. Hiatal hernia 2. Moderate reflux esophagitis 3. Healing prepyloric gastric ulcer 4. Normal sigmoidoscopy
Findings:	Endoscopy was performed with the Olympus video panendoscope, which was easily introduced into the esophagus. This was normal to the proximal midportion of the esophagus, but at the GE junction, there was evidence of a moderate degree of reflux esophagitis with several small superficial erosions at the location and also isolated erosions several centimeters above. The endoscope was advanced into the stomach and turned in a retrograde direction. The cardiac and fundic areas were examined and found to be otherwise normal. The antrum showed normal peristalsis and mucosa. In the immediate prepyloric area, a small defect was thought to represent scarring from a previous ulcer, which was still healing. Biopsies were obtained. The duodenum, including the second portion, was normal. Subsequently, the endoscope was withdrawn, and the patient turned onto his left side. Flexible sigmoidoscopy then was carried out to the lower descending colon. A biopsy of the sigmoid was obtained. Patient tolerated the procedure well.

Assign appropriate CPT code(s) for the preceding procedures and indicate the index entries that were used to identify the codes. Assign only CPT codes (no E/M codes) and append any applicable modifiers.

Code(s):____________________________________

Index entries:

____

____

Surgical Case #24

Operative Report

Procedure: Esophagogastroduodenoscopy

Instrument Used: Olympus GIF-100

Premedication: The patient was premedicated with a total of Fentanyl, 50 mcg, and Versed, 4 mg, intravenously.

Indications: The patient has presented with recurrent dysphagia. She has a history of a Schatzki's ring, which has been dilated in the past.

Procedure: The endoscope was inserted into the esophagus without difficulty. The esophageal mucosa was normal. A reformed Schatzki's ring was located at the Z line, which was at approximately 29 cm. The endoscope could be inserted through this area with no resistance. The ring was located above a 3-cm hiatal hernia. The stomach, duodenal bulb, and descending duodenum were all normal. After the endoscope was withdrawn, a #60 French Maloney dilator was passed with very mild resistance. The patient tolerated the procedure well, and there were no immediate complications.

Impression:
1. A reformed Schatzki's ring, which was dilated
2. A 3-cm hiatal hernia

Assign appropriate CPT code(s) for the preceding procedures and indicate the index entries that were used to identify the codes. Assign only CPT codes (no E/M codes) and append any applicable modifiers.

Code(s):______________________________

Index entries:

____

____

Surgical Case #25

Emergency Department Report

Chief Complaint:	Lacerations, left face
History of Present Illness:	Patient is a 26-year-old man who was driving a car with the window down when another car moving in the opposite direction hit his mirror. Glass from the broken mirror flew into his face, and he sustained two small lacerations. There were no other injuries.
Past Medical History:	Unremarkable
Medications:	None
Allergies:	None

Physical Examination:

General:	Alert male in no acute distress
HEENT:	Pupils are equal and reactive to light. Extraocular muscles intact. Nose is clear. Oropharynx negative. Two lacerations are on left cheek region. The uppermost laceration is about 2 cm below the eye laterally and is about 0.75 cm in length. Full-skin thickness. The second laceration is about 1.5 cm below the first and is 1.25 cm in length. Full-skin thickness. No palpable foreign bodies.
Procedure:	Local injection with a total of 3 cc 1% lidocaine with epinephrine. Prepped and routine exploration performed. The upper laceration is only about 5 mm deep. No foreign bodies noted. No neurovascular injuries. It was closed with three 6-0 nylon sutures. The lower laceration was approximately 12 to 15 mm deep. I could not palpate any foreign bodies. There are no obvious neurovascular injuries. Closed in single layer with five 6-0 nylon sutures. Polysporin ointment was applied.
Laboratory Data:	X-ray to rule out foreign body negative
Diagnosis:	1. Simple facial laceration, 1.25 cm 2. Simple facial laceration, 0.75 cm
Disposition and Plan:	Wound care instructions given; sutures out in five to seven days

Assign appropriate CPT code(s) for the preceding procedures and indicate the index entries that were used to identify the codes. Assign only CPT codes (no E/M codes) and append any applicable modifiers.

Code(s):______________________________

Index entries:

____

____

Surgical Case #26

Operative Report

Preoperative Diagnosis:	Dermal cyst of right breast
Postoperative Diagnosis:	Dermal cyst of right breast
Procedure Performed:	Excision of dermal cyst of right breast
Description of Procedure:	Erythematous dermal cystic area of the right breast was marked out with an elliptical incision, anesthetized with local anesthesia, and prepped and draped sterilely. Incision was made elliptically, including the whole cyst down through the fatty tissue. On palpation afterward, no abnormalities were noted. Then the area had hemostasis obtained with electrocautery. The incision was closed with interrupted 3-0 Vicryl sutures. The skin was closed with interrupted 5-0 nylon sutures. Steri-Strips and a sterile dressing were applied over it. The patient tolerated the procedure well and was sent to the recovery room with instructions to be discharged home with follow-up appointment given.

Assign appropriate CPT code(s) for the preceding procedures and indicate the index entries that were used to identify the codes. Assign only CPT codes (no E/M codes) and append any applicable modifiers.

Code(s):______________________________

Index entries:

____

____

Surgical Case #27

Operative Report

Preoperative Diagnosis:	Right arm lipoma
Postoperative Diagnosis:	Same
Procedure Performed:	Excision of right arm lipoma
Anesthesia:	Local
Indications for Procedure:	The patient is a 48-year-old woman who presents with a 4.0-cm mass on her right arm. She has had the mass for several months, and it is getting larger. She now presents for an excisional biopsy.
Description of Procedure:	The patient was brought to the OR and placed on the operating table in the supine position. Her right arm was prepared and draped in the usual sterile fashion, and anesthetized with 1% lidocaine with bicarbonate. A longitudinal incision was made measuring 3 cm and carried down through the skin and subcutaneous tissues, and the underlying lipoma was dissected away from the surrounding tissues and removed. Parts of the lipoma were intermingled with surrounding tissues, requiring these areas to be pulled out. Hemostasis then was ensured and the wound closed with layered Vicryl, followed by Benzoin, Steri-Strips, and a Tegaderm dressing. The patient tolerated the procedure well and was taken to the recovery room in stable condition.
Pathological Diagnosis:	Forearm, right: lipoma
Gross:	The specimen consists of nine pieces of soft, predominantly fatty yellow tissue ranging from 0.9 cm to 3 cm in greatest diameter; representative sections were submitted in one cassette.

Assign appropriate CPT code(s) for the preceding procedures and indicate the index entries that were used to identify the codes. Assign only CPT codes (no E/M codes) and append any applicable modifiers.

Code(s):____________________________________

Index entries:

____

____

Surgical Case #28

Operative Report

Preoperative Diagnosis:	Elevated PSA of 16.6 and bladder outlet obstruction
Postoperative Diagnosis:	Same
Procedure:	Cystoscopy and transrectal needle biopsy of the prostate
Anesthesia:	General
Procedure:	This man was taken to the operative suite, placed in the dorsolithotomy position after being administered anesthesia, and sterilely prepped and draped in the normal fashion. A needle was used to take multiple transrectal biopsies of his prostate. After this, a cystoscopy was performed and bladder outlet obstruction and BPH were noted. The urethra was normal, and the bladder was moderately trabeculated. There was no evidence of neoplasm, infection, or calculus; and the ureters were normal in position, effluxing clear urine. The bladder was emptied, and the patient was sent to the recovery room in satisfactory condition.

Assign appropriate CPT code(s) for the preceding procedures and indicate the index entries that were used to identify the codes. Assign only CPT codes (no E/M codes) and append any applicable modifiers.

Code(s):____

Index entries:

____

____

Surgical Case #29

Operative Report

Preoperative Diagnosis:	Incomplete abortion
Postoperative Diagnosis:	Same
Operation:	Dilatation & curettage
History:	This 22-year-old female, gravida IV, para II, AB I, comes in today because of abdominal pain and passing fetus on the sidewalk just outside the hospital. Apparently, her last menstrual period was two months ago. She had been doing well, and this problem just started today.
Procedure:	The patient was placed on the operating table in the lithotomy position, and prepped and draped in the usual manner. Under satisfactory intravenous sedation, the cervix was visualized by means of a weighted speculum and grasped in the anterior lip with a sponge forceps. Cord was prolapsed through the cervix and vagina, and a considerable amount of placental tissue was in the vagina and cervix. This was removed. A sharp curet was used to explore the endometrial cavity, and a minimal amount of curettings was obtained. The patient tolerated the procedure well.

Assign appropriate CPT code(s) for the preceding procedures and indicate the index entries that were used to identify the codes. Assign only CPT codes (no E/M codes) and append any applicable modifiers.

Code(s):____

Index entries:

____

____

Surgical Case #30

Operative Report

Procedure: Sigmoidoscopy

Indications for Procedure: The patient is 75 years old. She has had an alteration in her bowel pattern and is being evaluated with a sigmoidoscopy.

Description of Procedure: She was given Fleet's enema preparation. She required no sedation. The CF100L video colonoscope was inserted and passed without difficulty to 50 cm. The mucosa were normal. No diverticulosis was observed. Some scybalous stool was present, but this was minimal. The patient tolerated the procedure well.

Assign appropriate CPT code(s) for the preceding procedures and indicate the index entries that were used to identify the codes. Assign only CPT codes (no E/M codes) and append any applicable modifiers.

Code(s):____

Index entries:

____

____

Surgical Case #31

Operative Report

Diagnosis: Hodgkin's disease, nonsclerosing type

Operation: Placement of right subclavian Hickman catheter

Indications: The patient is a 35-year-old woman with the diagnosis of Hodgkin's disease. Her indication for a Hickman catheter was chemotherapy infusion.

Procedure: The patient was taken to the operating room and placed in the supine position. The right chest and subclavian area, neck, and shoulder were prepped and draped in routine manner. A total of 48 cc of 1% Carbocaine without epinephrine was used for anesthesia. The subcutaneous area below the right clavicle was numbed with the lidocaine down to the periosteum. The subclavian vein was stuck with the needle. Good blood flow was returned. The guide wire was passed. At this time, a 2-cm incision was made below the clavicle at the middle aspect. The Hickman catheter was then placed over the guide wire into the superior vena cava. This was documented with fluoroscopy. A second incision was made 3 cm below the first distance of 2 cm transverse. The area between the two incisions was then tunneled with a curved six. The distal aspect of the catheter was brought out through the second inferior incision. The Teflon Hickman catheter was trimmed to the appropriate length with Teflon coating at the skin incision. The superior skin incision was closed with interrupted #3-0 nylon, as was the inferior skin incision. The patient tolerated the procedure well.

Assign appropriate CPT code(s) for the preceding procedures and indicate the index entries that were used to identify the codes. Assign only CPT codes (no E/M codes) and append any applicable modifiers.

Code(s):____

Index entries:

____

____

Surgical Case #32

Operative Report

Preoperative Diagnosis: Ventral hernia

Postoperative Diagnosis: Ventral hernia

Operation Performed: Laparoscopic repair of ventral hernia

Anesthesia: General

Details of Procedure: The patient was taken to the operating room, placed in the supine position. The abdomen was prepped and draped in the usual sterile fashion. A Veress needle was then inserted in the left lateral abdominal wall. The abdomen was insufflated with CO_2 gas. A 10-mm Surgiport was then placed. The laparoscopic camera was then inserted. Additional 5-mm Surgiports were placed under direct vision, one in the left lower quadrant of the abdomen, the other in the left upper quadrant of the abdomen.

The 5-mm harmonic scalpel was used along with the dissecting forceps to take down the adhesions from within and around the hernia sac. There were a number of adhesions, primarily involving the omentum. These were all removed.

Two hernia defects were noted, one just above the umbilicus, perhaps 3 to 4 cm in diameter, and another toward the upper aspect of the midline incision, that had not been previously recognized.

It was elected to place an 18 × 24-cm segment of Gore-Tex dual mesh. #1 Prolene was sewn at each of the corners of this as well as in between, at the midpoint of each of the sides. Suitable locations were chosen for tying the anchoring sutures. The patch then was rolled around a grasper and inserted into the abdominal cavity through the 10-mm port. The patch was then unrolled and the orientation placed with the smooth side down against the bowel. An endoclose device was used to grasp each of the sutures and bring out through the previously placed incisions for the anchoring sutures. The patch was anchored at each of the six locations as noted previously. Then, an auto suture Protac was placed around the periphery of the patch. Additional staples were placed within the inner aspect of the patch using an Ethicon tacking stapler. The patch was noted to be quite taut and applied closely to the abdominal wall to prevent any movement of the patch. The abdomen was then desufflated and the ports withdrawn. Each of the skin incisions was closed with 4-0 clear PDS subcuticular suture and Steri-Strips. Tegaderm dressings were then applied. The patient tolerated the procedure well with no apparent difficulty. She was then taken to the postanesthesia recovery room for further postoperative care.

Assign appropriate CPT code(s) for the preceding procedures and indicate the index entries that were used to identify the codes. Assign only CPT codes (no E/M codes) and append any applicable modifiers.

Code(s):____

Index entries:

____

____

Surgical Case #33

Operative Report

Preoperative Diagnosis: Right breast mammographic abnormality

Postoperative Diagnosis: Same

Indications: This is a 53-year-old woman who presented with a nonpalpable right breast mammographic abnormality. A stereotactic biopsy showed columnar cell hyperplasia without evidence of obvious malignancy; however, excision was recommended. Possible perioperative risks and complications and alternatives were discussed with her prior to surgery.

Details of Procedure: After informed consent was obtained from the patient, she was taken to the OR and placed on the table in the supine position. The right breast was noted to contain a localization wire. The films were reviewed. The breast was prepped with Betadine solution and draped sterilely. Sedation was administered by anesthesia. Local anesthesia was achieved with 1% lidocaine and 0.5% Marcaine with epinephrine. An incision was made over the course of the localization needle, and the underlying core of tissue surrounding the localization needle was excised using electrocautery. This was forwarded to the radiology department, which confirmed the presence of the previously marked mammographic abnormality within the specimen. It was then forwarded to pathology.

Wound was inspected for hemostasis, which was excellent. The deep tissues were approximated with interrupted 3-0 Vicryl, and a running 4-0 Monocryl subcuticular stitch was used to approximate the skin edges. Benzoin, Steri-Strips, and dry sterile dressing were applied. The patient was then awakened from anesthesia and returned to the recovery room in stable condition.

Assign appropriate CPT code(s) for the preceding procedures and indicate the index entries that were used to identify the codes. Assign only CPT codes (no E/M codes) and append any applicable modifiers.

Code(s):______________________________

Index entries:

____

____

Surgical Case #34

Operative Report

Preoperative Diagnosis: Chalazion, left lower lid

Postoperative Diagnosis: Same

Operation: Excision of mass, left lower lid

Procedure: Under adequate topical anesthesia and block anesthesia, the eye was prepared and draped in the usual manner. Chalazion speculum was applied. The left lower lid was everted and a vertical incision made. Excision of the mass was performed using curet, and a biopsy of the capsule of this 9-mm mass was made, as requested. Patient tolerated the procedure well and left the operating room in good condition after application of Cortisporin ointment and pressure patch.

Assign appropriate CPT code(s) for the preceding procedures and indicate the index entries that were used to identify the codes. Assign only CPT codes (no E/M codes) and append any applicable modifiers.

Code(s):____

Index entries:

____

____

Surgical Case #35

Operative Report

Preoperative Diagnosis: Carpal tunnel compression, left, severe

Postoperative Diagnosis: Same

Operation: Release, left carpal tunnel

Procedure: After successful axillary block was placed, the patient's left arm was prepared and draped in the usual sterile manner. Tourniquet was inflated. A curvilinear hypothenar incision was made and the palmaris retracted radially. The carpal tunnel and the transverse carpal ligament were then opened and completely freed in the proximal directions. It was noted to be severely tight in the palm with flattening and swelling of the median nerve. The carpal tunnel was opened distally in the hand and noted to be clear, out to the transverse palmar crease. The wound was then closed with 4-0 Dexon in subcuticular tissues. Sterile bulky dressing was applied, and the patient was awakened and taken to the recovery room in satisfactory condition.

Assign appropriate CPT code(s) for the preceding procedures and indicate the index entries that were used to identify the codes. Assign only CPT codes (no E/M codes) and append any applicable modifiers.

Code(s):____

Index entries:

____

____

Surgical Case #36

Operative Report

Preoperative Diagnosis:	Keratosis of glans penis
Postoperative Diagnosis:	Same
Procedure:	The penis was prepared and draped in the usual manner. Along the distal portion of the penis on the right side and adjoining the urinary meatus was a well-defined, firm area suggesting a keratosis. The entire lesion was excised and submitted for pathological examination. The pathologist confirmed the diagnosis of keratosis. The glans penis was then approximated with black silk. The patient returned to the recovery room in satisfactory condition.

Assign appropriate CPT code(s) for the preceding procedures and indicate the index entries that were used to identify the codes. Assign only CPT codes (no E/M codes) and append any applicable modifiers.

Code(s):____________________________

Index entries:

____

____

Surgical Case #37

Operative Report

Preoperative diagnosis:	Herniated disc at L4-L5, L5-S1; good relief with previous two epidural blocks
Postoperative diagnosis:	Same
Operation:	Therapeutic epidural block
Procedure:	The patient is kept on the left lateral side. The back is prepared with Betadine solution, and 1% Xylocaine is infiltrated at the L5-S1 interspace. Deep infiltration is carried out with a 22-gauge needle, and a 17-gauge Touhy needle is used and an epidural is performed. After careful aspiration, which was negative for blood as well as for cerebrospinal fluid, about 80 mg of Depo-Medrol then were injected along with 5 cc of 0.25% Marcaine and 1 cc of 50 mcg of fentanyl citrate. The injection was done in a fractionated dose in a slow fashion. The patient was examined and evaluated following the block and found to have excellent relief of pain. The patient is advised to continue physical therapy and to come back in one month for further evaluation.

Assign appropriate CPT code(s) for the preceding procedures and indicate the index entries that were used to identify the codes. Assign only CPT codes (no E/M codes) and append any applicable modifiers.

Code(s):____________________________

Index entries:

____

____

Surgical Case #38

Operative Report

Procedure: Excision of left axillary lymph nodes

Indications for Procedure: This female patient had a lumpectomy for a breast lesion approximately 2.5 years ago. She presents with palpable adenopathy in the left axilla.

Description of Procedure: The patient was brought into the operating room and placed on the OR table in the supine position. The left axilla was prepared and draped in the usual sterile fashion. After an adequate level of general anesthesia had been achieved, a knife with a #10 blade was used to make a curvilinear incision in the skin overlying the adenopathy.

This incision was carried down deep through the subcutaneous tissue using a Bovie knife. Babcock forceps were used to grasp the area of tissue surrounding the lymph node, which was carefully dissected from the surrounding tissues using a Bovie knife and scissors. All vessels encountered were either Bovied or clipped.

The wound was irrigated and carefully examined for bleeders. The subcutaneous tissue was closed using a Vicryl suture placed in interrupted fashion, and the skin was reapproximated using staples. Drainage was achieved with a Jackson-Pratt drain brought out through a separate wound. Sterile dressings were applied, and the patient was taken to the recovery room in a stable postoperative condition.

Assign appropriate CPT code(s) for the preceding procedures and indicate the index entries that were used to identify the codes. Assign only CPT codes (no E/M codes) and append any applicable modifiers.

Code(s):______________________________

Index entries:

____

____

Surgical Case #39

Operative Report

Preoperative Diagnosis: Subepidermal nodular 1.5-cm lesion of the left side of the nose

Operation: Excision, lesion of nose

Procedure: Under local anesthesia, we excised the 1.5-cm lesion with 0.5 cm margins on all sides of the defect. The lesion was excised in fragments and submitted to pathology along with an ellipse of skin margins. Bleeding was controlled with electrocautery, and the wound was closed with four vertical mattress sutures of 5-0 nylon. Polysporin and dressing were applied.

Pathological Diagnosis: Well-organized basal cell carcinoma with no significant increase in activity or dysplasia of the cells

Assign appropriate CPT code(s) for the preceding procedures and indicate the index entries that were used to identify the codes. Assign only CPT codes (no E/M codes) and append any applicable modifiers.

Code(s):______________________________

Index entries:

____

____

Surgical Case #40

Emergency Department Physician Report

Chief Complaint: Left eye, foreign body × two days

History of Present Illness: The patient is a 29-year-old man who presents to the emergency room after having a piece of metal fly into his left eye yesterday. Since that time, he still continues to have the metal present. He denies any major disturbance in vision, although he states that his vision is slightly more blurry and irritated. He does complain of some pain.

Past Medical History: Hypertension

Allergies: None

Immunizations: Unknown for tetanus

Social and Family History: Noncontributory

Physical Examination of Eyes: Reveals the left eye to have some periorbital erythema, but minimal swelling of the lids. PERRLA: No papilledema. EOMs intact. Vision intact. Inspection of the left eye shows a foreign body that resembles a piece of metal at the 6 o'clock position. At this time, Tetracaine was applied. The foreign body was successfully removed with the bevel of a 22-gauge needle. Two more drops of Tetracaine were applied, followed by Homatropine and Polysporin ophthalmic ointment.

Assessment: Foreign body of left eye, removed. The patient understood all instructions and agreed with the plan, at which time he was discharged.

Assign appropriate CPT code(s) for the preceding procedures and indicate the index entries that were used to identify the codes. Assign only CPT codes (no E/M codes) and append any applicable modifiers.

Code(s):____________________

Index entries:

____

____

Surgical Case #41

Operative Report

Preprocedure Diagnosis: Left lower lobe lung nodule

Postprocedure Diagnosis: Left lower lobe lung nodule

Operations Performed:
1. Left video-assisted thoracoscopy
2. Wedge resection biopsy, left lower lobe times two
3. Bronchoscopy with the right upper lobe, transbronchial biopsy times two

Indications for Procedure: The patient, who has been followed by both the pulmonary services as well as seen in the thoracic surgery clinic, had had a long history of smoking. His chest CT had a nodule in the left lower lobe as well as an area in the right upper lobe that was consistent with some consolidation that had not increased in size. It was decided to perform a wedge biopsy of the left lower lobe lung nodule since this is a discrete mass, and bronchoscopy for the right upper lobe. Patient understood the previously mentioned procedures and approach. Informed consent was obtained.

Procedure: Patient was brought into the operating room, placed on the operating table in the supine position. After smooth induction of general anesthesia and endotracheal intubation, a Foley catheter was placed. The double-lumen endotracheal tube was placed. Patient was then turned to the left lateral decubitus position with the left side up and right side down. We prepared and draped with Hibiclens, alcohol, and Loban. We then made a small incision in the posterior space with a scalpel, dissected down, bluntly entered into the chest cavity, and placed a 5-mm port.

We then placed an additional port and moved the camera to the anterior inferior portion and placed another 5-mm trocar posterior inferior. We then used gross inspection of the chest. There were no adhesions and no pleural fluid to sweep out. No gross masses. Using a blunt grasper, we were able to palpate the left lower lobe posteriorly and feel the mass. We then used graspers retracted to the lung specimen up, used the EndoGIA staplers to perform wedge biopsies or initial wedge biopsy. We did not have the specimen. In this second wedge biopsy, we were able to get around from the green staple load and perform the biopsy and wedge out the mass lesion. This was then placed in a EndoCatch bag and removed. We were then able to palpate the mass, but the scalpel we opened had an appearance of an infectious etiology. Gram staining was sent and then it was sent for further dissection.

We then placed a #9 French pneumocatheter anteriorly under direct vision. There was no bleeding to speak of. We removed our trocars under direct vision. Lung was allowed to reinflate. Chest tube was placed to suction 10 cm to close the 10 × 12 site with 2-0 Vicryl and 4-0 Vicryl followed by Dermabond. Other trocar sites were closed with 4-0 Monocryl and Dermabond. Once this was completed, the patient was turned supine. We then performed a bronchoscopy. During bronchoscopy, the trachea at the right appeared normal. On the right side, the bronchus intermedius appeared normal. We were able to cannulate the right upper lobe. We were able to then use the biopsy forceps to cannulate the apical segment of the right upper lobe. We sent several specimens with biopsy forceps for cytology as well as performed a biopsy with fluoroscopic guidance times two. We then removed the biopsy forceps.

We inspected the bronchus intermedius, the right medial lobe and right lower lobe orifices appeared normal. We then removed, pulled the scope back, advanced down the left main stem bronchus. All segments and lobes appeared normal. Through the bronchoscope, this point of procedure was terminated. Patient was extubated, transferred off the operating room table, awakened stable to the SICU. Dr. Howard was present for the entire procedure. There were no complications.

Assign appropriate CPT code(s) for the preceding procedures and indicate the index entries that were used to identify the codes. Assign only CPT codes (no E/M codes) and append any applicable modifiers.

Code(s):______________________________

Index entries:

____

____

Surgical Case #42

Operative Report

Preoperative Diagnosis:	Arthritis of right acromioclavicular joint
Postoperative Diagnosis:	Same
Operation:	Mumford procedure, right shoulder
Procedure:	The patient was brought to the operating room after general anesthesia. The patient was placed in the lounge chair position, the right shoulder was sterilely scrubbed and draped in the usual manner. Routine incision was taken down to the distal clavicle. The distal clavicle was identified subperiosteally. Retractors were put in place. At this time the clavicle was osteotomized using a saw, and the distal end of the clavicle was removed. The wound was then irrigated. Marcaine with epinephrine was injected. The periosteum was closed with 0 Vicryl, subcutaneous, with 2-0 Vicryl, and the skin with staples. Dry sterile dressings were applied, and the patient was sent to the recovery room in good condition.

Assign appropriate CPT code(s) for the preceding procedures and indicate the index entries that were used to identify the codes. Assign only CPT codes (no E/M codes) and append any applicable modifiers.

Code(s):______________________________

Index entries:

____

____

Surgical Case #43

Operative Report

Preoperative Diagnosis:	Epidermal cyst
Postoperative Diagnosis:	Awaiting permanent section by pathology
Operation:	Excision of the area
Procedure:	This 91-year-old woman who resides in the Sunnybrook Nursing Home presented with a 1.25 × 1.25-cm enlarging tender granulomatous type lesion over the dorsum of the MCP joint of the left ring finger. Because of the patient's arthritis, she was left in the wheelchair while the procedure was done. The left hand was scrubbed for 10 minutes with sterile soap solution with Betadine, prepared with Betadine. The patient was draped with sterile towels and drapes exposing the area and then the area about the lesion was blocked with 1% lidocaine without epinephrine. Then an ellipse was outlined with long axis vertical, and the lesion was excised and submitted to pathology. The total excised lesion including margins was 2.0 cm. It was closed with five sutures of 5-0 Prolene and dressed with Polysporin and a Band-Aid. The family was instructed that the Band-Aid could be changed, and she was discharged to the home where I will follow her and remove the sutures in one to two weeks.
Pathological Diagnosis:	Skin lesion, left ring finger: epidermal cyst, excised and actinic keratosis with extensive atypical basosquamous cell hyperplasia

Assign appropriate CPT code(s) for the preceding procedures and indicate the index entries that were used to identify the codes. Assign only CPT codes (no E/M codes) and append any applicable modifiers.

Code(s):________________________________

Index entries:

____

____

Emergency Department Case #44

Emergency Department Record

Chief Complaint:	Injury to right fourth and fifth toes
History of Present Illness:	Patient states that he was running for the phone when he stubbed his toes on a piece of furniture. Did this yesterday and has marked ecchymosis noted in the fourth and fifth toes of the right foot, slight swelling also. He states he has been able to ambulate and that his foot does not hurt, except for when he walks. Denies any numbness, tingling, or loss of sensation. He does also have an abrasion noted to the distal aspect of the fourth toe. He denies any further injury.
Past Medical History:	Noncontributory
Allergies:	Patient has no known medication allergies
Current Medications:	None
Review of Systems:	Negative

Physical Examination

Vital Signs:	Blood pressure is 145/89. Temperature is 97.7° F, pulse of 76, respirations 16.
General:	Patient is alert, oriented, in no acute distress.
Extremities:	Shows marked ecchymosis noted in the fourth and fifth toes and in the dorsal aspect of the foot adjacent to the fourth and fifth toes on the right foot. The patient is tender to palpation over the fourth and fifth digits proximal. Right foot is neurovascularly intact. Sensation is intact. Patient has an abrasion noted to the distal aspect of the right fourth digit. Range of motion is intact. Patient is able to ambulate with a slight limp due to pain. Remainder of physical examination is normal.
Emergency Department Course:	An x-ray was taken of the patient's right foot with attention to the fourth and fifth toes. X-ray showed a fracture of the fourth and fifth proximal phalanx. X-ray was also reviewed by Dr. Smith, who agreed with this assessment. The patient's right fourth and fifth toes were digitally blocked with 2.5 cc of 2% lidocaine each. Abrasion on the fourth digit was prepared per protocol. Fractures were reduced in the fourth and fifth digits and buddy taped. Patient's right foot was again x-rayed. His postreduction film showed that the fractures were in better alignment. X-rays were also reviewed by Dr. Blevins, who agreed with this assessment. Patient was fitted for a postoperative shoe.
Impressions/Diagnosis:	Patient has fractured right fourth and fifth toes.
Plan:	1. Rest, ice, compress, and elevate the right foot. 2. Buddy tape × two weeks. 3. Follow-up with family medical doctor as needed. 4. Return if condition worsens. Patient refused any pain medication.
Disposition:	Home

Assign appropriate CPT code(s) for the preceding procedures and indicate the index entries that were used to identify the codes. Assign only CPT codes (no E/M codes) and append any applicable modifiers.

Code(s):______________________________

Index entries:

____

____

Surgical Case #45

Operative Report

Preoperative Diagnosis: Lipoma of the right shoulder

Postoperative Diagnosis: Same

Procedure: Removal of lipoma

Description of Procedure: The patient was taken to the operating room and prepared and draped in the usual manner. A longitudinal incision was made centered over the palpable and visible mass, carried down through the skin. The subcutaneous layer was noted to be large lobulations, and dissection was begun around the obvious palpable 3.0 cm mass. This was dissected free and carried down through the deltoid muscle down to the level of the subscapularis tendon of the shoulder joint. Did not seem to have any major neurovascular attachments otherwise. Mass was dissected free through the muscle-slitting incision. The cephalic vein was retracted laterally. Bleeding was controlled with hemostats and Bovie cautery. Estimated blood loss: 30 cc. The wound was then copiously irrigated after total removal was verified, and the fascia was closed with 2-0 chromic catgut, subcutaneous layer with 2-0 plain catgut and skin with 2-0 Dermalon. The patient tolerated the procedure well and left the OR in good condition after dressing was applied.

Assign appropriate CPT code(s) for the preceding procedures and indicate the index entries that were used to identify the codes. Assign only CPT codes (no E/M codes) and append any applicable modifiers.

Code(s):____

Index entries:

____

____

Surgical Case #46

Operative Report

Preoperative Diagnosis:	Ptosis, left upper eyelid
Postoperative Diagnosis:	Same
Procedure:	Frontalis ptosis, left upper eyelid
Anesthesia:	Local
Description of Procedure:	Topical Tetracaine was applied to both eyes. The left upper lid and brow were infiltrated with Xylocaine with epinephrine and Marcaine with Wydase. The patient was prepared and draped in the usual fashion for oculoplastic surgery. Incisions were made in the medial and lateral thirds of the lid, 3 mm above the lash line. Stat incisions were made at the medial and lateral thirds of the brow, approximately 5 mm above the brow and a single incision was made in the middle of the brow, approximately 1 cm higher than the previous two incisions. A 3-0 Prolene suture was passed from the lateral lid incision to the medial lid incision beneath the orbicularis, just above the tarsus. Suture was then passed beneath the brow and frontalis to emerge from the medial and lateral brow incisions respectively. Each end of the suture was then passed beneath the frontalis to emerge through the central brow incision. The suture was tied and tension was adjusted so that the lid level was just above the papillary border. The brow incisions were closed with interrupted sutures of 6-0 Prolene, the eye was dressed with Ocumycin ointment. The patient tolerated the procedure well and left the OR in good condition.

Assign appropriate CPT code(s) for the preceding procedures and indicate the index entries that were used to identify the codes. Assign only CPT codes (no E/M codes) and append any applicable modifiers.

Code(s):______________________________

Index entries:

____

____

Surgical Case #47

Operative Report

Preoperative Diagnosis:	Displaced, rotated fractures of left index and long metacarpal shafts
Postoperative Diagnosis:	Same
Procedure:	Closed reduction and percutaneous pin fixation of displaced fractures of the left index and long metacarpal shafts
Description of Procedure:	The patient is a 22-year-old, right-hand-dominant man who sustained left index and long metacarpal shaft fractures while playing soccer. He was referred to my office and was found to have internal rotation and shortening deformities through the index and long metacarpal shaft fractures and subsequently is scheduled for closed, possibly open, reduction and percutaneous pin fixation or possible internal fixation of the previously-mentioned fractures. The patient was placed in the supine position on the OR table and general anesthesia was administered. Left proximal arm tourniquet was placed, and the left upper extremity was prepared and draped in the usual sterile fashion. The arm was exsanguinated with an Esmarch bandage and the tourniquet inflated to 250 mm Hg. Sterile finger traps and ropes were then applied to the left index and long fingers, and 10 lb of weight were then applied over the end of the hand table. The fractures were then gently manipulated and multiple fluoroscopic views were obtained, which revealed satisfactory alignment. Attention was then turned to the index metacarpal shaft fracture, which was percutaneously pinned from its radial to ulnar aspect with excellent purchase being obtained on both sides. X-rays were then taken and revealed anatomic alignment. Attention was then turned to the long metacarpal shaft fracture, which was still slightly distracted and displaced. Additional manipulation was performed. A pin was initially inserted from radial to ulnar, which resulted in further distraction of the fracture. The pin was removed, and another pin was inserted from ulnar to radial. This appeared to close the fracture gap and held the fracture in better alignment. A second pin was then placed just proximal and parallel to the original pin with resultant satisfactory alignment. There was still some slight gapping at the fracture site, but the rotation and angulation were corrected. The finger traps were removed, and the fingers were flexed to the same degree. All fingertips appeared to point to the distal pole of the scaphoid without any evidence of angulation or rotation malalignment. The pins were trimmed and bent over at 90-degree angles. The pin sites were irrigated, and Xeroform dressings were applied. Sterile gauze, lightly compressive hand dressing was then applied, reinforced with plaster splint with the hand placed in the intrinsic plus position and the PIP joint left free. The patient tolerated the procedure well and was sent to recovery in satisfactory condition.

Assign appropriate CPT code(s) for the preceding procedures and indicate the index entries that were used to identify the codes. Assign only CPT codes (no E/M codes) and append any applicable modifiers.

Code(s):____

Index entries:

____

____

Surgical Case #48

Operative Report

Preoperative Diagnosis:	Symptomatic third-degree heart block
Postoperative Diagnosis:	Same
Operation:	Placement of permanent pacemaker with transvenous electrode
Anesthesia:	Local infiltration of lidocaine 1%, total volume 13 cc
Complications:	None
Indications:	This 74-year-old man was admitted with a diagnosis of third-degree heart block complicated by congestive cardiac failure. Patient is scheduled for placement of a permanent pacemaker today.
Procedure:	With the patient supine on the operating table with a shoulder roll placed beneath the thoracic spine, the chest was prepared and draped in a sterile fashion. In the right infraclavicular region, a subcutaneous pocket was created for containing the pulse generator. Using an introducer guide wire, a sheath technique bipolar-targeted lead was introduced into the right subclavian vein. Under fluoroscopy control, this was directed into the right ventricle. Two initial locations were not satisfactory for pacing parameters. Finally, the pacemaker was positioned in satisfactory position with the following parameters: at the threshold 0.4 volts, current 1.5 milliamps, and R wave 15. The pacing system analyzer was then turned to 10 volts output and the diaphragm observed for pulsations, which were not proven. The lead was then secured under the clavicle with a single suture of 2-0 Ethibond. It was then attached to a 5794 Medtronic low-profile VVI pacemaker programmed at 70 beats per minute. The pulse generator was then anchored in the subcutaneous pocket with a single 0 PDS suture. The subcutaneous tissue was then approximated with 2-0 PDS and the skin approximated with 4-0 Maxon. Sterile dressing was applied. A chest x-ray was obtained, which showed no pneumothorax and satisfactory position of the lead. The patient was then returned to the coronary care unit in good condition.

Assign appropriate CPT code(s) for the preceding procedures and indicate the index entries that were used to identify the codes. Assign only CPT codes (no E/M codes) and append any applicable modifiers.

Code(s):______________________________

Index entries:

____

____

Surgical Case #49

Operative Report

Preoperative Diagnosis:	Nasolacrimal duct obstruction, right eye
Postoperative Diagnosis:	Same
Operation:	1. Probing right nasolacrimal duct 2. Balloon dilation, right nasolacrimal duct
Procedure:	The patient was taken to the operating room and given general anesthesia by mask. The right upper punctum was then dilated and a #0 Bowman probe passed from the upper punctum into the lacrimal sac and down through the nasolacrimal duct with a small amount of resistance. A second probe was then passed under the right inferior turbinate and definite metal-on-metal contact established. The original probe was then withdrawn, and a #2 Lacricath was inserted from the upper punctum into the lacrimal sac and down through the nasolacrimal duct. Its position was confirmed in the nose. The balloon was inflated eight atmospheres for 90 seconds. It was then withdrawn 5 mm and again inflated eight atmospheres for 60 seconds. At this point, the Lacricath was withdrawn. A lacrimal cannula attached to a syringe containing normal saline dyed with fluorescein was then inserted from the upper punctum into the lacrimal sac and fluid freely irrigated into the nose and recovered with a suction catheter. A drop of a steroid antibiotic combination was then applied to the right eye, and the patient awakened and returned to the recovery room in good condition.

Assign appropriate CPT code(s) for the preceding procedures and indicate the index entries that were used to identify the codes. Assign only CPT codes (no E/M codes) and append any applicable modifiers.

Code(s):____________________________

Index entries:

____

____

Emergency Department Case #50

Emergency Department Record

Chief Complaint:	A laceration to the left lower leg
History of Present Illness:	The patient is a 33-year-old man who presents to the ER today with a chief complaint of a laceration to his left lower leg. The patient states that he came to Cincinnati for a mountain bike competition, which he was in today. The patient stated that he was practicing before the competition when he accidentally cut the posterior aspect of his left leg on the pedal of his bike. The patient stated that the pedal was clean and that he had this accident on the pavement. There was no grass or dirt around at that time. The patient currently complains of pain to the area of the laceration. He is ambulatory with a limp. The patient stated that the accident happened approximately one hour prior to arrival at the emergency room. The patient denies any left calf pain. Denies any left knee pain. The patient did not have any head injury or any loss of consciousness. The patient's tetanus is up to date. The patient also denies any neck or back injury. The patient has no other complaints.
Review of Systems:	See HPI; otherwise negative
Past Medical History:	Unremarkable
Medications:	None
Allergies:	No known drug allergies

Physical Examination:

Vital Signs:	Blood pressure is 128/68; temperature is 97.8° F; pulse 77; respirations 18
General:	The patient is a 33-year-old man who is in no acute distress. The patient is alert and oriented × 3.
Skin:	Pink, warm. Patient currently has a 5-cm gaping laceration to the posterior aspect of his left leg that is just inferior and medial to the left knee.
HEENT:	Within normal limits
Neck:	Supple, no cervical tenderness; no cervical adenopathy
Musculoskeletal:	The patient has full active range of motion of his left knee at this time. There is no edema, ecchymosis, or erythema noted to the left knee. However, the patient's posterior aspect of his left knee is indurated somewhat. The patient is nontender with palpation over the left gastrocnemius muscle. The patient's dorsalis pedis and posterior tibialis pulses are present and strong. Doppler was then used to pick up the patient's left popliteal pulse. This was present and strong, and when compared to the popliteal pulse of the right leg, it was the same strength. The patient is nontender with palpation of the left quadriceps as well as over the left hamstring muscles.
ED Course:	The patient was discussed with Dr. Ferguson. Dr. Ferguson also examined the patient. X-rays were then obtained of the patient's left tib/fib as well as the patient's left knee. X-rays were reviewed by both myself and Dr. Ferguson and were unremarkable. The patient was then given Keflex 1 g p.o. The patient was then given Lortab 5 mg p.o.
ED Procedure:	The patient's laceration was anesthetized using 15 cc of 1% lidocaine plain. The area was then cleansed using Betadine and normal saline solution. The wound was then explored for any evidence of foreign bodies. No foreign bodies were noted. Wound edges were then well approximated and brought together using three deep-layered sutures of 4-0 Vicryl and seven mattress sutures of 4-0 nylon as well as one simple suture of 4-0 nylon. The area was then cleansed again using normal saline. Xeroform was applied as well as a 2 × 2 Keflex wrap and Ace wrap. The patient was informed to remove the Ace wrap prior to sleeping in the evening. The patient was also given a Lortab starter pack and informed to fill his antibiotic prescription. Patient was also informed to watch for any pain to his left calf. The patient understood this and stated that he would return if any pain occurred.

Emergency Department Case #50 (Continued)

Impression/Diagnosis: 1. A 5-cm laceration, left posterior leg, which was repaired

Plan:

1. Keep area clean and dry
2. Suture removal 10 to 12 days by primary care physician
3. Wound care instructions: Watch for infection
4. Keflex 500 mg #20 no refills
5. Lortab 5 mg #10 no refills
6. Return with any worsening symptoms

Assign appropriate CPT code(s) for the preceding procedures and indicate the index entries that were used to identify the codes. Assign only CPT codes (no E/M codes) and append any applicable modifiers.

Code(s):______________________________

Index entries:

____

____

Surgical Case #51

Operative Report

Preoperative Diagnosis: Rule out bladder tumor

Postoperative Diagnosis: Same

Procedures: Cystoscopy, biopsy, and fulguration of bladder

Anesthesia: Spinal

Indications: This is a 68-year-old white woman with a history of grade II superficial transitional cell carcinoma of the bladder. Cystoscopy showed a suspicious erythematous area on the right trigone. She presented today for cystoscopy, biopsy, and fulguration.

Findings: The urethra was normal, the bladder was 1+ trabeculated, the mid and right trigone area were slightly erythematous and hypervascular, no papillary tumors were noted, no mucosal abnormalities were noted.

Description of Procedure: The patient was placed on the table in supine position, satisfactory spinal anesthesia was obtained. She was placed in the dorsolithotomy position and prepared and draped in the usual manner. A #22 French cystoscopy sheath was passed per urethra in atraumatic fashion. The bladder was resected with a 70-degree lens with findings as noted previously. Cup biopsy forceps were placed and three biopsies were taken of the suspicious areas of the trigone. For hemostasis, these areas were fulgurated with the Bugby electrode. There was no active bleeding seen. The scope was removed, and the patient was returned to recovery in satisfactory condition.

Pathology Report:

Bladder biopsy: chronic cystitis (cystica) with squamous metaplasia

Assign appropriate CPT code(s) for the preceding procedures and indicate the index entries that were used to identify the codes. Assign only CPT codes (no E/M codes) and append any applicable modifiers.

Code(s):______________________________

Index entries:

____

____

Surgical Case #52

Operative Report

Preoperative Diagnosis:	Thrombosis, right forearm, Gore-Tex graft
Postoperative Diagnosis:	Same
Operation:	Thrombectomy
Indications:	This 73-year-old woman has a right forearm graft that has developed an arterial occlusion.
Procedure:	The patient was placed in the supine position and prepared and draped in the normal fashion. A transverse incision was made at the outflow tract of the vein and the Gore-Tex graft anastomosis. A complete thrombectomy was performed. The area was fully irrigated with saline and heparin lock. There was satisfactory pulse through the graft, and the incisions were closed with 3-0 Dexon and running 4-0 Prolene. The patient tolerated the procedure well.

Assign appropriate CPT code(s) for the preceding procedures and indicate the index entries that were used to identify the codes. Assign only CPT codes (no E/M codes) and append any applicable modifiers.

Code(s):____________________

Index entries:

____

____

Surgical Case #53

ENDOSCOPY REPORT

Procedure:	Gastroenterology consultation/gastroscopy/esophageal dilatation
Indications:	This is a 72-year-old woman who has had dysphagia for solids for some time. Barium swallow showed a smooth stricture at the LES. She is generally in good health otherwise except for hypertension. Because of her dysphagia, upper GI endoscopy is done today. She was premedicated with Versed. Conscious sedation was monitored in the usual fashion. The Olympus video endoscope was introduced into the esophagus. The distal esophagus has a tight stricture at the LES. The stomach, pyloric channel, duodenal bulb, and second part of the duodenum were normal. The scope was withdrawn, and she was serially dilated using Maloney dilators.

Assign appropriate CPT code(s) for the preceding procedures and indicate the index entries that were used to identify the codes. Assign only CPT codes (no E/M codes) and append any applicable modifiers.

Code(s):____________________

Index entries:

____

____

Surgical Case #54

Operative Report

Preoperative Diagnosis:	Squamous cell carcinoma of the left forearm, 8 mm
Postoperative Diagnosis:	Same
Procedure:	Excision of the same with layered primary closure, 4 cm in length
Anesthetic:	Local
Brief Clinical History:	The patient had a biopsy-proven squamous cell carcinoma of the left forearm. After explanation of the risks, benefits, and alternatives, she agreed to re-excision and closure. She understood that there would be a scar as a result.
Details of Procedure:	The patient was taken to the outpatient operating area. An ellipse was taken around the primary lesion with 5-mm margins for excision around the lesion. The area was infiltrated with 0.5% Xylocaine with 1:200,000 epinephrine and approximately 5 cc was used. The area was prepared with Betadine paint and draped in a sterile manner. The lesion was elliptically excised and closed in layers with 4-0PDS. The deep subcutaneous layer was closed separately and then a running subcuticular layer was performed. She tolerated the procedure well. She was given instructions for local care and will return in nine days for a checkup and suture removal.

Assign appropriate CPT code(s) for the preceding procedures and indicate the index entries that were used to identify the codes. Assign only CPT codes (no E/M codes) and append any applicable modifiers.

Code(s):____

Index entries:

____

____

Surgical Case #55

Operative Report

Preoperative Diagnosis: Right true vocal cord lesion

Postoperative Diagnosis: Same

Operative Procedure: Direct laryngoscopy with excision of right true vocal cord lesion

Findings: Firm right true vocal cord lesion and some scarring on the right true vocal cord, otherwise normal laryngoscopy

Indication for the Procedure: This is a 51-year-old man who had a history of anterior commissure nodule that was biopsied in 2001 and came back as benign. He was lost to follow-up, but returned with increasing hoarseness and was found on flexible laryngoscopy to have a mid-right-sided true vocal cord lesion. He was brought to the operating room today for laryngoscopy and removal of this lesion.

Details of the Procedure: He was placed in the supine position on the operating room table and mask anesthesia was induced. Once deeper anesthesia had been achieved, the table was turned toward the laryngoscopy instrumentation. A Dedo laryngoscope was placed carefully into the mouth after the upper gums were protected using wet gauze. The lingual surface of the epiglottis appeared normal as did the vallecula. The laryngeal surface of the epiglottis also appeared completely normal as did the arytenoids and false vocal cords bilaterally. The true vocal cords were bilaterally mobile. They were slightly edematous and there was an approximately 1.5 cm whitish nodule on the right vocal cord in the middle third of the cord. There was a small area of heaped mucosa near the anterior commissure that was slightly hard, but deemed normal and another one at the vocal process that again had normal mucosa, but was slightly firm as if some scarring was present. Again, the left true vocal cord was completely normal except for slight edema. The posterior commissure area appeared normal. Again, the arytenoids were visualized and were thought to be completely normal. At this point, an LTA was sprayed and the patient was intubated. Completion of the direct laryngoscopy revealed a normal piriform sinus on the left normal postcricoid area and a normal right piriform sinus. At this point, the laryngoscope was replaced such that the right vocal cord was easily visualized and palpated. It was suspended at this time. Next, the operating microscope was brought into place, through the #400 lens, and the vocal cord was easily inspected and palpated. A right biting forceps was used to retract the mid third of the right vocal cord and a leftward scissors was used to dissect the area where this lesion was noted on the vocal cord. This did include the medial aspect of the true cord on that side. Once this was excised in toto, it was sent off for permanent pathology. There was minimal bleeding at the site. The microscope and Dedo laryngoscope were taken out of the field, and the patient was returned to the anesthesia department for reawakening, extubation, and transported to the postanesthesia care unit in a stable condition. Dr. Fowler was present for this entire case.

Pathology Report

Specimen: Right true vocal cord lesion

Gross description: One specimen is received in formalin labeled with demographics and "right true vocal cord." It consists of a 0.2 × 0.1 × 0.1 cm white tissue fragment. The specimen is stained with eosin and entirely submitted in one cassette.

Microscopic Examination/ Diagnosis: Squamous mucosa with focal moderate dysplasia

Assign appropriate CPT code(s) for the preceding procedures and indicate the index entries that were used to identify the codes. Assign only CPT codes (no E/M codes) and append any applicable modifiers.

Code(s):____________________________________

Index entries:

____

____

Surgical Case #56

Operative Report

Preoperative Diagnosis:	Previous history of polyps
Postoperative Diagnosis:	Descending colon polyp
Operation:	Colonoscopy total and polypectomy of descending colon polyp
Procedure:	Patient was placed in the left lateral position. After adequate sedation the 168-cm videoscope was passed through the rectum, through the sigmoid colon, through the descending colon, through the transverse colon to the right colon. The position of the cecum was confirmed. The cecum and the right colon were found to be normal. The transverse colon was found to be normal. In the descending colon there was a small 3-mm polyp. This was removed with use of cold knife forceps. The polyp was then given out for histopathology. The base of the polyp was electrocoagulated. The remainder of the colon was found to be normal except for diverticulosis involving sigmoid colon. The rectum was found to be normal except for hypertrophied anal polyp. The scope was removed. The patient tolerated the procedure well and was transferred to the recovery room in fair condition.

Assign appropriate CPT code(s) for the preceding procedures and indicate the index entries that were used to identify the codes. Assign only CPT codes (no E/M codes) and append any applicable modifiers.

Code(s):____

Index entries:

____

____

Emergency Department Record Case #57

Operative Report (Emergency Room)

Preoperative Diagnosis:	Multiple lacerations to both ears
Preoperative Diagnosis:	Multiple lacerations to both ears, a laceration to the left ear and a series of four lacerations to the right ear
Anesthetic:	Local anesthetic was used, 1% carbocaine plain
Indications:	The patient sustained the above-named lacerations when she was involved in a hay wagon accident.
Procedure:	The patient was treated in the emergency department. The right ear was treated first. The two smaller, more superficial lacerations, measuring 1.0 cm each, were closed after the wound had been infiltrated with 1% carbocaine and then cleaned copiously with Betadine, saline, and peroxide. They were closed with simple interrupted #6-0 Prolene sutures. The two other lacerations on the right ear, total of 3 cm in length, and two different lacerations were closed in the deep layer with #5-0 Vicryl suture after they had been infiltrated with 1% carbocaine, prepared and draped in the appropriate fashion using Betadine, peroxide, and saline. The superficial layers were closed with interrupted #6-0 Prolene suture. After the right ear was completed the wounds were covered with polysporin. The left ear was then treated after the 2.0-cm wound was infiltrated with 1% carbocaine. After the wound was cleaned with Betadine, saline, and peroxide, the superficial layers were closed with interrupted #6-0 Prolene suture. The wounds were then covered with polysporin.
Follow-Up:	The patient was instructed to follow up and take the sutures out in six to seven days.

Assign appropriate CPT code(s) for the preceding procedures and indicate the index entries that were used to identify the codes. Assign only CPT codes (no E/M codes) and append any applicable modifiers.

Code(s):____

Index entries:

____

____

Surgical Case #58

Operative Report

Preprocedure: Diagnosis(es):	1. Backache, unspecified 2. Related back and leg pain
Procedure(s) Performed:	Lumbar epidural steroid injection L5-S1 interspace
Indications for Procedure:	The patient is a 41-year-old man with severe work-related back and leg pain, more left than right. The patient understands the reasons for the procedure and the risk associated with it. The patient is anxious and needed IV sedation and tolerated the pain associated with injection.
Details of Procedure:	For the procedure, the patient was sedated with 2 mg of Versed and 1,250 mg of Alfenta. The patient was monitored throughout the procedure and afterward with pulse oximeter and Dinamap. The pulse oximetry ranged in the lower and upper 90 range. The patient tolerated the IV well; therefore, the procedure went well. For the procedure, the patient was placed prone on the fluoroscopy table with a pillow under his abdomen. We identified the sacral hiatus. We prepared the skin with alcohol and DuraPrep and applied drapes and anesthetized the skin with xylocaine. Next, we used fluoroscopy to guide the 17-gauge needle into the spinal canal through the sacral hiatus. This was advanced under AP and lateral fluoroscopic guidance with loss of resistance. We verified proper depth and placement with myelography injection. The lumbar myelography injection was extradural in the lumbosacral area and consisted of 2 cc of Isovue 300. This showed we were in the spinal canal and highlighting the nerve roots at the lumbosacral region. Next, we placed the catheter to the L5-S1 interspace. Through the catheter we injected steroid solution that contained 80 mg of Depo-Medrol, 3 cc of 0.75% marcaine, and 4 cc of Omnipaque 300. This was injected under fluoroscopy, visualizing the nerve roots well throughout the lower lumbar area, more left than right. We cleared the catheter and needle of solution and removed them from the back. Permanent films were taken, and the patient was taken to the recovery room where he recovered in good condition.
Interpretation of Permanent Films:	The permanent films afterward verified the myelography and steroid solution were in the proper areas. On AP and lateral views, the solution highlighted the nerve roots at the lower lumbar area but scar tissue is preventing the spread of medication throughout the entire region. Nerve roots do highlight in the lower lumbar spine. No evidence of dural puncture.

Assign appropriate CPT code(s) for the preceding procedures and indicate the index entries that were used to identify the codes. Assign only CPT codes (no E/M codes) and append any applicable modifiers.

Code(s):____

Index entries:

____

____

Surgical Case #59

Operative Report

Preoperative Diagnosis: Bladder neck contracture, status post radical retropubic prostatectomy

Postoperative Diagnosis: Same

Procedure: Cystoscopy with dilation

Indications for Procedure: The patient is a 58-year-old man who underwent a radical prostatectomy in 2004. Postoperatively, he has had problems with bladder neck contractures requiring dilation. His last dilation was done in November 2004. He had been performing intermittent catheterization following this with good results of continence. Unfortunately, over the past several months, he had been unable to pass this catheter and appeared to be in urinary retention. He was scheduled for cystoscopy and dilation of bladder neck contracture accordingly. All alternative treatment options as well as risks and benefits and expected outcomes of the procedure were explained to the patient prior to the procedure and he understood these and wished to proceed.

Findings: Severe bladder neck contracture was noted. It was approximately #5 French in diameter.

Details of Procedure: After informed consent was obtained and the patient received 1 g of ampicillin and 100 mg of gentamicin IV, the patient was brought to the operating theater and placed in supine fashion. After adequate sedation, the patient was placed in the dorsal lithotomy position; his genitalia and perineum were prepared and draped in the usual sterile fashion. Using a #22.5 French sheath, a scope was inserted into the patient's urethra and subsequently into the bladder. A long filiform was passed through the bladder neck contracture. Subsequent dilation from #8 French to #20 French was carried out. After approximately #16 French, it is very difficult to pass the dilator and therefore this was determined at the #20 French dilation. Another attempt at placing the filiform or followers was discontinued at approximately #14 French because of difficulty in passing the followers.

The filiform was then removed, and under direct visualization, an Amplatz super stiff guide wire was inserted into the bladder with the aid of a Pollack catheter to the #5 French open-ended catheter. The renal Amplatz dilators were then used to dilate the bladder neck contracture to #18 French. A #18 French Councill catheter was then inserted over the guide wire into the bladder. 10 cc was inflated into the balloon and the wire was removed. Irrigation confirmed that this was in the bladder. Patient was taken to the recovery room in satisfactory condition.

Assign appropriate CPT code(s) for the preceding procedures and indicate the index entries that were used to identify the codes. Assign only CPT codes (no E/M codes) and append any applicable modifiers.

Code(s):____

Index entries:

____

____

Surgical Case #60

Operative Report

Preoperative Diagnosis:	Stab wound, left thigh
Postoperative Diagnosis:	Stab wound, left thigh with arterial bleeders secondary to branches off the deep femoral artery
Procedures Performed:	Exploration of left thigh stab wound with control of bleeding and repair of rectus femoris muscle
Indications for Procedure:	This 24-year-old man was stabbed in the left anteromedial thigh earlier this morning. He presented to the emergency department, and the examination revealed a 1-cm stab wound about 20 cm below the inguinal ligament in the mid-thigh anteromedial. Posterior tibial pulses were equal bilaterally. There was no swelling in his foot or calf. The wound was explored in the emergency room, and it was obvious that there was a huge cavity within the rectus femoris muscle. Nothing further was done there and he was brought to the operating room.
Details of Procedure:	The patient was placed on the operating table in the supine position. General endotracheal anesthesia was induced, and endotracheal tube was used. Left leg was prepared with Betadine and then draped. Enlarged the stab wound medial and laterally in oblique fashion, carried it down to the muscle, opened up the anterior fascia of the rectus femoris, got into a large cavity within it that went down almost to the femur. At the base of this there were two small pumping vessels that were electrocoagulated, which pretty much controlled the bleeding. There were then multiple small bleeders within the muscle belly itself that we coagulated. The wound was copiously irrigated, rechecked, and little bleeders Bovied and the bleeding was controlled. We evacuated all the hematoma that was present. Cleaned it out, irrigated it again, rechecked it, and no further bleeding was noted. The anterior fascia was closed with interrupted 2-0 Vicryl, and subcutaneous tissue was irrigated and the skin closed with staples, 4 × 4 Kerlix and Ace wrap over that. The patient tolerated the procedure well. Estimated blood loss of the actual procedure was only about 50 cc. He was extubated, and taken to the recovery room in stable condition.

Assign appropriate CPT code(s) for the preceding procedures and indicate the index entries that were used to identify the codes. Assign only CPT codes (no E/M codes) and append any applicable modifiers.

Code(s):______________________________

Index entries:

____

____

Surgical Case #61

Operative Report

Preoperative Diagnosis: Neurogenic bladder with an implanted sacral nerve stimulator

Postoperative Diagnosis: Neurogenic bladder with an implanted sacral nerve stimulator

Procedure Performed: Removal of InterStim sacral nerve stimulator

Indications for Procedure: This patient is a 96-year-old female with a history of neurogenic bladder with recurrent urinary tract infections due to poor emptying. She is here for removal of her sacral nerve stimulator, which had subsequently quit working. After all the risks, benefits, and expected outcomes were explained, she agreed to proceed.

Details of Procedure: The patient was brought to the operative suite, given a light intravenous anesthetic, and laid in the prone position. The area overlying the InterStim neurostimulator was infiltrated using 1% lidocaine mixed with 0.35% Marcaine. Once this was done, an incision was made over this and dissection was carried down to the InterStim neurostimulator. The device was removed from its pouch. The leads, which were tunneled down to the S3 foramina, were identified and with careful manipulation we were able to remove in their entirety. Once this was done, hemostasis was obtained. The wound was copiously irrigated using antibiotic solution. The 3-0 Vicryl pop-offs were used to close the subcutaneous tissue, 4-0 Monocryl was used to close the skin. Benzoin, Steri-Strips, and Tegaderm were applied. She tolerated the procedure well and was taken to the recovery room in stable condition.

Assign appropriate CPT code(s) for the preceding procedures and indicate the index entries that were used to identify the codes. Assign only CPT codes (no E/M codes) and append any applicable modifiers.

Code(s):________________________________

Index entries:

____

____

Surgical Case #62

Operative Report

Preoperative Diagnosis: Left third finger, trigger finger

Postoperative Diagnosis: Left third finger, trigger finger

Procedure Performed: Release of the left third finger, trigger finger

Indications for Procedure: Patient is an 84-year-old male who presented to our clinic with complaint of the left third finger locked up on extension. He was diagnosed with a trigger finger and was scheduled for repair.

Procedure: Patient was placed in supine position. After prep and draping, approximately 20 cc of local anesthetic consisting of 2% lidocaine, without epinephrine, was injected over the palmar aspect of the left third finger over the MCP, followed by tight wrap over the forearm and blood pressure cuff over the left forearm, then it inflated to 215 mmHg and tight wrap was then released and with the blood pressure cuff remained inflated for hemostasis. An incision was made over the palmar aspect of the left third finger at the MCP, and this incision was then carried down through the fascia to expose the tendon sheath, and the tendon sheath was then opened using sharp dissection. Hemostasis, meanwhile, obtained using electrocautery. After release was done, patient was asked to flex and extend the finger and his symptoms subsequently resolved. Compression was used for hemostasis while the tourniquet was deflated. Before closure, approximately 3 cc of Kenalog was used for steroid treatment. For closure, a #5-0 nylon was used in an interrupted fashion to approximate the skin edges in a nontension fashion. For dressing with Bacitracin was applied over the finger and the hand was wrapped and finally Ace bandage was applied. The patient tolerated the procedure well and was subsequently transferred to recovery.

Assign appropriate CPT code(s) for the preceding procedures and indicate the index entries that were used to identify the codes. Assign only CPT codes (no E/M codes) and append any applicable modifiers.

Code(s):____

Index entries:

____

____

Surgical Case #63

Operative Report

Preoperative Diagnosis: Menometrorrhagia and anemia

Postoperative Diagnosis: Same

Procedures: Dilatation and curettage, Hysteroscopy.

Indications for Procedure: The patient is a 53-year-old female who reports that she has had extremely heavy periods for several months. The patient had two periods lasting 10 each for the past two months.

Based on the patient's history of simple hyperplasia, anemia, and menometrorrhagia, the risks, benefits and alternatives of the D&C, hysteroscopy were thoroughly discussed with the patient who agreed to the procedure.

Description of Operation: The patient was taken to the operating room where under the effects of adequate general anesthesia, was prepped and draped in the usual sterile fashion for vaginal surgery.

A weighted speculum was placed posteriorly and the Sims anteriorly to allow visualization of the cervix. The cervix was noted to descend to the introitus. The uterus was then sounded to 10 cm. On examination under anesthesia, she had no appreciable adnexal masses. Her uterus was slightly enlarged, anteverted, mobile.

The patient's cervix was dilated to a #15 dilator. The hysteroscope was then introduced into the cervix. The endocervical canal appeared without lesions. Advancing to the uterus, there appeared to be a desynchronous endometrium with lush endometrium posteriorly and somewhat atrophic appearing anteriorly. Tissue sample were taken for pathological diagnosis.

The right tubal ostia was visualized; the left was obscured by lush endometrium. The hysteroscope was then removed.

The cervix was then dilated to #20 dilator. The sharp curet was then removed. All instruments were then removed from the patient.

All sponge, needle and instrument counts were correct at the end of the procedure.

The patient tolerated the procedure well, was taken to the postoperative recovery room in good condition.

Assign appropriate CPT code(s) for the preceding procedures and indicate the index entries that were used to identify the codes. Assign only CPT codes (no E/M codes) and append any applicable modifiers.

Code(s):____

Index entries:

____

____

Appendix D

Answers to Chapter Review Exercises

Chapter 1: Introduction to Clinical Coding

Exercise 1.1 Introduction

1. The American Medical Association (AMA) updates the CPT codes, and the Centers for Medicare and Medicaid Services (CMS) updates the HCPCS National Codes (Level II).
2. Four
3. ICD-9-CM and HCPCS
4. a. Diagnosis: ICD-9-CM
   Procedure: HCPCS
   b. Diagnosis: ICD-9-CM
   Procedure: HCPCS
   c. UB-04 (CMS-1450)
5. ICD-9-CM
6. Procedure code 11440 is linked with diagnosis code #1 (216.3). Procedure code 82951 is linked with diagnosis code #3 (790.29).

   Note: Depending on the carrier, you may link more than one reference number in block 24E, whereas some payers require just one. When reporting more than one code on a CMS-1500 claim, enter the code with the highest fee in line 1 of block 24 and the remaining in descending order of charges.

Chapter 2: Application of the CPT System

Exercise 2.1 Organization of CPT

1. Surgery
2. Evaluation and Management
3. Pathology and Laboratory
4. Category II codes
5. Medicine
6. Radiology
7. Anesthesia
8. Category III codes
9. Maternity Care and Delivery
10. Prolonged Services
11. Radiation Oncology
12. Surgical Pathology

Exercise 2.2 CPT Conventions

1. Repair blood vessel, direct; hand, finger
2. Two
3. Revised descriptor
4. Esophagoscopy, rigid or flexible, with insertion of plastic tube or stent
5. New descriptor
6. No

7. No
8. 13152, 13153
9. 40814
10. 31578, 31576

Exercise 2.3 Use of the Alphabetical Index

1. 23400 Green operation, *see* scapulopexy
2. 10021 Fine Needle Aspiration
3. 35556 Graft, *see* Bypass graft, Femoral Artery or Popliteal Artery
4. 49555 Hernia repair, femoral, recurrent
5. 26991 Incision and drainage, bursa, hip
6. 01680 Anesthesia, shoulder
7. 31525 Laryngoscopy, direct
8. 72149 MRI, *see* magnetic resonance imaging, spine, lumbar
9. 11055 Paring, skin lesion, benign hyperkeratotic, single lesion
10. 86701 HIV-1, antibody

Note: Answers to exercises 11 through 20 are located in the Instructor's Guide and available to faculty of educational programs.

Exercise 2.4 CPT Coding Process

1. Colonoscopy and polypectomy
2. 45384–45385
3. How was the polyp removed (hot biopsy forceps, snare, and so on)?
4. "Was removed with hot biopsy forceps and retrieved"
5. 45384

Exercise 2.5 CPT Coding Process

1. Excision
2. Can be located under Excision, lesion, skin; or Lesion, skin, excision

Selections:	Benign	11400–11471
	Malignant	11600–11646

3. Pathologic diagnosis indicates that the lesion was malignant (11600–11646).
4. Documentation is needed to code malignant lesion, size of lesion + margins (or size of excision) (2.0 cm + 0.5 cm + 0.5 cm = 3.0 cm excision site) and site (arm).
5. 11603

Exercise 2.6 CPT Coding Process

1. Hernia repair
2. Index entries: Hernia repair, umbilicus; Repair, hernia, umbilical. Codes to review: 49580–49587
3. Age of patient; incarcerated or strangulated hernia
4. Review of documentation (38-year-old patient and no documentation for incarcerated/strangulated hernia). Using the abstracted documentation and process of elimination, the correct code would be 49585.
5. Wound closure would be an integral part of the procedure and would not be assigned a CPT code.

Exercise 2.7 Coding References

1. 45380
2. *CPT Assistant,* January 1996, page 7, instructs the coder to assign 45385. *CPT Assistant,* January 2004, states that if a small polyp is removed via cold knife biopsy, the appropriate code is 45380. This is a good example of the need to research the most current coding advice.

Exercise 2.8 Coding References

1. When a biopsy of a lesion is obtained and the remaining portion of the *same* lesion is then excised/fulgurated, only the code for the excision/fulguration should be used. When the biopsy is taken from a *different* lesion than the one excised, the biopsy code and an additional code for the removal of the separate lesion are reported. It would be appropriate to append modifier 59 to the code reported for the biopsy procedure.
2. Reference: *CPT Assistant,* October 2004, Skin Biopsy Coding Guidelines.

Exercise 2.9 Chapter 2 Review

1. Bullet
2. 11100 and 11101
3. Category III
4. 42320
5. 40843

Note: Answers to exercises 6 through 10 are located in the Instructor's Guide and available to faculty of educational programs.

Chapter 3: Modifiers

Exercise 3.1 Chapter 3 Review

1. 55
2. 77
3. 22
4. 62
5. 53
6. 64721–50 Carpal tunnel syndrome, decompression
7. 11730–FA Avulsion, nails
8. 11043–73 Debridement, muscle
9. 64611–52 Chemodenervation, salivary glands
10. 19102–LT Biopsy, breast
11. 28485–RT Fracture, metatarsal, open treatment

    Note: –T9 is not applicable in this case because the procedure refers to the bones of the foot, not the toes.

Chapter 4: Surgery

Exercise 4.1 Integumentary System—Debridement

1. 11042 Debridement, skin, subcutaneous tissue
2. 11010 Debridement, skin, with open fracture
3. 11005 Debridement, skin, infected

    11008 Removal, mesh, abdominal wall

Exercise 4.2 Integumentary System—Lesions

1. 11421 Excision, skin, lesion, benign; or

    11402 Lesion, skin, excision, benign
2. 17110 Lesion, skin, destruction, benign
3. 11642 Excision, skin, lesion, malignant; or Lesion, skin, excision, malignant
4. 11200 Skin, tags, removal

Note: Answers to exercises 5 through 7 are located in the Instructor's Guide and available to faculty of educational programs.

Exercise 4.3 Integumentary System

1. 11442 Excision, skin, lesion, benign; or Lesion, skin, excision, benign

Exercise 4.4 Integumentary System

1. 11308 Lesion, skin, shaving

Exercise 4.5 Integumentary System—Wound Repairs

1. 12002 Wound, repair; or Repair, wound, simple
2. 12032 Wound, repair; or Repair, wound, intermediate
3. 12041 Wound, repair; or Repair, wound, intermediate

    12002 Wound, repair; or Repair, wound, simple (sum of repairs)

Exercise 4.6 Integumentary System

1. 12001 Wound, repair; or Repair, wound, simple

Exercise 4.7 Integumentary System

1. 12032 Wound, repair; or Repair wound (simple and intermediate)

    12005

Exercise 4.8 Integumentary System

1. 13121 Wound, repair (complex)

    13122

Exercise 4.9 Integumentary System

1. 11603 Lesion, skin, excision, malignant
   12031 Wound, repair (intermediate)

Exercise 4.10 Integumentary System—Skin Grafts

1. 14021 Skin Graft and Flap, tissue transfer
2. 15150 Skin Graft and Flap, tissue-cultured
   15151
3. 15220 Skin Graft and Flap, free skin graft, full thickness

Exercise 4.11 Integumentary System

1. 15120 Autograft, skin, epidermal
   11646 Excision, skin, lesion, malignant; or Lesion, skin, excision, malignant

Exercise 4.12 Integumentary System

1. 15100 Skin, grafts, free

Exercise 4.13 Integumentary System

1. 19000–LT Breast, cyst, puncture aspiration

Exercise 4.14 Integumentary System

1. 19125–LT Excision, breast, cyst; or Breast, excision, lesion by needle localization

   Note: The hospital also would assign 19290 for placement of the wire. The surgeon would not assign this code because the radiologist performed the procedure. In addition, a radiology code would be submitted for both the facility and the radiologist. Radiology is introduced in chapter 5.

Exercise 4.15 Integumentary System

1. 19120–RT Breast, excision, cyst; or Excision, breast, cyst

   Note: The entire nodule was excised, not just a piece of tissue, which is implied with the term *biopsy.*

Exercise 4.16 Integumentary System Review

1. 16020 Burns, dressings
2. 14020 Skin Graft and Flap, tissue transfer

   Note: Excision of lesion is included and should not be assigned an additional code.
3. 12032 Wound, repair, intermediate

   Note: Anatomic modifiers (LT, RT) are not appropriate.
4. 19102–LT Breast, biopsy
   19295–LT Breast, metallic localization clip placement
5. 11606 Lesion, skin, excision, malignant

Note: Answers to exercises 6 through 10 are located in the Instructor's Guide and available to faculty of educational programs.

Exercise 4.17 Musculoskeletal System—Fractures

1. 25545–LT Fracture, ulna, shaft, open treatment
2. 21800 Fracture, rib, closed treatment
   21800
3. 23605–RT Fracture, humerus, closed with manipulation
4. 27532–RT Fracture, tibia, closed treatment (initial cast application included with treatment code)

Note: Answers to exercises 5 through 7 are located in the Instructor's Guide and available to faculty of educational programs.

Exercise 4.18 Musculoskeletal System

1. 29515–RT Splint, leg, short

   Note: E/M code 99283–25 is applicable in this case.

Exercise 4.19 Musculoskeletal System

1. 27788–LT Fracture, fibula, closed treatment; or Fracture, fibula, with manipulation

Exercise 4.20 Musculoskeletal System—Arthroscopy

1. 29875–LT Arthroscopy, surgical, knee
2. 29827–RT Arthroscopy, surgical, shoulder
3. 29846–LT Arthroscopy, surgical, wrist
4. 29837–LT Arthroscopy, surgical, elbow

Exercise 4.21 Musculoskeletal System

1. 29882–RT Arthroscopy, surgical, knee

Exercise 4.22 Musculoskeletal System Review

1. 28475–LT 28475–LT Fracture, metatarsal, closed
2. 28285–T1 Hammertoe repair
3. 27766–RT Fracture, ankle, medial
4. 20101 Wound, exploration, penetrating, chest
5. 23030 Hematoma, shoulder, drainage

Note: Answers to exercises 6 through 10 are located in the Instructor's Guide and available to faculty of educational programs.

Exercise 4.23 Respiratory System—Endoscopy

1. 31255–50 Ethmoidectomy, endoscopic
2. 31238–LT Endoscopy, nose, surgical; or Nose, endoscopy, surgical
3. 31233–50 Sinusoscopy, sinus, maxillary

Exercise 4.24 Respiratory System

1. 30520 Septoplasty
   31267–50 Endoscopy, nose, surgical
   30140–50 Turbinate, excision

Exercise 4.25 Respiratory System—Laryngoscopy

1. 31540 Laryngoscopy, direct
2. 31577 Laryngoscopy, fiberoptic
3. 31510 Laryngoscopy, indirect
4. 31541 Laryngoscopy, direct

Exercise 4.26 Respiratory System

1. 31536 Laryngoscopy, direct

Exercise 4.27 Respiratory System—Bronchoscopy

1. 31628 Bronchoscopy, biopsy
2. 31641 Bronchoscopy, removal, tumor
3. 31625 Bronchoscopy, biopsy
   31623 Bronchoscopy, brushing

Exercise 4.28 Respiratory System

1. 31623 Bronchoscopy, brushing

Exercise 4.29 Respiratory System Review

1. 32666 Thoracoscopy, surgical with wedge resection of lung
2. 30110 Polyp, nose, excision, simple
3. 31625 Bronchoscopy, biopsy
4. 30300 Removal, foreign body, nose
5. 31237 Endoscopy, nose, surgical

Note: Answers to exercises 6 through 10 are located in the Instructor's Guide and available to faculty of educational programs.

Exercise 4.30 Cardiovascular System

1. 33207 Pacemaker, heart, insertion; or Insertion, pacemaker, heart

Exercise 4.31 Cardiovascular System

1. 36590 Removal, venous access device

Exercise 4.32 Cardiovascular System

1. 36556 Insertion, venous access device, central

Exercise 4.33 Cardiovascular System Review

1. 33222 Pacemaker, heart, revise pocket, chest
2. 36833 Arteriovenous Fistula, Revision, with thrombectomy
3. 33824 Ductus Arteriosus, repair
4. 36215 Catheterization, brachiocephalic artery
5. 36582 Venous Access Device, replacement

Note: Answers to exercises 6 through 10 are located in the Instructor's Guide and available to faculty of educational programs.

Exercise 4.34 Digestive System—Endoscopy

1. 43202 Endoscopy, esophagus, biopsy

   43217 Endoscopy, esophagus, removal, polyp

   Note: Modifier 59 would apply.
2. 45305 Proctosigmoidoscopy, biopsy
3. 43258 Endoscopy, gastrointestinal, upper, destruction of lesion
4. 45380 Endoscopy, colon, biopsy
5. 43264 Bile Duct, endoscopy, removal, calculi

Exercise 4.35 Digestive System

1. 43247 Endoscopy, gastrointestinal, upper, foreign body

Exercise 4.36 Digestive System

1. 45384 Colonoscopy, removal, polyp; or Endoscopy, colon, removal, polyp

Exercise 4.37 Digestive System

1. 45330 Sigmoidoscopy, exploration

Exercise 4.38 Digestive System—Hernia Repairs

1. 49500 Hernia, repair, inguinal
2. 49561–RT Hernia, repair, incisional, incarcerated

   49568 Implantation, mesh
3. 49651 Laparoscopy, hernia repair, inguinal, recurrent

Note: Answers to exercises 4 through 6 are located in the Instructor's Guide and available to faculty of educational programs.

Exercise 4.39 Digestive System

1. 49505–LT Hernia, repair, inguinal

   Note: Mesh code is only coded with incisional and ventral hernia repairs.

Exercise 4.40 Digestive System Review

1. 46930 Hemorrhoids, destruction
2. 43644 Laparoscopy, gastric restrictive procedures
3. 43245 Endoscopy, gastrointestinal, upper, dilation
4. 42200 Palatoplasty
5. 45383 Colonoscopy, destruction, lesion

Note: Answers to exercises 6 through 10 are located in the Instructor's Guide and available to faculty of educational programs.

Exercise 4.41 Urinary System—Cystoscopy

1. 52332 Cystourethroscopy, insertion, indwelling ureteral stent
2. 52234 Cystourethroscopy, with fulguration, tumor
3. 52353 Cystourethroscopy, lithotripsy
4. 52282 Cystourethroscopy, insertion, urethral stent

Exercise 4.42 Urinary System

1. 52352 Cystourethroscopy, removal, calculus

   52332–51–RT Insertion, stent, ureteral

   Note: Because the stent was inserted at the conclusion of the procedure, one can presume it is an indwelling ureteral stent.

Exercise 4.43 Urinary System

1. 52234 Cystourethroscopy, with fulguration, tumor

Exercise 4.44 Urinary System Review

1. 51992 Sling Operation, stress incontinence
2. 53260 Excision, polyp, urethra
3. 52235 Cystourethroscopy, with fulguration, tumor
4. 51525 Cystotomy, excision, bladder diverticulum
5. 50200 Kidney, biopsy

Note: Answers to exercises 6 through 10 are located in the Instructor's Guide and available to faculty of educational programs.

Exercise 4.45 Male Genital System

1. 54057 Lesion, penis, destruction, laser surgery
2. 10060 Incision and drainage, abscess, skin
3. 55845 Prostatectomy, retropubic, radical
4. 54861 Epididymectomy, bilateral
5. 54150 Circumcision, surgical excision, newborn

Exercise 4.46 Male Genital System

1. 55875 Prostate, brachytherapy, needle insertion

Exercise 4.47 Male Genital System

1. 54520–LT Orchiectomy, simple

Exercise 4.48 Male Genital System Review

1. 54840 Spermatocele, excision
2. 54415 Penile Prosthesis, removal, inflatable
3. 54690 Orchiectomy, laparoscopic
4. 54322 Hypospadias, one stage, meatal advancement
5. 54865 Epididymis, exploration, biopsy

Note: Answers to exercises 6 through 10 are located in the Instructor's Guide and available to faculty of educational programs.

Exercise 4.49 Female Genital System

1. 58670 Laparoscopy, oviduct surgery
2. 58120 Dilation and curettage, corpus uteri
3. 59812 Abortion, incomplete
4. 49322 Laparoscopy, aspiration
5. 58545 Laparoscopy, removal, leiomyomata
6. 58262 Hysterectomy, vaginal, removal tubes/ovaries

Exercise 4.50 Female Genital System

1. 57461 LEEP Procedure

Exercise 4.51 Female Genital System

1. 58558 Hysteroscopy, surgical with biopsy

Exercise 4.52 Female Genital System Review

1. 57455 Colposcopy, biopsy (range of codes)
2. 56620 Vulvectomy, simple, partial (use definitions at beginning of section)
3. 58662 Laparoscopy, destruction, lesion
4. 58150 Hysterectomy, abdominal, total
5. 57023 Incision and Drainage, hematoma, vagina

Note: Answers to exercises 6 through 10 are located in the Instructor's Guide and available to faculty of educational programs.

Exercise 4.53 Endocrine System Review

1. 60280 Thyroglossal Duct, cyst, excision
2. 60650 Laparoscopy, adrenal gland, excision

   Note: There are several misleading index entries for this example. Adrenalectomy, laparoscopic, leads to 50545. Same is true for Laparoscopy, adrenalectomy.
3. 60260–50 Thyroid Gland, excision, total, removal of all thyroid tissue
4. 60300 Thyroid gland, cyst, aspiration
5. 60500 Parathyroid Gland, excision

Exercise 4.54 Nervous System

1.	64445	Injection, nerve, anesthetic
2.	64702–F8	Neuroplasty, digital nerve
	69990	Operating microscope
3.	62281	Epidural, injection
4.	64831–F5	Neurorrhaphy
	64832–F8	

Exercise 4.55 Nervous System

1.	63075	Discectomy

Exercise 4.56 Nervous System Review

1.	62220	Creation, shunt, ventriculo
2.	64712	Neuroplasty, peripheral nerve
3.	64782	Excision, neuroma
4.	64840	Suture, nerve
5.	63272	Laminectomy

Note: Answers to exercises 6 through 10 are located in the Instructor's Guide and available to faculty of educational programs.

Exercise 4.57 Eye and Ocular Adnexa

1.	66984–LT	Phacoemulsification, removal, extracapsular cataract

Exercise 4.58 Eye and Ocular Adnexa Review

1.	65222	Removal, foreign body, cornea with slit lamp
2.	67810–E1	Biopsy, eyelid
3.	68110	Lesion, conjunctiva, excision
4.	67800–E3	Chalazion, excision, single
5.	67311	Strabismus, repair, one horizontal muscle

Note: Answers to exercises 6 through 10 are located in the Instructor's Guide and available to faculty of educational programs.

Exercise 4.59 Auditory System

1.	69436–50	Tympanostomy (–50 for bilateral)

Exercise 4.60 Auditory System Review

1.	69910	Labyrinthectomy with mastoidectomy
2.	69205–LT	Removal, foreign body, auditory canal, external, with anesthesia
3.	69636	Tympanoplasty, with mastoidotomy, with ossicular chain reconstruction
4.	69005–LT	Abscess, ear, external, complicated (would expect to see documentation to explain why the procedure took an extensive amount of time)
5.	69401	Eustachian Tube, inflation, without catheterization

Exercise 4.61 Chapter 4 Review: Coding for Facility

1.	42305	Incision and drainage, abscess, parotid gland
2.	69436–50	Tympanostomy
3.	57455	Colposcopy, biopsy
4.	52234	Cystourethroscopy, with fulguration, tumor
5.	19101–LT	Biopsy, breast
6.	12051	Repair, wound, intermediate
7.	26750–F5	Fracture, phalanges, closed treatment, distal
8.	31536	Laryngoscopy, direct
9.	36569	Catheter, venous, central line
10.	45333	Sigmoidoscopy, removal, polyp

Note: Answers to exercises 11 through 20 are located in the Instructor's Guide and available to faculty of educational programs.

Exercise 4.62 Chapter 4 Review: Coding for Physician Services

1.	61520–62	(physician #1)
		Cerebellopontine angle tumor, *see* brain, tumor, excision
	61520–62	(physician #2)
2.	59840	Abortion, induced by dilation & curettage
3.	29821–RT	Arthroscopy, surgical, shoulder
4.	#1: 33208–55 #2: 33208–56	Pacemaker, heart, insertion
5.	43268	ERCP, *see* Pancreatic duct, endoscopy, tube placement

Note: Answers to exercises 6 through 11 are located in the Instructor's Guide and available to faculty of educational programs.

Chapter 5: Radiology

Exercise 5.1 Diagnostic Radiology

1.	74182	MRI, *see* magnetic resonance imaging, abdomen
2.	72131	CT scan without contrast, spine, lumbar
3.	72170	X-ray, pelvis
4.	74241	X-ray, gastrointestinal
5.	74430	Cystography
6.	74261	CT scan, without contrast, colon, colonography
7.	74177	CT scan, with contrast, abdomen

(**Note**: The note under code 74170 directs the coder to assign a code for a combined CT of abdomen and pelvis)

Exercise 5.2 Diagnostic Ultrasound

1.	76831	Hysterosonography, *see* Ultrasound; Sonohysterography
2.	76815	Ultrasound, pregnant uterus
3.	76645	Ultrasound, breasts

Exercise 5.3 Chapter 5 Review

1.	73090–26	X-ray, arm, lower
2.	72142–26	MRI, *see* magnetic resonance imaging, spine, cervical
3.	74430	Cystography
4.	78451	Myocardial, Perfusion imaging
5.	77057	Mammography, screening
6.	74178	CT scan, without and with Contrast, Abdomen
7.	70460–TC	CT scan, with contrast, head
8.	76817	Ultrasound, pregnant uterus
9.	76942	Ultrasound, guidance, needle biopsy
10.	78306	Bone, nuclear medicine, imaging

Note: Answers to exercises 11 through 25 are located in the Instructor's Guide and available to faculty of educational programs.

Chapter 6: Pathology and Laboratory Services

Exercise 6.1 Chapter 6 Review

1.	88305	Pathology, gross and micro exam
2.	83880	Natriuretic peptide
3.	80402	ACTH, *see* adrenocorticotropic hormone, stimulation panel
4.	81003	Urinalysis, automated
5.	85055	Platelet assay
6.	88309	Pathology, surgical, gross and micro exam
7.	86485	*Candida* skin test
8.	86689	Antibody, HTLV-1
9.	80061	Organ- or disease-oriented panel, lipid panel
	80051	Organ- or disease-oriented panel, electrolyte
10.	80198	Drug assay, theophylline

Note: Answers to exercises 11 through 15 are located in the Instructor's Guide and available to faculty of educational programs.

Chapter 7: Evaluation and Management Services

Exercise 7.1 Evaluation and Management (History)

1. HPI is brief (location, quality, and duration). Review of system(s) is problem specific. No PFSH documented. The history component of this visit would be expanded problem-focused (brief HPI, problem-specific ROS, and expanded problem-focused PFSH including past, family, and social history). The history component is equal to the lowest category documented.
2. HPI is brief (location, severity, and duration). Review of system(s) is extended (two to nine systems), and PFSH is pertinent (medications). The history is determined by the lowest level from all three categories; therefore, the history level would be expanded problem-focused.
3. HPI is extended (location, severity, duration, and context). Review of systems is extended (two to nine systems). The PFSH is complete (two history areas documented). The history level is detailed; all three categories met this level.

Exercise 7.2 Evaluation and Management (Physical Examination)

1. Comprehensive examination: eight body systems were reviewed.
2. Expanded problem-focused examination: two systems reviewed (constitutional and integumentary)
3. Detailed examination. Note that the criteria for expanded problem-focused and the detailed category are the same except in the level of specificity in the examination. Decisions on the level of specificity can be somewhat subjective.

Exercise 7.3 Evaluation and Management (Medical Decision Making)

1. Moderate complexity		
Category	**Documentation**	**Tabulation**
Number of Diagnosis or Treatment Options	New problem; no additional workup planned	3 points = multiple (moderate complexity)
Amount and/or Complexity of Data Reviewed	Review and order clinical laboratory tests (1 point) Review and order test in radiology section of CPT (1 point)	2 points = limited (low complexity)
Level of Risk	Undiagnosed new problem with uncertain prognosis (presenting problem) Documentation of prescription drug management (management options)	Moderate complexity
Final Tabulation	Note that medical decision making is determined by the highest two of three	Moderate complexity
2. Low complexity		
Number of Diagnosis or Treatment Options	Established problem; worsening	2 points = limited
Amount and/or Complexity of Data Reviewed	No data to be reviewed; no tests ordered	0 = minimal/low complexity
Risk Factors	Prescription drug management	Moderate complexity
Final Tabulation	One from each category—choose the middle	Low complexity
3. Straightforward		
Number of Diagnosis or Treatment Options	Self-limited or minor	1 point = minimal
Amount and/or Complexity of Data Reviewed	No data	Minimal/low complexity
Risk Factors	Acute uncomplicated injury (presenting problem) and over-the-counter medication (management options)	Low complexity
Final Tabulation	Two out of three from straightforward category	Straightforward

Exercise 7.4 Evaluation and Management Case Study

Established Patient History		
Elements of History	**Documentation**	**Category**
History of Present Illness	Location, duration, associated signs/ manifestations, severity	Extended
Review of Systems	Extended (2 to 9)	Detailed
PFSH	Complete (2 areas)	Complete
Result (equal to lowest category documented)	Extended is lowest category documented	Detailed history
Medical Decision Making		
Category	**Documentation**	**Tabulation**
Number of Diagnosis or Treatment Options	New problem; no additional workup planned	3 points = multiple
Amount and/or Complexity of Data Reviewed	Chest x-ray	1 point = minimal/low complexity
Risk Factors	Prescription drug management	Moderate complexity
Final Tabulation	Highest two of three categories	Moderate complexity

1. Review the code descriptions for 99211–99215. Need two out of the three key components. The case study revealed a detailed history and comprehensive examination, and the medical decision making was of moderate complexity. The correct E/M code selection is 99214.

Exercise 7.5 Evaluation and Management

1. True
2. False
3. False
4. False
5. False
6. Extended—Four elements: yesterday (duration); getting ready to go to church (context); vomited bile (quality); deafness at the start (associated signs/symptoms)
7. Expanded problem-focused—Systems reviewed: respiratory, integumentary, ENT (ears, nose, throat), cardiovascular, gastrointestinal. Expanded problem-focused (two to nine systems)
8. Pertinent—One area (past history)

Exercise 7.6 Chapter 7 Review

1. 99211
2. 99203
3. 99245
4. 99202
5. 99291

Note: Answers to exercises 6 through 11 are located in the Instructor's Guide and available to faculty of educational programs.

Chapter 8: Medicine

Exercise 8.1 Immunizations

1. 90460 Immunization administration, one vaccine/toxoid, with counseling
   90461 × 3 (each additional vaccine/toxoid component)
   90710 Vaccines, Measles, Mumps, Rubella and Varicella
2. 90471 Immunization administration, one vaccine/toxoid
   90703 Vaccines, tetanus toxoid
3. 90471 Immunization administration, one vaccine/toxoid
   90472 (add-on code) Immunization administration, each additional vaccine/toxoid
   90632 Vaccines, hepatitis A
   90658 Vaccines, influenza
4. 90470 Immunization administration, one vaccine/toxoid
   90650 Vaccine, Human Papilloma Virus
5. 90471 Immunization administration
   90472 each additional vaccine
   90748 Vaccines, hepatitis B and *Haemophilus influenzae B*

Exercise 8.2 Psychiatry

1. 90885 Psychiatric diagnosis, evaluation of records or reports
2. 90847 Psychotherapy, family
3. 90806 Psychiatric treatment, individual, insight-oriented, office or outpatient

Exercise 8.3 Dialysis

1. 90962 Dialysis, end-stage renal disease
2. 90945 Dialysis, peritoneal
3. 90969 Dialysis, end-stage renal disease
   90969 (per day)

Exercise 8.4 Ophthalmology

1. 92018 Gonioscopy (See note under code 92020)
2. 92004 Ophthalmology, Diagnostic, Eye Exam, New patient

Exercise 8.5 Cardiovascular Services

1. 93025 Cardiology, electrocardiogram, Microvolt T-wave Alternans
2. 93452 Catheterization, cardiac, left heart, with ventriculography
3. 92977 Thrombolysis, coronary vessels
4. 93015 Stress Tests, cardiovascular
5. 92995–LC Artery, coronary, atherectomy
   92996–LD
   Note: Do not report angioplasty because it was performed on the same vessel.
6. 92982–LD Percutaneous Transluminal Angioplasty, artery, coronary
   92984–RC
7. 93293 Telephone, Pacemaker Analysis

Exercise 8.6 Pulmonary Services

1. 94060 Spirometry, *see* Pulmology, diagnostic, spirometry, evaluation
2. 94660 CPAP, *see* Continuous Positive Airway Pressure
3. 94450 Hypoxia, breathing response

Exercise 8.7 Allergy and Clinical Immunology

1. 95010 Allergy Tests, skin tests, venoms
2. 95120 Allergen Immunotherapy, allergen, prescription/supply/injection

Exercise 8.8 Injections and Infusions

1. 96372 Injection, intramuscular, therapeutic (Also, J3420 would be assigned for specific substance.)
2. 96360 Infusion, Intravenous, Hydration
3. 96413 Chemotherapy, intravenous
   96415 (add-on code)
   Note: J code for Cisplatin would also be assigned.
4. 96420 Chemotherapy, intra-arterial

Exercise 8.9 Physical Medicine and Rehabilitation

1. 97032 × 2 TENS, *see* Physical Medicine, modalities, electric stimulation, attended, manual
2. 97113 × 2 Physical Medicine, aquatic therapy
3. 97006 Physical Medicine, athletic training, re-evaluation
4. 97602 Wound debridement, nonselective

Exercise 8.10 Chapter 8 Review

1. 90966 Dialysis, end-stage renal disease
2. 90471 Immunization administration, one vaccine/toxoid
   90719 Vaccines, Diphtheria Toxoid
3. 93010 EKG, *see* electrocardiography, evaluation
4. 96413 Chemotherapy, intravenous
   96415 × 2
5. 93600 Electrophysiology Procedure
6. 92556 Audiometry, speech
7. 96372 Injection, intramuscular
   99070 supply, materials
8. 90812 Psychiatric treatment, individual, interactive, office or outpatient
9. 92995 Atherectomies, coronary, *see* Artery, coronary, atherectomy
   92996 (additional vessel)
10. 92014–25 Ophthalmology, diagnostic, eye exam, established patient
    92283 Opththalmology, diagnostic, color vision exam

Note: Answers to exercises 11 through 21 are located in the Instructor's Guide and available to faculty of educational programs.

Chapter 9: Anesthesia

Exercise 9.1 Chapter 9 Review

1. 00406–P2 Anesthesia, breast
2. 01730–P1 Anesthesia, arm, upper
   99100
3. 00567–P4 Anesthesia, heart, coronary artery bypass grafting
4. 00540–P3 Anesthesia, lungs
5. 00350–P1 Anesthesia, neck

Note: Answers to exercises 6 through 10 are located in the Instructor's Guide and available to faculty of educational programs.

Chapter 10: HCPCS Level II

Exercise 10.1 HCPCS Level II Codes

1. A4611 Battery, heavy duty; replacement for patient-owed ventilator
2. H1010 Family Planning Education
3. J8520 Capecitabine, oral, 150 mg
4. M0076 Prolotherapy
5. Q0113 Pinworm Examination

Exercise 10.2 Chapter 10 Review

1. E0196 Mattress, gel pressure
2. A4550 Surgical, tray
3. J3420 Vitamin, B_{12}
4. A4490 Surgical, stocking
5. J1710 Hydrocortisone-sodium phosphate

Note: Answers to exercises 6 through 10 are located in the Instructor's Guide and available to faculty of educational programs.

Chapter 11: Reimbursement in the Ambulatory Setting

Exercise 11.1 Chapter 11 Review and Optional ICD-10-CM Coding Exercise

1. **Incorrect.** Because all repairs were of the same type (simple) and same site classification, the lacerations may be added together. The correct CPT code is 12014. Note that the use of modifiers is not appropriate with these codes.

   ICD-10-CM Codes:
   S01.81xA (Laceration, forehead)
   S01.112A (Laceration, eyelid)

   (an addition external cause code would also be assigned to the specific nature of the injury)

2. **Incorrect.** The CPT codebook provides codes 11200–11201 to report any type of removal of skin tags. The correct code is 11200.

   ICD-10-CM Code: L91.8 (Tag, skin)

3. **Incorrect.** A diagnostic colonoscopy is included in a surgical colonoscopy; only the code for the surgical colonoscopy is assigned (45385).

   ICD-10-CM Code: D12.0 (Polyp, cecum)

4. **Incorrect.** Code 52214 is in the urethra and bladder section and does not correctly identify the procedure. The correct code is 52354.

   ICD-10-CM Code: N28.89 (Polyp, ureter)

5. **Incorrect.** Code 58720 is identified as a separate procedure and thus should not be used with 58150.

   ICD-10-CM Code:
   D25.0 (Leiomyoma, uterus, submucous)

Note: Answers to exercises 6 through 10 are located in the Instructor's Guide and available to faculty of educational programs.

Glossary

Abstracting: 1. The process of extracting information from a document to create a brief summary of a patient's illness, treatment, and outcome. 2. The process of extracting elements of data from a source document or database and entering them into an automated system

Ambulatory care: Preventive or corrective healthcare services provided on a nonresident basis in a provider's office, clinic setting, or hospital outpatient setting

Ambulatory payment classification (APC) relative weight: A number reflecting the expected resource consumption of cases associated with each APC, relative to the average of all APCs, which is used in determining payment under the Medicare hospital outpatient prospective payment system (OPPS)

Ambulatory payment classification (APC) system: The Medicare reimbursement methodology system referred to as the hospital outpatient prospective payment system (OPPS). Hospital providers subject to the OPPS utilize the ambulatory payment classification (APC) system, which determines payment rates

Ambulatory surgery: An elective surgical procedure performed on a patient who is classified as an outpatient and who is usually released from the surgical facility on the day of surgery

Ambulatory surgery center or ambulatory surgical center (ASC): Under Medicare, an outpatient surgical facility that has its own national identifier; is a separate entity with respect to its licensure, accreditation, governance, professional supervision, administrative functions, clinical services, record keeping, and financial and accounting systems; has as its sole purpose the provision of services in connection with surgical procedures that do not require inpatient hospitalization; and meets the conditions and requirements set forth in the Medicare Conditions of Participation

Ambulatory surgical center (ASC) list: The Medicare ASC list that indicates procedures that are covered and paid if performed in the ASC setting

Ambulatory surgical center (ASC) services: ASC diagnostic and therapeutic procedures that can be safely performed outside a hospital setting

American Health Information Management Association (AHIMA): The professional membership organization for managers of health record services and healthcare information systems as well as coding services; provides accreditation, certification, and educational services

American Hospital Association (AHA): The national trade organization that provides education, conducts research, and represents the hospital industry's interests in national legislative matters; membership includes individual healthcare organizations as well as individual healthcare professionals working in specialized areas of hospitals, such as risk management; one of the four cooperating parties on policy development for the use of ICD-9-CM

Ancillary services: 1. Tests and procedures ordered by a physician to provide information for use in patient diagnosis or treatment 2. Professional healthcare services such as radiology, laboratory, or physical therapy

Attending physician: The physician primarily responsible for the care and treatment of a patient

Balanced Budget Act (BBA) of 1997: Public Law 105-33 enacted by Congress on August 5, 1997, which mandated a number of additions, deletions, and revisions to the original Medicare and Medicaid legislation; the legislation that added penalties for healthcare fraud and abuse to the Medicare and Medicaid programs and also affected the hospital outpatient prospective payment system (HOPPS) and programs of all-inclusive care for elderly (PACE)

Balanced Budget Refinement Act (BBRA) of 1999: The amended version of the Balanced Budget Act of 1997, which authorizes implementation of a per-discharge prospective payment system for care provided to Medicare beneficiaries by inpatient rehabilitation facilities

Bundled: The grouping of CPT codes related to a procedure when submitting a claim

Carrier, Medicare: An organization under contract with the Centers for Medicare and Medicaid Services to serve as the financial agent that works with providers and the federal government to locally administer Medicare eligibility and payments

Category I codes: Procedures or services identified by a five-digit CPT code and organized within the six sections of CPT

Category II codes: Codes located in the CPT codebook that represent performance measurement tracking; use is optional

Category III codes: Temporary emerging technology codes located within the CPT codebook

Centers for Medicare and Medicaid Services (CMS): The division of the Department of Health and Human Services that is responsible for developing healthcare policy in the United States and for administering the Medicare program and the federal portion of the Medicaid program; and maintaining the procedure portion of the International Classification of Diseases, 9th revision, Clinical Modification (ICD-9-CM); called the Health Care Financing Administration (HCFA) prior to 2001

Certified Coding Associate (CCA): An AHIMA credential awarded to entry-level coders who have demonstrated skill in classifying medical data by passing a certification exam

Certified Coding Specialist (CCS): An AHIMA credential awarded to individuals who have demonstrated skill in classifying medical data from patient records, generally in the hospital setting, by passing a certification examination

Certified Coding Specialist—Physician based (CCS–P): An AHIMA credential awarded to individuals who have demonstrated coding expertise in physician-based settings, such as group practices, by passing a certification examination

Charge code: The numerical identification of a service or supply that links the item to a particular department within the charge description master

Chargemaster: A financial management form that contains information about the organization's charges for the healthcare services it provides to patients; *see* **Charge description master (CDM)**

Chief complaint: A concise statement, usually stated in the patient's words, describing the symptom, problem, condition, diagnosis, physician-recommended return, or other factor that is the reason for a healthcare encounter

Claim: An itemized statement of healthcare services and their costs provided by a hospital, physician office, or other healthcare provider; submitted for reimbursement to the healthcare insurance plan by either the insured party or by the provider

Claims processing: The process of accumulating claims for services, submitting claims for reimbursement, and ensuring that claims are satisfied

Classification system: 1. A system for grouping similar diseases and procedures and organizing related information for easy retrieval. 2. A system for assigning numeric or alphanumeric code numbers to represent specific diseases and procedures

Clean claim: A completed insurance claim form that contains all the required information (without any missing information) so that it can be processed and paid promptly

Clinic: An outpatient facility providing a limited range of healthcare services and assuming overall healthcare responsibility for patients

Clinical abstract: A computerized file that summarizes patient demographics and other information, including reason for admission, diagnoses, procedures, physician information, and any additional information deemed pertinent by the facility

Clinical coding: The process of assigning numeric or alphanumeric classifications to diagnostic and procedural statements

Clinical data: Data captured during the process of diagnosis and treatment

CMS-1450: A Medicare form used for standardized uniform billing (also known as the Uniform Bill-04 (UB-04). The claim form is used by hospitals, nursing homes, hospice agencies, home health agencies, and other institutional providers.

CMS-1500: The universal insurance claim form developed and approved by the American Medical Association and the Centers for Medicare and Medicaid Services. Physicians use it to bill Medicare, Medicaid, and private insurers for professional services provided

Code: In information systems, software instructions that direct computers to perform a specified action; in healthcare, an alphanumeric representation of the terms in a clinical classification or vocabulary

Code editor: Software that evaluates the clinical consistency and completeness of health record information and identifies potential errors that could affect accurate prospective payment group assignment

Code of Federal Regulations (CFR): The official collection of legislative and regulatory guidelines that are mandated by final rules published in the *Federal Register*

Coded data: Data that are translated into a standard nomenclature of classification so that they may be aggregated, analyzed, and compared

Coder: A person assigned solely to the function of coding

Coder/biller: A person in an ambulatory care or a physician office setting who is generally responsible for processing the superbill

Coding: The process of assigning numeric or alphanumeric representations to clinical documentation

Coding Clinic: A publication issued quarterly by the American Hospital Association. Coding guidelines are clarified through unanimous agreement of the Cooperating Parties of the ICD-9-CM Coding Clinic. The Cooperating Parties include Centers for Medicare and Medicaid Services (CMS), National Center for Health Statistics (NCHS), American Health Information Management Association (AHIMA), and American Hospital Association (AHA)

Coding specialist: The healthcare worker responsible for assigning numeric or alphanumeric codes to diagnostic or procedural statements

Community of Practice (CoP): A Web-based electronic network for communication among members of the American Health Information Management Association

Consolidation: The process by which the ambulatory patient group classification system determines whether separate payment is appropriate when a patient is assigned multiple significant procedure groups

Consultation: The response by one healthcare professional to another healthcare professional's request to provide recommendations and/or opinions regarding the care of a particular patient/resident

Conversion factor: A national dollar amount that Congress designates to convert relative value units to dollars; updated annually

Correct Coding Initiative (CCI): A national initiative designed to improve the accuracy of Part B claims processed by Medicare carriers

CPT Assistant: The official publication of the American Medical Association that addresses CPT coding issues

CPT-5 Project: The AMA initiative to improve CPT to address the needs of hospitals, managed care organizations, and long-term care facilities

***Current Procedural Terminology, Fourth Edition* (CPT):** A comprehensive, descriptive list of terms and associate numeric and alphanumeric codes used for reporting diagnostic and therapeutic procedures and other medical services performed by physicians; published and updated annually by the American Medical Association

Denial: The circumstance when a bill has been accepted, but payment has been denied for any of several reasons (for example, sending the bill to the wrong insurance company, patient not having current coverage, inaccurate coding, lack of medical necessity, and so on)

Department of Health and Human Services (HHS or DHHS): The cabinet-level federal agency that oversees all the health- and human-services–related activities of the federal government and administers federal regulations

Diagnosis: A word or phrase used by a physician to identify a disease from which an individual patient suffers or a condition for which the patient needs, seeks, or receives medical care

Diagnosis chiefly responsible for services provided (outpatient): The diagnosis, condition, problem, or reason for an encounter/visit that is chiefly responsible for the services provided

Diagnosis-related groups (DRGs): A unit of case-mix classification adopted by the federal government and some other payers as a prospective payment mechanism for hospital inpatients in which diseases are placed into groups because related diseases and treatments tend to consume similar amounts of healthcare resources and incur similar amounts of cost; in the Medicare and Medicaid programs, one of more than 500 diagnostic classifications in which cases demonstrate similar resource consumption and length-of-stay patterns. Under the prospective payment system (PPS), hospitals are paid a set fee for treating patients in a single DRG category, regardless of the actual cost of care for the individual

Diagnostic codes: Numeric or alphanumeric characters used to classify and report diseases, conditions, and injuries

Diagnostic services: All diagnostic services of any type, including history, physical examination, laboratory, x-ray or radiography, and others that are performed or ordered pertinent to the patient's reasons for the encounter

Discharge diagnosis: Any one of the diagnoses recorded after all the data accumulated during the course of a patient's hospitalization or other circumscribed episode of medical care have been studied

Discharge status: The disposition of the patient at discharge (that is, left against medical advice, discharged to home, transferred to skilled nursing facility, or died)

Documentation: The recording of pertinent healthcare findings, interventions, and responses to treatment as a business record and form of communication among caregivers

Durable medical equipment (DME): Medical equipment designed for long-term use in the home, including eyeglasses, hearing aids, surgical appliances and supplies, orthotics and prostheses, and bulk and cylinder oxygen; *see* **Home medical equipment (HME)**

Durable medical equipment regional carrier (DMERC): A fiscal intermediary designated to process claims for durable medical equipment

Edit: A condition that must be satisfied before a computer system can accept data

E/M coding: *See* **Evaluation and management codes**

Emergency: A situation in which a patient requires immediate medical intervention as a result of severe, life-threatening, or potentially disabling conditions

Emergency patient: A patient who is admitted to the emergency services department of a hospital for the diagnosis and treatment of a condition that requires immediate medical, dental, or allied health services in order to sustain life or to prevent critical consequences

Encoder: Specialty software used to facilitate the assignment of diagnostic and procedural codes according to the rules of the coding system

Encounter: The professional, direct personal contact between a patient and a physician or other person who is authorized by state licensure law and, if applicable, by medical staff bylaws, to order or furnish healthcare services for the diagnosis or treatment of the patient; face-to-face contact between a patient and a provider who has primary responsibility for assessing and treating the condition

Episode of care: 1. A period of relatively continuous medical care performed by healthcare professionals in relation to a particular clinical problem or situation 2. One or more healthcare services given by a provider during a specific period of relatively continuous care in relation to a particular health or medical problem or situation 3. In home health, all home care services and nonroutine medical supplies delivered to a patient during a 60-day period; the episode of care is the unit of payment under the home health prospective payment system (HHPPS)

Established patient: A patient who has received professional services from the physician or another physician of the same specialty in the same practice group within the past three years

Evaluation and management (E/M) codes: CPT codes that describe patient encounters with healthcare professionals for assessment counseling and other routine healthcare services

Facilities, health: Buildings, including physical plant, equipment, and supplies, necessary in the provision of health services (for example, hospitals, nursing homes, and ambulatory care centers)

***Federal Register*:** The daily publication of the U.S. Government Printing Office that reports all changes in regulations and federally mandated standards, including HCPCS and ICD-9-CM codes

Fee schedule: A list of healthcare services and procedures (usually CPT/HCPCS codes) and the charges associated with them developed by a third-party payer to represent the approved payment levels for a given insurance plan; also called table of allowances

Fee-for-service (FFS) reimbursement: A method of reimbursement through which providers retrospectively receive payment based on either billed charges for services provided or on annually updated fee schedules

Fiscal intermediary (FI): An organization that contracts with the Centers for Medicare and Medicaid Services to serve as the financial agent between providers and the federal government in the local administration of Medicare Part A or Part B claims; usually, but not necessary, an insurance company

Fraud: 1. An intentional misrepresentation of facts to deceive or mislead in order to unjustly gain from another party 2. Intentionally making a claim for payment that one knows to be false

Fraud and abuse: The intentional and mistaken misrepresentation of reimbursement claims submitted to government-sponsored health programs

Freestanding facility: In Medicare terminology, an entity that furnishes healthcare services to beneficiaries and is not integrated with any other entity as a main provider, a department of a provider, or a provider-based entity

Geographic adjustment factor (GAF): Adjustment to the national standardized Medicare fee schedule relative value components used to account for differences in the cost of practicing medicine in different geographic areas of the country

Geographic practice cost index (GPCI): An index developed by the Centers for Medicare and Medicaid Services to measure the differences in resource costs among fee schedule areas compared to the national average in the three components of the relative value unit (RVU): physician work, practice expenses, and malpractice coverage; separate GPCIs exist for each element of the RVU and are used to adjust the RVUs, which are national averages, to reflect local costs

Global payment: A form of reimbursement used for radiological and other procedures that combines the professional and technical components of the procedures and disperses payments as lump sums to be distributed between the physician and the healthcare facility

Global surgery package: A CPT code denoting a normal surgical procedure with no complications that includes all the elements needed to perform the procedure

Group practice: An organization of physicians who share office space and administrative support services to achieve economies of scale, often a clinic or ambulatory care center

Grouping: A system for assigning patients to a classification scheme via a computer software program

Hard code: A code applied through a healthcare organization's chargemaster

Hard coding: 1. The process of attaching a CPT/HCPCS code to a procedure located on the facility's chargemaster so that the code will automatically be included on the patient's bill 2. Use of the charge description master to code repetitive services

HCFA-1450: Previous name for **CMS-1450;** *See* **CMS-1450**

HCFA-1500: Previous name for **CMS-1500;** *See* **CMS-1500**

HCFA Common Procedural Coding System (HCPCS): Previous name for the **Healthcare Common Procedure Coding System**

Health Care Financing Administration (HCFA): Previous name for the **Centers for Medicare and Medicaid Services**

Health Insurance Portability and Accountability Act of 1996 (HIPAA): The federal legislation enacted to provide continuity of health coverage, control fraud and abuse in healthcare, reduce healthcare costs, and guarantee the security and privacy of health information; limits exclusion for preexisting medical conditions, prohibits discrimination against employees and dependents based on health status, guarantees availability of health insurance to small employers, and guarantees renewability of insurance to all employees regardless of size; requires covered entities (most healthcare providers and organizations) to transmit healthcare claims in a specific format; develop, implement, and comply with the standards of the Privacy Rule and the Security Rule, and mandates that covered entities apply for and utilize national identifiers in HIPAA transactions. Also known as Public Law 104-191 and the Kassebaum-Kennedy Law

Health record: 1. A paper- or computer-based tool for collecting and storing information about the healthcare services provided to a patient in a single healthcare facility; also called a patient record, medical record, resident record, or client record, depending on the healthcare setting 2. Individually identifiable data, in any medium, that are collected, processed, stored, displayed, and used by healthcare professionals; documents the care rendered to the patient and the patient's healthcare status

Healthcare Common Procedure Coding System (HCPCS): An alphanumeric classification system that identifies healthcare procedures, equipment, and supplies for claim submission purposes; the three levels are as follows: I, *Current Procedural Terminology* codes, developed by the AMA; II, codes for equipment, supplies, and services not covered by *Current Procedural Terminology* codes, as well as modifiers that can be used with all levels of codes, developed by CMS; and III (eliminated December 31, 2003 to comply with HIPAA), local codes developed by regional Medicare Part B carriers and used to report physicians' services and supplies to Medicare for reimbursement

Healthcare provider: A provider of diagnostic, medical, and surgical care as well as the services or supplies related to the health of an individual and any other person or organization that issues reimbursement claims or is paid for healthcare in the normal course of business. A provider is legally responsible for the patient's diagnosis and treatment

HIPAA: *See* **Health Insurance Portability and Accountability Act of 1996**

History: The pertinent information about a patient, including chief complaint, past and present illnesses, family history, social history, and review of body systems

Home health prospective payment system (HHPPS): The reimbursement system developed by the Centers for Medicare and Medicaid Services to cover home health services provided to Medicare beneficiaries

Hospital: A healthcare entity that has an organized medical staff and permanent facilities that include inpatient beds and continuous medical/nursing services and that provides diagnostic and therapeutic services for patients as well as overnight accommodations and nutritional services

Hospital ambulatory care: All hospital-directed preventive, therapeutic, and rehabilitative services provided by physicians and their surrogates to patients who are not hospital inpatients

Hospital-based ambulatory care center: An organized hospital facility that provides nonemergency medical or dental services to patients who are not assigned to a bed as inpatients during the time services are rendered (an emergency department in which services are provided to nonemergency patients is not considered an ambulatory care center)

Hospital-based ambulatory surgery center: A department of an inpatient facility that provides same-day surgical services using the facility's equipment, staff, and support services

Hospital-based outpatient care: A subset of ambulatory care that utilizes a hospital's staff, equipment, and resources to render preventive and/or corrective healthcare services

Hospital outpatient: A hospital patient who receives services in one or more of a hospital's facilities when he or she is not currently an inpatient or a home care patient

Hospital outpatient care unit: An organized unit of a hospital that provides facilities and medical services exclusively or primarily to patients who are generally ambulatory and who do not currently require or are not currently receiving services as inpatients of the hospital

Hospitalization insurance (Medicare Part A): A federal program that covers the costs associated with inpatient hospitalization as well as other healthcare services provided to Medicare beneficiaries

Individual provider: A health professional who delivers, or is professionally responsible for delivering services to a patient, is exercising independent judgment in the care of the patient, and is not under the immediate supervision of another healthcare professional

Inpatient prospective payment system (IPPS): The reimbursement system for inpatient hospital services provided to Medicare and Medicaid beneficiaries, which is based on the use of diagnosis-related groups (DRGs) as a classification tool

***International Classification of Diseases, Ninth Revision, Clinical Modification* (ICD-9-CM):** A coding and classification system used in the United States to report diagnoses in all healthcare settings and inpatient procedures and services as well as morbidity and mortality information

***International Classification of Diseases, Tenth Revision* (ICD-10):** The most recent revision of the disease classification system developed and used by the World Health Organization to track morbidity and mortality information worldwide. ICD-10 will be implemented in the United States on October 1, 2013.

Item description: An explanation of a service or supply listed in the chargemaster

Level of service: 1. The relative intensity of services given when a physician provides one-on-one services for a patient (such as minimal, brief, limited, or intermediate). 2. The relative intensity of services provided by a healthcare facility (for example, tertiary care); also called level of significance

Line item: A service- or item-specific detail of a budget, bill, or reimbursement claim

Local medical review policies (LMRPs): Documents that define Medicare coverage of outpatient services via lists of diagnoses defined as medically reasonable and necessary for the services provided

Managed care: A generic term for reimbursement and delivery systems that integrate the financing and provision of healthcare services by means of entering contractual agreements with selected providers to furnish comprehensive healthcare services and developing explicit criteria for the selection of healthcare providers, formal programs of ongoing quality improvement and utilization review, and significant financial incentives for members to use providers associated with the plan

Managed fee-for-service reimbursement: A healthcare plan that implements utilization controls (prospective and retrospective review of healthcare services) for reimbursement under traditional fee-for-service insurance plans

Medicaid: An entitlement program that oversees medical assistance for individuals and families with low incomes and limited resources; jointly funded between state and federal governments and legislated by the Social Security Act

Medical care unit: An assemblage of inpatient beds (or newborn bassinets), related facilities, and assigned personnel that provide service to a defined and limited class of patients according to their particular medical care needs

Medical consultation: *See* **Consultation**

Medical history: A record of previous information provided by a patient to his or her physician to explain the patient's chief complaint, present and past illnesses, and personal and family medical problems; includes a description of the physician's review of systems

Medical nomenclature: A recognized system of preferred terminology for naming disease processes

Medical record: *See* **Health record**

Medicare: A federally funded health program established in 1965 to assist with the medical care costs of Americans 65 years of age and older as well as other individuals entitled to Social Security benefits owing to their disabilities

Medicare Advantage (Medicare Part C): Optional managed care plan for Medicare beneficiaries who are entitled to Part A, enrolled in Part B, and live in an area with a plan; types include health maintenance organization, point-of-service plan, preferred provider organization, and provider-sponsored organization; formerly **Medicare+Choice**

***Medicare Carriers Manual* (MCM): Provides direction about services and procedures to be reimbursed by the Medicare administrative contractor**

Medicare economic index (MEI): An index used by the Medicare program to update physician fee levels in relation to annual changes in the general economy for inflation, productivity, and changes in specific health-sector expense factors including malpractice, personnel costs, rent, and other expenses

Medicare fee schedule (MFS): A feature of the resource-based relative value system that includes a complete list of the payments Medicare makes to physicians and other providers

***Medicare National Coverage Determinations Manual*:** Indicates whether a service is covered or excluded under the Medicare program

Medicare Part A: The portion of Medicare that provides benefits for inpatient hospital services; *see* **hospitalization insurance**

Medicare Part B: An optional and supplemental portion of Medicare that provides benefits for physician services, medical services, and medical supplies not covered by Medicare Part A; *see* **Supplemental medical insurance**

Medicare Part C: Also known as Medicare Advantage, this is a managed care option that includes services under Parts A, B, and D and additional services that are not typically covered by Medicare; Medicare Part C requires an additional premium. Formerly known as Medicare+ Choice; *see* **Medicare Advantage**

Medicare Part D: Medicare drug benefit created by the Medicare Modernization Act of 2003 (MMA) that offers outpatient drug coverage to beneficiaries for an additional premium

Medicare prospective payment system: The reimbursement system for inpatient hospital services provided to Medicare and Medicaid beneficiaries that is based on the use of diagnosis-related groups (DRGs) as a classification tool; *see* **Acute care prospective payment system, Home health prospective payment system, Outpatient prospective payment system,** and **Skilled nursing facility prospective payment system**

National Codes (HCPCS Level II codes): (or Level II HCPCS codes): Codes, consisting of one alpha character (A through V) followed by four digits, created by the Centers for Medicare and Medicaid Services to supplement CPT codes by describing nonphysician procedures, durable medical equipment, or specific supplies

National Correct Coding Initiative (NCCI): A series of coding regulations to prevent fraud and abuse in Medicare Part B claims; specifically addresses unbundling and mutually exclusive procedures

New patient: An individual who has not received professional services from the physician or any other physician of the same specialty in the same practice group within the past three years

Nomenclature: A recognized system of terms used in a science or art that follows pre-established naming conventions; a disease nomenclature is a listing of the proper name for each disease entity with its specific code number

Observation patient: A patient who presents with a medical condition with a significant degree of instability and disability and who needs to be monitored, evaluated, and assessed to determine whether he or she should be admitted for inpatient care or discharged for care in another setting

Omnibus Budget Reconciliation Act (OBRA) of 1989: The federal legislation that mandated important changes in the payment rules for Medicare physicians; specifically, the legislation that requires nursing facilities to conduct regular patient assessments for Medicare and Medicaid beneficiaries. The Act implemented the resource-based relative value scale (RBRVS) system, which is used to reimburse physician services

Operating room (OR) procedure: Procedure that the physician panel classifies as occurring in the operating room in most hospitals; presence of an OR procedure groups a case to a surgical diagnosis-related group (DRG)

Operation: *See* **Surgical operation**

Operative report: A formal document that describes the events surrounding a surgical procedure or operation and identifies the principal participants in the surgery

Other diagnoses: All conditions (recorded to the highest documented level of specificity) that coexist at the time of admission, develop subsequently, or affect the treatment received or length of stay

Outpatient: A patient who receives ambulatory care services in a hospital-based clinic or department

Outpatient code editor (OCE): A software program linked to the Correct Coding Initiative that applies a set of logical rules to determine whether various combinations of codes are correct and appropriately represent the services provided; *see* **Editor**

Outpatient coder: An individual responsible for assigning ICD-9-CM and CPT/HCPCS codes to ambulatory surgery, emergency department cases, or outpatient ancillary clinic visits

Outpatient prospective payment system (OPPS): The Medicare prospective payment system used for hospital-based outpatient services and procedures that is predicated on the assignment of ambulatory payment classifications

Outpatient unit: A hospital-based ambulatory care facility organized into sections (clinics) whose number depends on the size and degree of departmentalization of the medical or clinic staff, available facilities, type of service needed in the community, and the needs of the patients for whom it accepts responsibility

Outpatient visit: A patient's visit to one or more units located in the ambulatory services area (clinic or physician's office) of an acute care hospital

Packaging: A payment under the Medicare outpatient prospective payment system that includes items such as anesthesia, supplies, certain drugs, and the use of recovery and observation rooms

Partial hospitalization: A limited patient stay in the hospital setting, typically as part of a transitional program to a less intense level of service; for example, psychiatric and drug and alcohol treatment facilities that offer services to help patients reenter the community, return to work, and assume family responsibilities

Patient: A living or deceased individual who is receiving or has received healthcare services

Patient health record: *See* **Health record**

Physical examination report: Documentation of a physician's assessment of a patient's body systems

Primary care physician (PCP): 1. Physician who provides, supervises, and coordinates the healthcare of a member and who manages referrals to other healthcare providers and utilization of healthcare services both inside and outside a managed care plan. Family and general practitioners, internists, pediatricians, and obstetricians/gynecologists are primary care physicians.2. The physician who makes the initial diagnosis of a patient's medical condition; *see* **Primary care provider**

Primary care provider (PCP): Healthcare provider who provides, supervises, and coordinates the healthcare of a member; primary physicians can be family and general practitioners, internists, pediatricians, and obstetricians/gynecologists; other PCPs are nurse practitioners and physician assistants; *see* **Primary care physician**

Primary diagnosis: *See* **Principal diagnosis**

Principal diagnosis: The disease or condition that was present on admission, was the principal reason for admission, and received treatment or evaluation during the hospital stay or visit, or the reason established after study to be chiefly responsible for occasioning the admission of the patient to the hospital for care; *see* **Most significant diagnosis**

Principal procedure: The procedure performed for the definitive treatment of a condition (as opposed to a procedure performed for diagnostic or exploratory purposes) or for care of a complication

Procedural codes: The numeric or alphanumeric characters used to classify and report the medical procedures and services performed for patients

Procedures and services (outpatient): All medical procedures and services of any type (including history, physical examination, laboratory, x-ray or radiograph, and others) that are performed pertinent to the patient's reasons for the encounter, all therapeutic services performed at the time of the encounter, and all preventive services and procedures performed at the time of the encounter

Professional component (PC): 1. The portion of a healthcare procedure performed by a physician 2. A term generally used in reference to the elements of radiological procedures performed by a physician

Prospective payment system (PPS): A type of reimbursement system that is based on preset payment levels rather than actual charges billed after the service has been provided; specifically, one of several Medicare reimbursement systems based on predetermined payment rates or periods and linked to the anticipated intensity of services delivered as well as the beneficiary's condition; *see* **Acute care prospective payment system, Home health prospective payment system, Outpatient prospective payment system,** and **Skilled nursing facility payment system**

Provider: Physician, clinic, hospital, nursing home, or other healthcare entity (second party) that delivers healthcare services

Referral: A request by a provider for a patient under the provider's care to be evaluated or treated by another provider

Referred outpatient: An outpatient who is provided special diagnostic or therapeutic services by a hospital on an ambulatory basis but whose medical care remains the responsibility of the referring physician

Reimbursement: Compensation or repayment for healthcare services

Rejection: The process of having a submitted bill not accepted by the payer, although corrections can be made and the claim resubmitted

Relative value unit (RVU): A number assigned to a procedure that describes its difficulty and expense in relationship to other procedures. by assigning weights to such factors as personnel, time, and level of skill; *see* **Physician work, Practice expenses, Malpractice, Geographic practice cost index,** and **Resource-based relative value scale**

Resource-based relative value scale (RBRVS): A Medicare reimbursement system implemented in 1992 to compensate physicians according to a fee schedule predicated on weights assigned on the basis of the resources required to provide the services

Retrospective payment system: Type of fee-for-service reimbursement in which providers receive recompense after health services have been rendered; also called retrospective payment method

Revenue code: A three- or four-digit number in the chargemaster that totals all items and their charges for printing on the form used for Medicare billing

Significant procedure: A procedure that is surgical in nature or carries a procedural or an anesthetic risk or requires specialized training

Significant procedure ambulatory payment classification: A procedure that constitutes the reason for the visit, dominates the time and resources rendered during the visit, and is not subject to payment reduction/discounting

Skilled nursing facility prospective payment system (SNFPPS): A per diem reimbursement system implemented in July 1998 for costs (routine, ancillary, and capital) associated with covered skilled nursing facility services furnished to Medicare Part A beneficiaries

Special care unit: A medical care unit in which there is appropriate equipment and a concentration of physicians, nurses, and others who have special skills and experience to provide optimal medical care for critically ill patients or continuous care of patients in special diagnostic categories

Superbill: The office form used for physician office billing that is initiated by the physician and states the diagnoses and other information for each patient encounter

Supplemental medical insurance (SMI): A small independent insurance policy that consumers may take out independently of their primary insurance

Surgery: An umbrella term referring to the procedures of incision, excision, amputation, introduction, endoscopy, suture, and manipulation

Surgical operation: One or more surgical procedures performed at one time for one patient via a common approach or for a common purpose

Surgical procedure: Any single, separate, systematic process upon or within the body that can be complete in itself; is normally performed by a physician, dentist, or other licensed practitioner; can be performed either with or without instruments; and is performed to restore disunited or deficient parts, remove diseased or injured tissues, extract foreign matter, assist in obstetrical delivery, or aid in diagnosis

Tax Equity and Fiscal Responsibility Act of 1982 (TEFRA): The federal legislation that modified Medicare's retrospective reimbursement system for inpatient hospital stays by requiring implementation of diagnosis-related groups and the acute care prospective payment system

Technical component (TC): The portion of radiological and other procedures that is facility based or nonphysician based (for example, radiology films, equipment, overhead, endoscopic suites, and so on)

Third-party payer: An insurance company (for example, Blue Cross/Blue Shield) or healthcare program (for example, Medicare) that pays or reimburses healthcare providers (second party) and/or patients (first party) for the delivery of medical services

UB-04: *See* **Uniform Bill-04**

Unbundling: The practice of using multiple codes to bill for the various individual steps in a single procedure rather than using a single code that includes all the steps of the comprehensive procedure

Undercoding: A form of incomplete documentation that results when diagnoses or procedures that should be coded are not assigned

Uniform Bill-04 (UB-04): *See* **CMS-1450**

Unlisted procedure: Codes available in each section of CPT to describe procedures that have no specific procedure code assigned because the procedure is new or unusual

Upcoding: The practice of assigning diagnostic or procedural codes that represent higher payment rates than the codes that actually reflect the services provided to patients; *see* **Overcoding**

Usual, customary, and reasonable (UCR): Type of retrospective fee-for-service payment method in which the third party payer pays for fees that are usual, customary, and reasonable, wherein "usual" is usual for the individual provider's practice; "customary" means customary for the community; and "reasonable" is reasonable for the situation

Visit: A single encounter with a healthcare professional that includes all of the services supplied during the encounter

World Health Organization (WHO): The United Nations specialized agency created to ensure the attainment by all peoples of the highest possible levels of health; responsible for a number of international classifications, including *The International Statistical Classification of Diseases & Related Health Problems* (ICD-10) and *The International Classification of Functioning, Disability & Health* (ICF)

Index